Advances in Biliary Endoscopy

Editor

MOUEN KHASHAB

GASTROINTESTINAL ENDOSCOPY
CLINICS OF NORTH AMERICA

www.giendo.theclinics.com

Consulting Editor
CHARLES J. LIGHTDALE

July 2022 • Volume 32 • Number 3

ELSEVIER

1600 John F. Kennedy Boulevard • Suite 1800 • Philadelphia, Pennsylvania, 19103-2899

http://www.theclinics.com

GASTROINTESTINAL ENDOSCOPY CLINICS OF NORTH AMERICA Volume 32, Number 3
July 2022 ISSN 1052-5157, ISBN-13: 978-0-323-98683-0

Editor: Kerry Holland
Developmental Editor: Jessica Cañaberal

Gastrointestinal Endoscopy Clinics of North America (ISSN 1052-5157) is published quarterly by Elsevier Inc., 360 Park Avenue South, New York, NY 10010-1710. Months of issue are January, April, July, and October. Business and Editorial Offices: 1600 John F. Kennedy Blvd., Suite 1800, Philadelphia, PA, 19103-2899. Periodicals postage paid at New York, NY and additional mailing offices. Subscription prices are $370.00 per year for US individuals, $837.00 per year for US institutions, $100.00 per year for US and Canadian students/residents, $407.00 per year for Canadian individuals, $862.00 per year for Canadian institutions, $486.00 per year for international individuals, $862.00 per year for international institutions, and $245.00 per year for international students/residents. To receive student/resident rate, orders must be accompanied by name of affiliated institution, date of term, and the *signature* of program/residency coordinator on institution letterhead. Orders will be billed at individual rate until proof of status is received. Foreign air speed delivery is included in all *Clinics* subscription prices. All prices are subject to change without notice. **POSTMASTER:** Send address change to *Gastrointestinal Endoscopy Clinics of North America*, Elsevier Health Sciences Division, Subscription Customer Service, 3251 Riverport Lane, Maryland Heights, MO 63043. **Customer Service: 1-800-654-2452 (US). From outside the United States, call 1-314-447-8871. Fax: 1-314-447-8029. E-mail: JournalsCustomerService-usa@elsevier.com (for print support) or JournalsOnlineSupport-usa@elsevier.com (for online support).**

Reprints. For copies of 100 or more, of articles in this publication, please contact the Commercial Reprints Department, Elsevier Inc., 360 Park Avenue South, New York, NY 10010-1710. Tel. 212-633-3874; Fax: 212-633-3820; E-mail: reprints@elsevier.com.

Gastrointestinal Endoscopy Clinics of North America is covered in *Excerpta Medica, MEDLINE/PubMed (Index Medicus), and MEDLINE/MEDLARS.*

Contributors

CONSULTING EDITOR

CHARLES J. LIGHTDALE, MD
Professor of Medicine, Division of Digestive and Liver Diseases, Columbia University Medical Center, New York, New York, USA

EDITOR

MOUEN KHASHAB, MD, MASGE, FJGES
Professor of Medicine, Director of Therapeutic Endoscopy, Lead, Therapeutic Endoscopy Group, Johns Hopkins Enterprise, Johns Hopkins Hospital, Towson, Maryland, USA; Department of Gastroenterology and Hepatology, Johns Hopkins Medical Institutions, Baltimore, Maryland, USA

AUTHORS

VENKATA S. AKSHINTALA, MD
Division of Gastroenterology, Johns Hopkins Medical Institutions, Baltimore, Maryland, USA

MARIANNA ARVANITAKIS, MD, PhD
Department of Gastroenterology, Hepatopancreatology, and Digestive Oncology, CUB Hôpital Erasme, Université Libre de Bruxelles, Brussels, Belgium

IVO BOŠKOSKI, MD, PhD
Digestive Endoscopy Unit, Fondazione Policlinico Universitario Agostino Gemelli IRCCS, Centre for Endoscopic Research Therapeutics and Training (CERTT), Università Cattolica Del Sacro Cuore di Roma, Rome, Italy

MARCO J. BRUNO, MD, PhD
Department of Gastroenterology and Hepatology, Erasmus University Medical Center, Rotterdam, the Netherlands

SARA TELES DE CAMPOS, MD
Department of Gastroenterology, Digestive Unit, Champalimaud Foundation, Lisbon, Portugal

GUIDO COSTAMAGNA
Digestive Endoscopy Unit, Fondazione Policlinico Universitario Agostino Gemelli IRCCS, Centre for Endoscopic Research Therapeutics and Training (CERTT), Università Cattolica Del Sacro Cuore di Roma, Rome, Italy

VINAY DHIR, MD, FASGE
Division of Endosonography, Institute of Digestive and Liver Care, SL Raheja Hospital-A Fortis Associate, Mumbai, India

NIMA HAFEZI-NEJAD, MD
Interventional Radiology Resident, Division of Vascular and Interventional Radiology, Department of Radiology and Radiological Sciences, Johns Hopkins School of Medicine, Baltimore, Maryland, USA

ROBERT H. HAWES, MD
Orlando Health Digestive Health Institute, Orlando, Florida, USA; Medical Director, Center for Advanced Endoscopy, Research and Education (CARE), Professor of Medicine, University of Central Florida College of Medicine

SHAYAN IRANI, MD
Digestive Disease Institute, Virginia Mason Medical Center, Seattle, Washington, USA

MOUEN KHASHAB, MD, MASGE, FJGES
Professor of Medicine, Director of Therapeutic Endoscopy, Lead, Therapeutic Endoscopy Group, Johns Hopkins Enterprise, Johns Hopkins Hospital, Towson, Maryland, USA; Department of Gastroenterology and Hepatology, Johns Hopkins Medical Institutions, Baltimore, Maryland, USA

TAE HOON LEE, MD, PhD
Division of Gastroenterology and Hepatology, Department of Internal Medicine, SoonChunHyang University Cheonan Hospital, SoonChunHyang University School of Medicine, Cheonan, Republic of Korea

ROBERT P. LIDDELL, MD
Assistant Professor, Division of Vascular and Interventional Radiology, Department of Radiology and Radiological Sciences, Johns Hopkins School of Medicine, Baltimore, Maryland, USA

XIAOBEI, LUO, MD
Department of Gastroenterology, Nanfang Hospital, Southern Medical University, Guangzhou, China

JORGE D. MACHICADO, MD, MPH
Division of Gastroenterology and Hepatology, University of Michigan, Ann Arbor, Michigan, USA

JONG HO MOON, MD, FASGE, FJGES
Division of Gastroenterology and Hepatology, Department of Internal Medicine, SoonChunHyang University Bucheon Hospital, SoonChunHyang University School of Medicine, Bucheon, Republic of Korea

ZAHEER NABI, MD, DNB
Consultant Gastroenterologist, Asian Institute of Gastroenterology, Hyderabad, India

SIMON PHILLPOTTS, MBBS, MRCP
Endoscopy Fellow. Department of Gastroenterology, University College London Hospitals, London, England

ISAAC RAIJMAN, MD, FACG, AGAF, FACP
Texas Digestive Disease Consultants, Texas, USA

D. NAGESHWAR REDDY, MD, DM, DSc, FAMS, FRCP, FASGE, FACG, MWGO, MASGE, FAGA, FJGES, FAAAS
Chairman and Chief Gastroenterologist, Asian Institute of Gastroenterology, Hyderabad, India

TOMMASO SCHEPIS
Digestive Endoscopy Unit, Fondazione Policlinico Universitario Agostino Gemelli IRCCS, Rome, Italy

RAHUL SHAH, MRCP
Division of Endosonography, Institute of Digestive and Liver Care, SL Raheja Hospital-A Fortis Associate, Mumbai, India

RAJ J. SHAH, MD, MASGE, AGAF, FACG
Director, Pancreas and Biliary Endoscopy, Division of Gastroenterology and Hepatology, University of Colorado Anschutz Medical Campus, Aurora, Colorado, USA

REEM SHARAIHA, MD
Division of Gastroenterology and Hepatology, NewYork-Presbyterian Hospital/Weill Cornell Medical Centre, New York, New York, USA

ANMOL SINGH, MD
Division of Gastroenterology, Johns Hopkins Medical Institutions, Baltimore, Maryland, USA

VIKESH K. SINGH, MD, MSc
Division of Gastroenterology, Johns Hopkins Medical Institutions, Baltimore, Maryland, USA

SHERMAN STUART, MD, MASGE
Professor of Medicine and Radiology, Department of Medicine, Division of Gastroenterology/Hepatology, Indiana University School of Medicine, Indiana University Health-University Hospital, Indianapolis, Indiana, USA

ANTHONY YUEN BUN TEOH, FRCSED
Professor, Department of Surgery, Prince of Wales Hospital, The Chinese University of Hong Kong, Shatin, Hong Kong

ANDREA TRINGALI
Digestive Endoscopy Unit, Fondazione Policlinico Universitario Agostino Gemelli IRCCS, Centre for Endoscopic Research Therapeutics and Training (CERTT), Università Cattolica Del Sacro Cuore di Roma, Rome, Italy

PRIYANKA UDAWAT, MD
Division of Endosonography, Institute of Digestive and Liver Care, SL Raheja Hospital-A Fortis Associate, Mumbai, India

GEORGE WEBSTER, MD, FRCP
Consultant Gastroenterologist and Hepatologist, Department of Gastroenterology, University College London Hospitals, London, England

LINDA Y. ZHANG, MBBS
Department of Gastroenterology and Hepatology, Johns Hopkins Medical Institutions, Baltimore, Maryland, USA

Contents

Successful biliary cannulation of a native papilla is usually the rate-limiting step toward a successful ERCP. Standard cannulation techniques usually succeed, particularly when utilizing the wire-guided technique. There are, however, a myriad of confirmations of the major papilla as well as anatomic variants and certain pathologies which can make cannulation exceedingly difficult. For these cases, advanced cannulation techniques and techniques termed "access sphincterotomy" have been developed which should allow successful cannulation in >90% of cases. This article should help all those performing ERCP to improve their cannulation rate.

Endoscopic retrograde cholangiopancreatography (ERCP) is an essential procedure for the management of pancreaticobiliary disorders. ERCP is, however, associated with the risk of complications including pancreatitis, bleeding, perforation, infection, and instrument failure, which can often be fatal. It is, therefore, necessary to recognize the risk of ERCP-associated complications and understand the methods to prevent and treat such complications.

 Video content accompanies this article at http://www.giendo. theclinics.com.

Biliary strictures that remain unclassified after cross-sectional imaging and endoscopic retrograde cholangiopancreatography–based tissue sampling are defined as indeterminate biliary strictures (IDBS). A substantial proportion of biliary strictures fall into this category due to low sensitivity of brush cytology and intraductal biopsy. Over last few decades, several modalities have emerged for the evaluation of IDBS. Of these, cholangioscopy and endosonography are the frontrunners and have cemented their place for the evaluation of IDBS. Both of these modalities are widely available, and therefore, biliary strictures that remain uncharacterized after their utilization represent IDBS in the current era.

> Malignant hilar biliary obstruction (MHO), an aggressive perihilar biliary obstruction caused by cholangiocarcinoma, gallbladder cancer, or other metastatic malignancies, has a poor prognosis. Surgical resection is the only curative treatment method for biliary malignancies. However, most of the patients with MHO cannot undergo surgeries on presentation because of an advanced inoperable state or a poor performance state due to old age or comorbid diseases. Therefore, palliative biliary drainage is mandatory to improve symptomatic jaundice and quality of life. Among drainage methods, endoscopic biliary drainage is the current standard for the palliation of unresectable advanced MHO. The development of stents and various accessories and advances in endoscopic techniques including endoscopic ultrasonography have facilitated primary endoscopic intervention in difficult high-grade hilar strictures. However, some issues are still under debate, such as palliation methods, appropriate stents, the number of stents, deployment methods, and additional local ablation therapies. Therefore, this review presents currently optimal endoscopic palliation methods for advanced MHO based on the reported literature.

> Benign biliary strictures (BBS) can be associated with several causes, with postoperative and inflammatory strictures representing the most common ones. Endoscopy represents nowadays the first-line treatment in the management of BBS. Endoscopic balloon dilatation, plastic stents placement, fully covered metal stent placement, and magnetic compression anastomosis are the endoscopic techniques available for the treatment of BBS. The aim of this study is to perform a review of the literature to assess the role of endoscopy in the management of BBS and to evaluate the application of the different procedures in the different clinical settings.

 Video content accompanies this article at http://www.giendo. theclinics.com.

> Complex biliary stones may be challenging to remove with standard endoscopic techniques. Factors contributing to complexity include large stone size ($\geq$15 mm), multiple stones, high stone:distal duct ratio, stones above strictures and those in difficult anatomic position. In these cases, additional techniques may be needed, such as endoscopic papillary large balloon dilatation, mechanical lithotripsy, cholangioscopic visually directed lithotripsy, and extracorporeal shockwave lithotripsy. The choice of technique depends on local expertise and resources. Cases should be planned to identify the appropriate technique to avoid multiple procedures. This article describes the factors linked to difficulty and the steps to overcome them.

Percutaneous biliary interventions (PBIs) are commonly performed by interventional radiologists for a variety of clinical indications including biliary infections, strictures, leaks, and postoperative complications. PBIs have high technical and clinical success rates and are relatively safe when compared with more invasive surgical techniques. Percutaneous transhepatic cholangiography and percutaneous biliary drainage play an essential role in the management of common posthepatobiliary complications including biliary strictures and leaks. Percutaneous biliary endoscopy can be used for direct visualization of the biliary tree and a variety of interventions including tissue biopsy, lithotripsy, stone removal, as well as stent placement and removal.

Endoscopic ultrasound (EUS)–guided biliary interventions have evolved to become an integral part of advanced gastrointestinal endoscopy units. EUS-guided biliary drainage is an accepted alternative for patients with failed ERCP or altered surgical anatomy. The potential advantages of EUS-guided interventions include choice of biliary access from stomach or duodenum, choice of stent exit in stomach and duodenum, and possibility of avoiding traversing through the obstruction. A variety of procedures have been described depending on the level of obstruction. Maximum evidence is available for distal malignant obstruction, and more studies are needed for hilar obstruction and benign indications.

Endoscopic drainage of the gallbladder for acute cholecystitis can be performed with the transpapillary method or endoscopic ultrasound (EUS)-guided method. EUS-guided gallbladder drainage (EUS-GBD) is gaining popularity as the treatment of choice for acute cholecystitis in patients who are deemed high-risk for cholecystectomy (CCY). It provides an alternative to percutaneous drainage and laparoscopic CCY in these patients. With the development of lumen-apposing metal stents (LAMS), the procedure is associated with high rates of technical and clinical success with low rates of adverse events (AEs). The aim of this article is to provide an overview of the current status of EUS-GBD including the indications, techniques, stent systems in-use, and how the procedure compares to conventional techniques are outlined. Furthermore, the feasibility of cholecystoscopy and advanced gallbladder interventions is explored. Finally, a comparison in outcomes of EUS-GBD versus laparoscopic CCY is provided giving some initial data in support of the procedure as an alternative to surgery in a selected group of patients.

GASTROINTESTINAL ENDOSCOPY CLINICS OF NORTH AMERICA

RELATED CLINICS SERIES

Gastroenterology Clinics
(www.gastro.theclinics.com)
Clinics in Liver Disease
(www.liver.theclinics.com)

THE CLINICS ARE AVAILABLE ONLINE!
Access your subscription at:
www.theclinics.com

Foreword

Endoscopy for Biliary Disease Continues to Advance

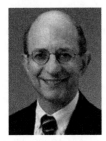

Charles J. Lightdale, MD
Consulting Editor

Endoscopic management of biliary disease, benign and malignant, has become widely available throughout the world. The major pillar of endoscopy for biliary disease is endoscopic retrograde cholangiopancreatography (ERCP), in which the papilla of Vater is identified with a duodenoscope and a flexible cannula is directed into the bile duct to inject radiographic contrast dye to visualize the biliary system. The first ERCP was performed by Dr William McCune in 1968. In 1972, Dr Peter Cotton in England published his experience with 60 diagnostic ERCP procedures, and in 1973, Dr Keiichi Kawai in Japan and Dr Meinhard Classen in Germany independently carried out biliary sphincterotomy, allowing endoscopic instruments to be passed into the biliary system for therapy. In recent years, ERCP has become used most frequently with therapeutic intent as less-invasive transabdominal ultrasonography, computed tomography, and magnetic resonance cholangiopancreatography have become the preferred modalities for diagnosis of biliary disease.

With the advent of more training programs in interventional endoscopy, endoscopic ultrasonography (EUS) has proved to be an important therapeutic modality for biliary disease, usually for more complex and difficult cases. There is an overall high level of success for the simplest biliary cases, for example, removal of small bile duct stones, placing stents for strictures, or bile leaks following laparoscopic cholecystectomy. However, large stones, complex strictures, or biliary disease associated with gastric bypass surgery are often best referred to academic medical centers, where highly skilled and experienced endoscopists are available with multimodality approaches, including therapeutic EUS and interventional radiology. The highlight of postgraduate courses featuring live endoscopy cases is usually the opportunity to observe master endoscopists take on difficult biliary cases.

Dr Mouen Khashab, a master interventional endoscopist at Johns Hopkins Hospital and a leader in the field of biliary endoscopy, has gathered an extraordinary

Gastrointest Endoscopy Clin N Am 32 (2022) xiii–xiv
https://doi.org/10.1016/j.giec.2022.03.004
1052-5157/22/© 2022 Published by Elsevier Inc.

international group of experts for this issue of the *Gastrointestinal Endoscopy Clinics of North America* devoted to "Advances in Biliary Endoscopy." This is a comprehensive state-of-the-art review featuring articles on basic and advanced bile duct cannulation techniques, removal of simple or complex biliary stones, the management of benign and malignant biliary obstruction, and approaches to indeterminant strictures of the bile duct. Other articles discuss the prevention and management of complications of biliary endoscopy, EUS and percutaneous approaches, endoscopic management of acute cholecystitis, biliary endoscopy in altered anatomy, and endoscopic papillectomy (the removal of an abnormal papilla). A final article explores the future of cholangioscopy, where a cannula-size endoscope is passed through a duodenoscope into the bile duct to directly observe abnormalities. Biliary endoscopists at all skill levels should read this issue.

Charles J. Lightdale, MD
Department of Medicine
Columbia University Medical Center
161 Fort Washington Avenue
New York, NY 10032, USA

E-mail address:
CJL18@columbia.edu

Preface

Advances in Biliary Endoscopy: Timely and Relevant

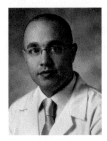

Mouen Khashab, MD, MASGE, FJGES
Editor

This issue of *Gastrointestinal Endoscopy Clinics of North America* on "Advances in Biliary Endoscopy" is a comprehensive summary of all aspects relevant to biliary endoscopy. Articles are practical and provide the reader with both expert and data-driven opinions on topics that span basic cannulation techniques to the future of cholangioscopy. Approaching a patient with biliary pathologic condition in need of an intervention requires a unique skillset and collaborative management with other disciplines, such as interventional radiology. In addition, we have seen an increasing role of endoscopic ultrasonography (EUS) in the diagnosis and interventional management of such patients. Integrating these disciplines and procedures into our daily practice is in the best interest of our patients. This issue is written by world experts on endoscopic retrograde cholangiopancreatography, EUS, and interventional radiology. I hope it will be a reference to all interested in this topic for years to come.

Mouen Khashab, MD, MASGE, FJGES
Therapeutic Endoscopy Group
Johns Hopkins Enterprise
Johns Hopkins Hospital
1800 Orleans Street
Baltimore, MD 21287, USA

E-mail address:
mkhasha1@jhmi.edu

Basic and Advanced Biliary Cannulation: How Do I Do It?

Robert H. Hawes, MD[a,b,c,*]

KEYWORDS

- Cannulation • Sphincterotomy • Access sphincterotomy • Guidewire-assisted
- Advanced techniques • Pancreatic stent • Post-ERCP pancreatitis

KEY POINTS

- Successful biliary cannulation is more art than science and there is no substitution for experience and failure.
- Standard cannulation attempts fail up to 20% of the time even in experienced hands.
- Application of advanced techniques to failed cannulation should raise the overall cannulation rate to 90%–95%.
- With the advent of wire-guided cannulation, advanced cannulation techniques and pancreatic stenting, severe post-ERCP pancreatitis (PEP) should be rare.

INTRODUCTION

Selective cannulation during ERCP is an art guided by experience and science. It is interesting to note that the general technique of ERCP has not fundamentally changed over the last 50 years and deep cannulation of the desired duct is still the rate-limiting step that determines a successful or failed procedure. Becoming a good ERCP artist requires experience. Science can be applied to ERCP cannulation but an individual's experience strongly influences how the "science" is applied to one's individual practice. The first part of this article is heavy on experience and short on science. The nuances of cannulation and the myriad confirmations of the major papilla prevent the application of rigorous scientific research. The general principles of cannulation can be taught along with the advantages and disadvantages of various accessories but cannulation itself is a fluid process combining an almost infinite number of subtle maneuvers of the endoscope in concert with the accessories and this process cannot be rigorously evaluated in randomized trials.

There are also challenges to studying various "advanced techniques" applied to "difficult" cannulations. Even the definition of a "difficult" cannulation is not uniformly accepted. However, advanced techniques do lend themselves to more rigorous, albeit

[a] Orlando Health Digestive Health Institute, 1335 Sligh Boulevard, 3rd Floor, Orlando, FL 33806, USA; [b] Center for Advanced Endoscopy, Research and Education (CARE); [c] University of Central Florida College of Medicine
* Orlando Health Digestive Health Institute, 1335 Sligh Blvd, 3rd Floor, Orlando, FL 33806.
E-mail address: robert.hawesmd@gmail.com

Gastrointest Endoscopy Clin N Am 32 (2022) 385–395
https://doi.org/10.1016/j.giec.2022.01.002
1052-5157/22/© 2022 Elsevier Inc. All rights reserved.

giendo.theclinics.com

imprecise, scientific study. The discussion on advanced cannulation techniques will present the science but ultimately the application of these advanced techniques will depend on the experience and bias of the individual endoscopist. Hopefully, this article will fully explain the art and science of cannulation in a clear and understandable way so that readers will be able to leverage this information to optimize their cannulation success and minimize complications.

BASIC CANNULATION TECHNIQUES

Despite improvements in endoscopes and accessories, deep cannulation of the desired duct in a native papilla remains the most challenging step to the successful completion of the procedure. No single technique is uniformly successful.

Important Components to Successful Cannulation Include

1. Taking the time to study the confirmation of the papilla.
2. Spending the necessary time to achieve proper positioning of the duodenoscope before touching the papilla.
3. Choosing your weapon.
4. When initiating cannulation, make sure that the leading edge of the accessory is perpendicular to the ampullary orifice
5. First obtaining a free "insinuation" of the ampullary orifice.
6. Use either the guidewire or a limited injection of contrast material (or both) as the first approach for deep cannulation
7. Never fight with the papilla.

Begin all ERCPs with a careful inspection of the papilla. What is the overall conformation of the major papilla including the intraduodenal length? Are there many surrounding folds and is the papilla semi-firm or very soft and mobile? In general, if the intraduodenal length is short, deep cannulation can be achieved by advancing the accessory in a single trajectory ("straight shot," no intrapapillary angles, single axis). Long intraduodenal segments, especially when associated with multiple folds and a soft texture will require careful, gentle, complex manipulation of the endoscope and accessory to negotiate and straighten angles.

An underappreciated aspect in achieving successful cannulation is the manipulation of the endoscope to obtain an optimal orientation to the papilla. We are taught to "shorten the scope" in the second portion of the duodenum and then begin cannulation. Although the "short scope" position provides the greatest maneuverability and keeps one close to the papilla, it is not a primary goal unto itself. The primary goal is to use whatever the confirmation of the scope is necessary to (1) allow the tip of the catheter to enter the papillary orifice at a perpendicular angle, (2) orient the papilla enface, (3) be acceptably close to the papilla, and (4) have the papilla in the center of the visual field (or slightly above). The radiographic scope position has no relevance to cannulation, but the fluoroscopic and endoscope positions must be coordinated to allow the radiographic observation of the shape of the distal, intrapapillary part of the duct. When this is suboptimal, consider repositioning the patient.

There are wide varieties of accessories available for initial cannulation. In the days of diagnostic ERCP, the procedure was often initiated with a standard catheter because many times the goal was to simply inject the appropriate duct (believe it or not, in the early days of ERCP, an accepted indication was to obtain a complete pancreatogram to determine if the patient had chronic pancreatitis using the Cambridge criteria.[1] At the NIH consensus conference on ERCP in 2002, it was concluded that diagnostic ERCP had been supplanted by CT, MRI and EUS.[2] There were no longer any indications for simply obtaining a cholangiogram or pancreatogram. Since the consensus confer- ence, the goal for cholangiopancreatography is to direct therapy. As a result, cannula- tion usually begins with a soft-tipped guidewire and a papillotome. There are of course exceptions if the patient has had a prior sphincterotomy or pancreas divisum. There is no universal best or perfect accessory. One should be inquisitive and gain experience with a broad spectrum of available accessories to enable the selection of the appro- priate ones for an individual case and to learn which ones you are most comfortable with.

The initial access for biliary cannulation is always cephalad (uphill). Whether using the wire or catheter tip at the initiation of cannulation, the tip should be perpendicular to the face of the papillary orifice with an uphill trajectory. Scope position and acces- sory orientation should be optimized before cannulation is initiated. Avoid forcefully engaging the papilla and then trying to reorient because this distorts the papilla and makes deep cannulation more difficult. Make every effort to stay reasonably close to the papilla. If the tip of the scope is too far from the papilla, the curvature of the cath- eter will inevitably cause the tip of the catheter to go into the roof of the papilla as it is advanced preventing deep cannulation. Operating far away from the papilla will also cause one to lose precision when making fine movements.

The first step to cannulation is to carefully and gently advance the tip of the acces- sory into the ampullary orifice; a maneuver that is termed "insinuation." The Miriam– Webster definition of insinuate is "to introduce something gradually or in a subtle, in- direct or covert way." Insinuation describes the deep seating of the catheter into the ampullary orifice. It is a "feel" thing. It is important to achieve a comfortable "seeding" of the accessory into the ampullary orifice before progressing to maneuvers to achieve deep cannulation. You will know when you are "seeded" when the guidewire or the catheter tip is deeply engaged without distorting the papilla. Do not force the catheter tip into the ampullary segment. This causes distortion and compression of the papilla. When the catheter tip is forced into the papillary orifice, attempts to advance a wire will cause progressive edema, rendering further attempts more difficult, or cause the disruption of the mucosa, creating a false tract. If you try injecting contrast material, it will either reflux into the duodenum lumen or you will cause a submucosal injection; further distorting the ampullary anatomy. Nothing good comes from what is called the "cram and squirt" maneuver; trying to deeply cannulate without first achieving a free insinuation.

Insinuation of the ampullary orifice can occur either with the catheter tip or with a guidewire. Once one achieves optimal seating into the ampullary orifice, there are several options for the next maneuver:

1. Insinuation with catheter tip
   a. Inject a small amount of contrast followed by the advancement of the guidewire
   b. Advance the guidewire alone (wire-guided technique)
2. Insinuation with guidewire
   a. Advance catheter tip to end of guidewire and inject contrast
   b. Advance the guidewire while adjusting the angle with the catheter (wire-guided technique)

If one insinuates with the catheter tip, whether this is followed by contrast injection or advancement of the guidewire, always release the pressure on the catheter before proceeding; it will be less traumatic and more effective.

Much has been written about wire-guided cannulation: cannulation of the desired duct with a guidewire under fluoroscopic control without contrast injection. It was initially conceived as a technique to reduce post-ERCP pancreatitis (PEP) by avoiding the injec- tion of contrast into the pancreatic duct.[3] Three meta-analyses concluded that the guidewire technique provided a significantly higher rate of biliary cannulation.[4–6] Four meta-analyses have compared wire-guided to contrast guided cannulation in terms of PEP and all 4 studies concluded that there is a lower risk of PEP associated with wire assisted biliary cannulation.[4–7] If a wire-guided technique is used, most endoscopists prefer a straight-tipped guidewire. Some believe that if wire-guided cannulation is failing with a straight-tipped guidewire, it is efficacious to switch to an angled-tipped guidewire. If using an angled-tipped guidewire, it is important that the guidewire is torque stable. In some circumstances, torquing and gently advancing an angled tip wire will successfully negotiate the papillary angles. The use of this technique should be a personal choice as randomized trials have not shown angle-tip guidewires to be superior to straight guidewires.[8]

Many experienced endoscopists feel there is too much emphasis placed on this approach. A gentle and limited injection of contrast material can provide a "roadmap" of the intra-ampullary segment, making it much easier to adjust the trajectory of the guidewire or catheter tip under fluoroscopic guidance to successfully negotiate tricky angles. The optimal approach is the careful use of either or both techniques depending on the circumstances. When there is an advanced pancreatic disease, there is no harm to limited pancreatic injections to achieve a radiographic roadmap. In these cases, ampullary distortion can be such that contrast guidance is indispensable in achieving a selective deep biliary cannulation. In the case of a normal pancreas, you may persist longer with a wire-guided method to avoid pancreatic injection (and the risk of pancreatitis). If an ampullary roadmap is desired, the injection should be slow, careful, under fluoroscopic guidance, and limited; the purpose is to understand the ampullary angles not to fill the biliopancreatic ducts.

No single technique is successful in all cases and it is important that one does not obstinately persist when a particular technique is not working. If you are trying to cannulate with the tip of the catheter, then switch to having a little guidewire protruding to more precisely engage at the 11 o'clock position. If you go into the pancreas, withdraw the catheter from the papilla and restart the cannulation from a slightly different angle. Do not forcefully engage the papilla and then try to redirect the catheter tip. If you are trying a wire-guided technique and it is not succeeding, inject a small amount of contrast material to obtain a roadmap.

One can examine the papilla and often predict what maneuvers will be required to cannulate. If the papilla faces downstream and there is a long intraduodenal segment, the scope tip will need to be positioned distal to the papilla so that the initial trajectory of the catheter/guidewire will be sufficiently "uphill." A distally oriented papilla may also require one to "hook" the papilla by engaging the elevator while pulling the scope shaft to straighten the ampulla and flatten the angle to facilitate deep cannulation. Remember that the tract to enter the bile duct is almost always some degree of an "S" shape; the acuteness of the angles is dependent on the individual anatomy and the pressure applied to the papilla by the accessory. The most common conformation of the papilla which can make cannulation difficult is what is called the "up and over" papilla (an accentuated "S" shape). On inspection, the papilla looks like a "camel's hump." It requires 3 distinct maneuvers to achieve deep cannulation. The first maneuver requires a cephalad trajectory, insinuation, and advancement to the apex of the hump. Then, one must direct the tip of the accessory downward and this requires: 1) turning left with the small dial of the scope and 2) pulling the shaft of the scope back. This will provide the downward trajectory needed to negotiate the angle at the top of the hump. This is also the time when your assistant can try to gently advance the guidewire. Once this is achieved, the scope shaft is pushed in (and the small dial gently turned back to the right) to re-achieve the cephalad trajectory needed to negotiate the second angle that is present at the ampullary duodenal junction. These angles are not only in the frontal but also in the anterior–posterior axis. Cannulation requires a 3–dimensional "vision" of what you are looking at.

A "shar-pei" papilla refers to one that has multiple redundant surrounding folds and no turgor (stiffness). This situation requires straightening the papilla by hooking it with the elevator and then turning left on a small dial while pulling back slightly on the scope shaft. With a shar-pei papilla, one will never achieve deep cannulation by simply pushing on the catheter or the guidewire.

ADVANCED TECHNIQUES

Despite the careful and persistent application of the cannulation principles outlined above, free cannulation may fail. Development of advanced techniques has been an important evolution in ERCP because data are now clear that prolonged papillary manipulation with repeated attempts to selectively cannulate the bile duct, particularly when inadvertent cannulation of the pancreas occurs, leads to an increased incidence of PEP.[9,10] In a study we published in 2016, we prospectively look at our cannulation rate of a native papilla using standard cannulation techniques. In a group of experienced pancreaticobiliary endoscopists, our cannulation rate was 87%.[11] However, we did not adhere to a uniform definition of "failure" using standard techniques. To understand and interpret the literature on difficult cannulation, one must understand the definition. The European Society of Gastrointestinal Endoscopy (ESGE)[12] defines "difficult biliary cannulation" by the presence of 1 or more of the following:

1. More than 5 contacts with the papilla while attempting to cannulate
2. More than 5 minutes spent attempting to cannulate the following visualization of the papilla
3. More than one unintended pancreatic duct cannulation or opacification

This definition is a consensus agreement with low-quality evidence to support it, but it provides readers some context to help understand when it may be appropriate to use "advanced techniques." It is a relatively conservative definition that was likely adopted to discourage prolonged manipulation of the papilla. In case of failed cannulation, the application of advanced cannulation techniques should be undertaken if the endoscopist has sufficient training and experience. In our study cited above, when we applied advanced techniques after failed standard techniques, our overall success rate for cannulation jumped to 98.3%.[11]

Advanced maneuvers have evolved to increase cannulation success when standard maneuvers fail. These can be organized into 2 categories:

1. Advanced cannulation techniques
2. Access sphincterotomy

ADVANCED CANNULATION TECHNIQUES

Advanced cannulation techniques primarily involve maneuvers to straighten the intra-ampullary angles. This is accomplished either by placing a guidewire into the pancreatic duct or by placing a small-caliber plastic stent. Placing a pancreatic guidewire is called "the double wire" technique. It involves achieving deep cannulation of the pancreatic duct with a soft-tipped guidewire, leaving the wire in place and then a cannula (usually a papillotome) loaded with a second guidewire is passed alongside the pancreatic wire and biliary cannulation is attempted. Theoretically, the guidewire "straightens" the ampullary segment providing more direct biliary access. Additionally, the endoscopist can now use fluoroscopy to adjust the trajectory angle of the catheter tip and/or guidewire toward the biliary direction. This technique is particularly popular in patients with a periampullary diverticulum which notoriously distorts and accentuates the angles of the distal bile duct and ampullary segment. Results from studies comparing the double wire technique to the persistence of standard cannulation techniques have been mixed. One study[13] showed no difference in successful cannulation and PEP, whereas another study showed a higher cannulation success rate but no difference in pancreatitis.[14] A Cochrane Systematic Review revealed that the sole use of the double wire technique was associated with an increased risk of PEP.[15] The review also concluded that the double guidewire technique was not superior to persistent attempts using standard cannulation techniques, precut sphincterotomy or a PD stent in achieving biliary cannulation. The ESGE clinical guidelines recommend that this should be the first maneuver attempted if standard cannulation techniques fail, especially if repeated unintentional pancreatic access has occurred.[12] If this maneuver is used, a prophylactic pancreatic stent should be placed before concluding the procedure.[12]

While the double wire technique is relatively straightforward conceptually, there are several cautionary points that are important. This maneuver is ideal if the course of the main pancreatic duct (MPD) is relatively straight because this makes the placement of the guidewire straightforward. However, if the MPD makes several acute turns within the head of the pancreas (sigmoid shaped) or the pancreatic duct makes a 360^0 curve (ansa pancreaticus), negotiating a guidewire around these angles to place the guidewire tip into the tail of the pancreas may be extremely difficult and may increase the risk of PEP. Another potential problem is that once a pancreatic guidewire is in place, the team must be diligent to monitor the tip of the guidewire. While concentrating on achieving biliary cannulation, the pancreatic guidewire can move. If the tip of the guidewire is forcefully passed into a side-branch of the pancreatic duct, it can cause perforation and subsequent acute pancreatitis.

If the double wire technique fails, one should place a small-caliber pancreatic stent and then try to cannulate alongside the stent. This can be cumbersome because many endoscopists will place a 5 French pancreatic stent. This caliber stent can completely fill the papillary orifice and make even guidewire cannulation alongside the stent quite difficult. Four French stents can be passed over an 0.025″ guidewire which may make this technique easier.

ACCESS SPHINCTEROTOMY

This section is termed "access sphincterotomy" because it is the best description of the maneuvers. Most readers are more familiar with the term "precut sphincterotomy." Historically, the term "precut" was coined by Kees Huibregtse to describe a technique that he conceived whereby a needle knife is used to initiate an incision at the ampullary orifice.[16] He used this technique to gain access to the biliary tree when standard cannulation attempts failed. Once access was achieved, the biliary orifice was often extended using a standard papillotome, hence the term "pre-cut." There are now several techniques that are variations on Professor Huibregtse's original description and all of them are used to gain access to the biliary tree after failed cannulation. The term "access sphincterotomy" is a better descriptor for this group of advanced sphincterotomy techniques used to gain access to the biliary tree because we often do not further extend the cut as originally described.

There are 4 techniques described in this section:

1. Free-hand sphincterotomy using a needle knife (Huibregtse technique)
2. Needle-knife sphincterotomy over a pancreatic stent
3. Fistulotomy

4. Pancreatic sphincterotomy

Which technique is applied in what circumstance should be determined by the personal preference of the endoscopist and taking into account the overall health of the pancreas. Free-hand (precut sphincterotomy) and pancreatic sphincterotomy should be reserved primarily for those patients with advanced pancreatic disease; either advanced chronic pancreatitis or pancreatic cancer. These 2 techniques can adversely affect pancreatic drainage and patients with a normal pancreas are at high risk of PEP, to begin with. The other 2 techniques either protect pancreatic drainage with a stent or avoid the pancreatic duct altogether.

Free-hand access sphincterotomy using a needle knife was developed and championed by Kees Huibregtse at the Academic Medical Center (AMC) in Amsterdam (now the Amsterdam University Medical Center - AUMC).[16] It involves using a needle knife, beginning the incision at the ampullary orifice, and working cephalad in the 11:00 direction. Most people apply a "layering" cut for which the initial incision is superficial and then continued at deeper and deeper levels until the biliary orifice are identified. In the early days, this technique was criticized because of the potential for causing PEP. If this technique is applied primarily to patients with common bile duct stones, chronic pancreatitis, or pancreatic cancer, it is generally safe because these are patients at very low risk of PEP. However, when this technique is used in patients at higher risk of PEP (abdominal pain, recurrent acute pancreatitis, or a low probability of bile duct stones), early studies showed a high risk of PEP, particularly before the advent of pancreatic stenting. Early on, the free needle-knife precut sphincterotomy was often applied after prolonged attempts using standard techniques. Multiple meta-analyses have now suggested that the PEP rate may be related to timing; early application after failed cannulation seems to minimize the PEP rate.[17–20]

Access sphincterotomy performed with a needle-knife over a pancreatic stent has several advantages and therefore is the preferred technique by many endoscopists. The pancreatic stent is placed immediately after failed cannulation and thus assures pancreatic drainage early on during the procedure. After placement, the stent serves 2 main purposes. First, it provides a direction for the incision. This was initially described in 1994 and is a useful tip for biliary, pancreatic, and minor papilla sphincterotomy.[21] Second, it serves as a stable platform and prevents the endoscopist from extending the incision too deeply. Finally, if something happens during the course of the procedure that requires the procedure to be suspended, the stent is securely in place to prevent PEP. A prospective randomized trial was conducted comparing access sphincterotomy alone to the placement of a prophylactic pancreatic stent.[22] This study of 151 patients concluded that placing and maintaining a pancreatic stent for needle-knife precut sphincterotomy reduces the frequency and severity of PEP. In rare cases, there is a transposition of the ducts such that the pancreatic duct initially takes off in the 11 o'clock position while the bile duct takes off at 5:00 o'clock. With this technique, the ampullary segment is exposed with the stent clearly identifying the pancreatic duct and the aberrant orientation of the bile duct can be relatively easily detected. This technique (or fistulotomy – see later in discussion) are the techniques that the ESGE recommends in cases of a difficult cannulation associated with a peri-ampullary diverticulum.[12]

Although it is not popular or often used, this article would be incomplete without describing the placement of a 3 French pancreatic stent to facilitate access sphincterotomy. One must use a 0.018″ guidewire in conjunction with a tapered tip catheter to place a 3 French pancreatic stent. The floppy coiled tip and the nitinol body of the 0.018″ guidewire make it relatively easy to advance to the pancreatic tail. The 3 French stent (Cook Medical, Winston-Salem, NC) comes in a 12 cm length with a single full pigtail on the duodenal and but no side flap. The stent can be cut to an optimal length but the stent should be passed beyond the genu to ensure that it stays in place for at least 72 hours. The advantage of the small stent is that it almost always spontaneously passes on its own (prevents the need for a second procedure for stent removal) but is stable in the pancreas during the course of the sphincterotomy and whatever additional maneuvers are performed to complete the ERCP. It is soft and flexible and therefore does not cause damage to the MPD. Similar advantages can probably be obtained with a 4 French stent (Boston Scientific, Natick, MA) which can be passed over the more popular 0.025″ guidewire.

Fistulotomy refers to a technique that uses a needle knife to make an incision on the dome of the intraduodenal segment of the ampulla. This technique was developed because the incision does not extend to the ampullary orifice and thus should reduce the risk of PEP. This was tested in a randomized trial which showed needle-knife fistulotomy to be as effective as conventional needle-knife precut sphincterotomy but had a lower rate of PEP.[23] However, this technique depends on the conformation of the papilla and cannot be applied when there is no significant intraduodenal segment of the papilla.[24] A superficial incision is made and then slowly extended layer by layer until the bile duct is identified (usually by the visualization of bile). Sometimes bile is not seen if there is upstream obstruction and in which case one has to gently probe within the incision bed aiming in the 11:00 direction of the bile duct.

The technique of pancreatic sphincterotomy involves accessing the pancreatic duct and advancing a guidewire deeply enough into the pancreatic duct to stabilize the papillotome and then performing a sphincterotomy in the biliary direction. This technique can be very successful with one study accomplishing a 97% biliary cannulation rate in 255 cases of failed standard cannulation.[25] This technique is safe in patients with pancreatic cancer and advanced chronic pancreatitis but can carry a high risk of PEP if applied and the patient with normal pancreas, especially if a prophylactic pancreatic stent is not placed.[26] The advantage of this technique is that it uses a standard accessory (papillotome) and a familiar technique of standard sphincterotomy.

Ideally, all the advanced techniques described above should be in the armamentarium of the endoscopist. Which ones are used and the sequence of utilization is at the discretion of the endoscopist. An example of how these techniques can be used algorithmically was described by Lee and colleagues[27] In this study of 711 patients with a naïve papilla, 140 were determined to be "difficult cannulation" by their established criteria. If they failed cannulation but had no unintentional cannulations of the pancreatic duct, they applied the fistulotomy technique. If they had ≥3 unintentional pancreatic cannulations, then they first tried the double wire technique and if this failed, they performed an access sphincterotomy over a pancreatic stent. Using this algorithm, of the 140 patients with failed standard cannulation, they were able to achieve biliary cannulation and 90% (126/140).[27]

It is difficult to compare advanced cannulation techniques. Individual comparative studies will differ in a myriad of important parameters including the definition of "difficult cannulation," variability in the patients studied, and variability in the skills of the endoscopist. Experienced endoscopists also develop personal bias with techniques and it is difficult to neutralize these biases in comparative studies. Nevertheless, a recent systematic review and network meta-analysis endeavored to evaluate the comparative efficacy of different methods for difficult biliary cannulation.[28] They compared advanced cannulation and access sphincterotomy techniques with their primary focus being: (1) success rate of biliary cannulation and (2) the incidence of PEP. The techniques studied included:

1. Persistence with standard cannulation techniques
2. Pancreatic guidewire-assisted technique
3. Pancreatic stent-assisted technique
4. Early needle knife techniques
5. Late needle knife techniques
6. Transpancreatic sphincterotomy

In addition to the issues mentioned above, another weakness of this article is that they lump all needle knife techniques together (free-hand needle knife, needle knife over a pancreatic stent, and fistulotomy). The results showed that in terms of the success rate of biliary cannulation, transpancreatic sphincterotomy was the most successful followed by early needle-knife techniques. In terms of the rate of PEP, early needle-knife techniques were superior followed by transpancreatic sphincterotomy. The significant conclusions were that transpancreatic sphincterotomy increases the success rate of biliary cannulation as compared with persistence with standard cannulation techniques and early needle-knife techniques and transpancreatic sphincterotomy were superior to other interventions and decreasing rates of PEP.

SUMMARY

In this article, we have reviewed standard techniques for selective cannulation. With experience, these techniques should result in successful cannulation in 75% to 85% of cases. However, some notes of caution should be expressed. A good endoscopist will always be gentle with the papilla. If initial cannulation attempts fail, ultimate success is never accomplished by becoming angry with the patient, the scope, the papilla, or your coworkers. Careful, precise technique always produces better outcomes than force and frustration. However, even the very best endoscopists using the optimal technique will fail using standard techniques. We know now that prolonged persistence with standard cannulation techniques increases the risk of PEP. All endoscopists should have a reasonable threshold for abandoning standard cannulation techniques and adopting advanced techniques. In experienced hands, the application of advanced cannulation/sphincterotomy techniques should increase the overall cannulation rate to ≥ 95%. Experience is a key term because the techniques described above cannot be applied by simply reading about them or watching videos.

CLINICS CARE POINTS

- In most circumstances, the wire-guided technique should be the initial approach to selective cannulation.
- Standard cannulation should be limited by time and unintended pancreatic cannulation/ injection to avoid an increased risk of PEP.
- Appropriate use of advanced cannulation and access sphincterotomy techniques will improve biliary cannulation success.

DISCLOSURE

Dr R.H. Hawes is a consultant for Olympus and Fuji and has stock in Apollo Endosurgery.

REFERENCES

1. Sarner M, Cotton PB. Classification of pancreatitis. Gut 1984;25:756–9.

2. Cohen S, Bacon BR, Berlin JA, et al. National Institutes of Health State–of–the–Science Conference Statement: ERCP for diagnosis and therapy. Gastrointest Endosc 2002;56(6):803–9.
3. Lella F, Bagnolo F, Colombo E, et al. a simple way of avoiding post–ERCP pancreatitis. Gastrointest Endosc 2004;59:830–4.
4. Cheung J, Tsoi KK, Quan WL, et al. Guidewire versus conventional contrast cannulation of the common bile duct for the prevention of post ERCP pancreatitis: A systematic review and meta-analysis. Gastrointest Endosc 2009;70:1211–29.
5. Tse F, Yuan Y, Moayyedi P, et al. Guidewire–assisted cannulation for the prevention of post–ERCP pancreatitis: A systematic review and meta-analysis. Endoscopy 2013;45:605–18.
6. Shao LM, Chen QY, Chen MY, et al. Can wire–guided cannulation reduce the risk of post endoscopic retrograde cholangiopancreatography pancreatitis? Meta-analysis of randomized control trials. J Gastroenterol Hepatol 2009;24:1710–5.
7. Cennamo V, Fuccio L, Zagari RM, et al. Can a wire guided cannulation technique increase bile duct cannulation rate and prevent post- ERCP pancreatitis? A meta-analysis of randomized control trials. Am J Gastroenterol 2009;104:2343–50.
8. Tsuchiya T, Itoi T, Maetani I, et al. Effectiveness of the J–tip guidewire for selective biliary cannulation compared to conventional guidewires (the JANGLE study). Dig Dis Sci 2015;60(8):2502–8.
9. Freeman ML, DiSario JA, Nelson DB, et al. Risk factors for post-ERCP pancreatitis: a prospective multicenter study. Gastrointest Endosc 2001;54:425–34.
10. Wang P, Li ZS, Liu F, et al. Risk factors for ERCP-related complications: a prospective multicenter study. Am J Gastroenterol 2009;104:31–40.
11. Holt BA, Hawes R, Hasan M, et al. Biliary drainage: role of EUS guidance. Gastrointest Endosc 2016;83(1):160–5.
12. Testoni PA, Mariani A, Aabakken L, et al. Papillary cannulation and sphincterotomy techniques in ERCP: European Society of Gastrointestinal Endoscopy (ESGE) clinical guideline. Endoscopy 2016;48:657–83.
13. Herreros de Tejada A, Calleja JL, Diaz G, et al. Double-guidewire technique for difficult bile duct cannulation: A multicenter randomized, controlled trial. Gastrointest Endosc 2009;70:700–9.
14. Maeda S, Hayashi H, Hosokawa O, et al. Prospective randomized pilot trial of selective biliary cannulation using pancreatic guide-wire placement. Endoscopy 2003;35:721–4.
15. Tse F, Yuan Y, Bukhari M, et al. Pancreatic duct guidewire placement for biliary cannulation for the prevention of post–endoscopic retrograde cholangiopancreatography (ERCP) pancreatitis. Cochrane Database Syst Rev 2016;(5):CD010571.
16. Huibregtse K, Katon RM, Tytgat GN. Precut papillotomy via fine-needle knife papillotome: a safe and effective technique. Gastrointest Endosc 1986;32(6):403–5.
17. Cennamo V, Fuccio L, Zagari RM, et al. Can early precut implementation reduce endoscopic retrograde cholangiopancreatography related complication risk? Meta-analysis of randomized control trials. Endoscopy 2010;42(5):381–8.
18. Gong B, Hao L, Bie L, et al. Does precut technique improved selective bile duct cannulation or increase post ERCP pancreatitis rate? A meta-analysis of randomized control trials. Surg Endosc 2010;24(11):2670–80.
19. Navaneethan U, Konjeti R, Venkatesh PG, et al. Early precut sphincterotomy and the risk of endoscopic retrograde cholangiopancreatography related complications: An updated meta-analysis. World J Gastrointest Endosc 2014;6(5):200–8.
20. Sundaralingam P, Masson P, Bourke MJ. Early precut sphincterotomy does not increase risk during endoscopic retrograde cholangiopancreatography in

patients with difficult biliary access: Meta-analysis of randomized control trials. Clin Gastroenterol Hepatol 2015;13(10):1722–9.

21. Siegel JH, Cohen SA, Kasmin FE, et al. Stent guided sphincterotomy. Gastrointest Endosc 1994;40(5):567–72.

22. Cha S-W, Leung WD, Lehman GL, et al. Does leaving a main pancreatic duct stent in place reduce the incidence of precut biliary sphincterotomy–associated pancreatitis? A randomized, prospective study. Gastrointest Endosc 2013;77(2):209–16.

23. Mavrogiannis C, Liatsos C, Romanos A, et al. needle-knife fistulotomy versus needle-knife precut papillotomy for the treatment of bile duct stones. Gastrointest Endosc 1999;50(3):334–92.

24. Zhang Q-S, Xu J-H, Dong Z-Q, et al. success and safety of needle-knife papillotomy and fistulotomy based on papillary anatomy: A prospective controlled trial. Dig Dis Sci 2021 [Online ahead of print].

25. Halttunen J, Keranen I, Udd M, et al. Pancreatic sphincterotomy versus a needle-knife precut and difficult biliary cannulation. Surg Endosc 2009;23(4):745–9.

26. Goff JS. Common bile duct pre-cut sphincterotomy: Transpancreatic sphincter approach. Gastrointest Endosc 1995;41(5):502–5.

27. Lee TH, Hwang SO, Choi HJ, et al. Sequential algorithm analysis to facilitate selective biliary access for difficult biliary cannulation in ERCP: A prospective clinical study. BMC Gastroenterol 2014;14:30.

28. Facciorusso A, Ramai D, Gkolfakis P, et al. Comparative efficacy of different methods for difficult biliary cannulation in ERCP: systematic review and network meta-analysis. Gastrointest Endosc 2022;95(1):60–71.

Prevention and Management of Complications of Biliary Endoscopy

Venkata S. Akshintala, MD, Anmol Singh, MD,
Vikesh K. Singh, MD, MSc*

KEYWORDS

- ERCP • Complications • Pancreatitis • Bleeding • Perforation

KEY POINTS

- Endoscopic retrograde cholangiopancreatography (ERCP) and biliary endoscopy-associated complications are common.
- Endoscopists must be aware of the techniques to prevent and manage such complications.
- The common complications include pancreatitis, bleeding, perforation, cholangitis, and instrument-associated complications.

INTRODUCTION

Endoscopic retrograde cholangiopancreatography (ERCP) or biliary endoscopy is used in the management of a variety of pancreaticobiliary disorders, and around 700,000 of these procedures are performed annually in the United States.[1] Over the past decade, ERCP has been less frequently pursued for the diagnostic indications and moved toward increasingly complex therapeutic indications, with a concurrent increase in the incidence of ERCP-associated complications.[2] It is, therefore, necessary to recognize the risk of ERCP-associated complications and familiarize oneself with the methods to prevent and treat such complications. In the current review, the authors discuss the prevention and the management of complications associated with ERCP, with emphasis on biliary endoscopy.

POSTENDOSCOPIC RETROGRADE CHOLANGIOPANCREATOGRAPHY PANCREATITIS

Post-ERCP pancreatitis (PEP) is the most frequent complication of ERCP. PEP occurs in 2% to 15% of cases and accounts for substantial morbidity, occasional mortality, and increased health care expenditures.[3] PEP adds more than $200 million annually

Division of Gastroenterology, Johns Hopkins Medical Institutions, Johns Hopkins University School of Medicine, 1830 East Monument Street, Suite 428, Baltimore, MD 21205, USA
* Corresponding author.
E-mail address: vsingh1@jhmi.edu

Gastrointest Endoscopy Clin N Am 32 (2022) 397–409
https://doi.org/10.1016/j.giec.2022.03.001
1052-5157/22/© 2022 Elsevier Inc. All rights reserved.

giendo.theclinics.com

to health care costs in the United States and was found to be the most common reason for lawsuits related to ERCP.[4,5] Interestingly, there was a 15.3% increase in the rate of PEP admissions from 2011 to 2017, as ERCP is less frequently pursued for diagnostic indications and moved toward increasingly complex therapeutic indications.[2]

Risk Factors for Postendoscopic Retrograde Cholangiopancreatography Pancreatitis

Numerous procedural and patient demographic features have previously been identified as risk factors for the development of PEP. ERCP procedures involving difficult or failed cannulation; guidewire cannulation; papillary, biliary, or pancreatic sphincterotomy; precut sphincterotomy; pancreatic duct (PD) brush cytology; pneumatic biliary dilation without biliary sphincterotomy; more than 2 PD guidewire passes; more than 2 PD contrast injections; pancreatic acinarization; and trainee involvement in the procedure have all been associated with an increased risk of developing PEP.[6–15] Patient-related risk factors have also been shown to increase the risk of PEP, such as female sex, age less than 50 years, pancreas divisum, sphincter of Oddi dysfunction, pancreaticobiliary malignancy, history of acute pancreatitis, history of PEP, and prior cholecystectomy.[16,17]

Contrast-assisted cannulation involving the engagement of a cannula into the papilla followed by injection of contrast in the direction of the desired duct has been the standard cannulation technique historically. However, over the past several years, guidewire-assisted cannulation into the desired duct without the aid of contrast injection has become the most widely practiced technique.[18] Guidewire-assisted cannulation has been associated with higher cannulation success.[19,20] However, the authors have identified a higher PEP rate when compared with contrast-assisted cannulation (odds ratio [OR] 0.14 [0.02–0.99]).[21] The PEP risk increased significantly when there were more than 2 guidewire passes into the PD, and the PEP risk increased with an increasing number of guidewire passes into the PD. Pancreatic brush cytology also increased the PEP risk significantly (OR 6.37 [1.1–36.9]). This suggests an important effect from the trauma from guidewire or ERCP accessories in the PD or its side branches in the etiopathogenesis of PEP (**Fig. 1**).

Given a large number of risk factors for PEP, with varying importance or weight of contribution to the overall PEP risk, it is challenging in a clinical situation to precisely

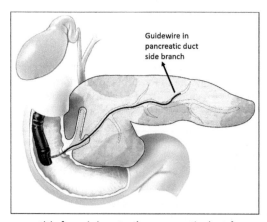

Guidewire in pancreatic duct side branch

Fig. 1. Post-ERCP pancreatitis from injury to the pancreatic duct from guidewire.

determine a patient's risk for PEP. Several prognostic scoring systems have therefore been developed to stratify patients based on their risk of developing PEP, primarily using multivariable linear regression models, although none are in widespread clinical use or endorsed by professional society guidelines.[22-27] These have however been limited due to the use of retrospective and nonrandomized data, incorporation of small numbers of risk factors, and limited ability to account for the interaction between risk factors.[23-25] Further, the previously described models were unable to predict risk reduction associated with PEP prophylaxis strategies such as rectal nonsteroidal anti-inflammatory drugs (NSAIDs), aggressive hydration, or prophylactic PD stenting.[28] However, there has been some promise in this regard, with the utilization of data from randomized controlled trials (RCTs) and application of novel machine learning–based statistical techniques.[29]

Prevention of Postendoscopic Retrograde Cholangiopancreatography Pancreatitis

Numerous prophylactic agents for PEP prophylaxis have been investigated in RCTs since 1977.[30] However, the strongest evidence is in favor of rectal NSAIDs,[31] high-volume intravenous fluid (IVF) administration,[32,33] and pancreatic stent (PS) placement–based prophylaxes.[34] More recently, the role of combinations of these prophylaxes has been with cumulative additive benefit has been recognized but few head-to-head RCTs exist.[28] The European Society of Gastrointestinal Endoscopy guidelines recommend the routine use of rectal NSAIDs for all patients, PS for those deemed high risk, and IVF for those unable to receive rectal NSAIDs.[35] In contrast, the ASGE guidelines recommend more restricted use of rectal NSAIDs to those at high risk of PEP, but IVF potentially for all patients.[36]

Within the United States, rectal indomethacin became widely used as prophylaxis following the publication of a landmark clinical trial in 2012.[37,38] In a recent comprehensive review and network meta-analysis (NMA), the authors have identified 11 different NSAID regimens, including diclofenac, indomethacin, celecoxib, naproxen, and ketoprofen, in various doses and routes of delivery.[28] There were 15 RCTs that evaluated rectal indomethacin, 100 mg, whereas another 9 RCTs evaluated rectal diclofenac, 100 mg. Interestingly, rectal diclofenac, 100 mg, may be more efficacious than rectal indomethacin, 100 mg, (OR 0.59; 95% confidence interval: 0.40–0.89) or at least as effective. The choice of which rectal NSAID to use varies across centers based on availability and practice.[4] Because of the exorbitant increase in the cost of rectal indomethacin in the United States (from $2 in 2005 to $340 for 100 mg in 2019), it is important to consider alternatives to rectal indomethacin such as rectal diclofenac, but this is currently commercially unavailable in the United States and will need to be compounded.[39]

Periprocedural IVF has a clear role in PEP prophylaxis with a clear pathophysiologic basis for its efficacy.[40] In a recent NMA, the authors found aggressive hydration with lactated Ringer solution or normal saline to be more efficacious for PEP prophylaxis compared with placebo or the standard volume hydration.[28] With regard to combinations of IVF and NSAIDs, there is conflicting evidence on the additive benefits of using these combinations.[41] Given the differing mechanisms of action, it is plausible that a combination of IVF and rectal NSAIDs would provide cumulative additive benefit.

PD stents have long been used for PEP prophylaxis and are thought to prevent PEP and reduce the severity of PEP by preserving PD outflow.[34] PD stents vary in diameter, length, presence of internal flanges, and type (straight or single pigtail). NMAs have compared various dimensions of PD stents and found that 5-Fr PD stent is superior to the 3-Fr PD stent.[42] There are clear advantages of pharmacologic over endoscopic methods such as PD stent placement for PEP prophylaxis, given the costs involved with follow-up imaging and repeat endoscopy for stent removal. In addition, attempting to place a PD stent with a subsequent failure increases the risk of PEP likely due to PD injury.[43] The authors' recent NMA did not identify a significant difference between the use of a 5- to 7-Fr PD stent and a combination of IVF and rectal NSAIDs.[28] This, however, needs to be answered with a prospective RCT, if a combination of NSAIDs and IVF can be used in lieu of PD stent, and is the topic of a large ongoing RCT.[44]

POSTENDOSCOPIC RETROGRADE CHOLANGIOPANCREATOGRAPHY CHOLANGITIS

Cholangitis after ERCP and biliary endoscopy can occur in 0.4% to 10% of the procedures but a review of 21 studies including 16,855 patients reported the incidence of cholangitis as 1.4% and associated mortality of 0.1%.[45] Biliary interventions are associated with disruption of the protective anatomic barriers and placement of foreign bodies including catheters, stents, and contrast, leading to enteric flora entering the biliary system causing cholangitis. Cross-infection through contaminated endoscopes and ERCP instruments has been a concern, with recent reports suggesting difficulty cleaning the elevator mechanism of duodenoscopes as the cause of such cross-contamination.[46] Endoscopic societies and manufacturers have now adopted new reprocessing protocols and the use of disposable caps to reduce the risk of cross-contamination.

The risk of cholangitis increases when there is a failure or incomplete drainage of the biliary system, due to an obstructive pathology. The location and type of the obstruction determine the risk of cholangitis, such as in primary sclerosing cholangitis (PSC) with multifocal stricturing, where it is often challenging to achieve complete drainage during ERCP. Other risk factors for cholangitis include low-volume endoscopy centers, delay in performing ERCP, clogged stents, and the use of combined percutaneous endoscopic procedures.[47] Novel biliary endoscopy techniques such as cholangioscopy have a higher risk of cholangitis, with reports of around 7% incidence especially when concurrent stone therapy is performed with electrohydraulic lithotripsy.[48]

Strategies to reduce risk of cholangitis: limiting the volume of contrast used during ERCP reduces pressure within the bile duct and also reduces the risk of contrast entrapment from incomplete drainage. Societal guidelines recommend the use of cross-sectional imaging to plan the ERCP, especially among patients with PSC and hilar obstruction, to reduce the risk of incomplete biliary drainage.[49] Balloon dilation was found to be equivalent to stent placement in patients with PSC, which limits the foreign body presence within the bile duct and migration of enteric flora into the biliary system.[50] Periprocedural antibiotics controlling cholangitis and associated biliary sepsis should be considered before stone therapy, which will allow adequate instrumentation and contrast injection during lithotripsy.[51] Antibiotic prophylaxis should also be considered during procedures with incomplete biliary drainage and those involving high-pressure injection within the bile duct such as during cholangioscopy and among immunocompromised patients.

ENDOSCOPIC RETROGRADE CHOLANGIOPANCREATOGRAPHY–ASSOCIATED ACUTE CHOLECYSTITIS

ERCP-associated cholecystitis must be recognized early and distinguished from cholangitis. The incidence of cholecystitis is, however, relatively low, with studies reporting the rates to be anything from 0.1% to 8.6%, with a large series reporting an incidence of less than or equal to 0.5%.[13,15] The etiopathogenesis is likely from nonsterile contrast media entering poorly emptying gallbladder or debris or stent obstructing the cystic duct. Large-diameter, covered metal stents were suspected to be leading to cystic duct obstruction but interestingly, 2 meta-analyses showed no difference in the rate of acute cholecystitis between covered and uncovered metal stents when treating distal malignant biliary disease.[52,53]

Prevention and management: adequate care should be taken to limit the injection of contrast into the gall bladder during ERCP. Early or same admission cholecystectomy after choledocholithiasis treatment, along with sphincterotomy, reduces the risk of acute cholecystitis.[54] The management of acute cholecystitis is otherwise similar to those from other causes.

ENDOSCOPIC RETROGRADE CHOLANGIOPANCREATOGRAPHY–ASSOCIATED BLEEDING

ERCP-associated bleeding is reported after 1% to 2% of the procedures, and in a large review, the bleeding was seen in 1.3% ERCPs, with 29% of them being severe.[45] Immediate bleeding after ERCP is seen in up to 50% of the procedures, and delayed bleeding can occur up to 2 weeks after ERCP, which is especially concerning for outpatient ERCPs.[15,55] Postsphincterotomy bleeding is the most common site of ERCP-associated bleeding but bleeding can also occur from the bile duct after therapies such as dilation, especially in the setting of malignant stricture. Risk factors for bleeding include patient-related factors such as coagulopathy, cirrhosis, renal failure, use of anticoagulant, and antiplatelet drugs and procedure-related factors such as the use of needle-knife sphincterotomy, rapid cutting, type of electrocautery used, and papillectomy.[56]

Strategies to reduce risk of bleeding: identifying the patients at risk for bleeding and correcting the coagulopathy and transfusing to goal platelet and International normalized ratio (INR) counts reduce the risk of bleeding. Societal guidelines provide recommendations for the timing of discontinuation of the antiplatelet and anticoagulant medications.[57] The common recommendation has been to continue aspirin while discontinuing clopidogrel and prasugrel. Patients at high risk of thrombotic events require bridging of anticoagulant therapy or short duration for which the anticoagulant and antiplatelet can be held and warrants modifications to the ERCP techniques. Attention must be paid to the anatomy of the papilla, focusing the sphincterotomy along the 11 to 1′ o clock directions, which has the least concentration of vessels, avoidance of long or "zipper" cuts, limiting the need for precut sphincterotomy, and judicious use of electrocautery current reduces the risk of post-sphincterotomy bleeding.[58] Among patients at higher risk of bleeding, a combination of small sphincterotomy with balloon dilation should be considered to reduce the risk of bleeding. Prophylactic submucosal injections were studied in an RCT, which is promising, but further evidence is needed if this technique can be routinely applied.[59]

Treatment of ERCP-associated bleeding: fortunately, ERCP-associated bleeding is most commonly self-limited and stops spontaneously. Endoscopic therapy must be considered in the setting of immediate bleeding and for bleeding prophylaxis among high-risk patients. Spraying epinephrine and injection of dilute epinephrine (1:10,000) at the bleeding site is effective.[56] When injection therapy fails, hemostat clip should be considered to be applied at the bleeding site (**Fig. 2**).[60] It is, however, challenging to apply the hemostat clip using a duodenoscope, as the plastic sheath on the clip may bend and kink passing over the elevator, preventing deployment. Gastroscope with cap can be considered in this situation to visualize the site better. Thermal ablation using argon plasma coagulation or cautery probes can be considered but attention must be paid to avoid the PD orifice that is located at around 5′o clock position.

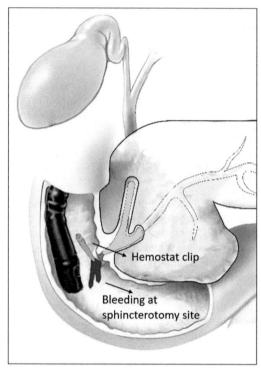

Fig. 2. ERCP-associated bleeding at the sphincterotomy site with hemostat clip placed.

Tamponade effect from a fully covered self-expandable metal stent controls bleeding at the sphincterotomy site and from within the bile duct and can be considered when the traditional methods are unsuccessful.[61]

ENDOSCOPIC RETROGRADE CHOLANGIOPANCREATOGRAPHY–ASSOCIATED PERFORATION

Perforation is a feared complication of the ERCP procedure and is classified based on the location as free bowel wall perforation, retroperitoneal duodenal perforation secondary to periampullary injury, and perforation in the bile duct.[62] Among these, retroperitoneal duodenal perforations are the most common that occur when the sphincterotomy extends beyond the intramural portion of the bile duct (**Fig. 3**). Perforations of the bile duct can occur during dilation of stricture or direct mechanical injury from the instruments used. Intraparenchymal bile duct injury can occur during guidewire manipulation and may lead to biloma formation. Free bowel wall perforation of the duodenum is rare and can occur in the presence of stricture or altered anatomy, which needs additional care.[63] Of note, free air following ERCP can be seen in up to 30% of asymptomatic patients and does not warrant further interventions.[64] In a large series, ERCP-associated perforation was noted in 0.6% of the procedures, resulting in a mortality of 0.06%.[45]

Strategies to prevent and treat perforation: ERCP-associated perforation must be promptly identified and treated. Most of the bile duct perforations and papillary perforations can be treated conservatively and with endoscopic therapies; however, duodenal perforations may often need surgical intervention. Patients identified to

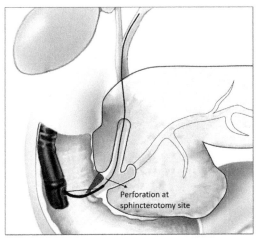

Fig. 3. ERCP-associated perforation at the sphincterotomy site.

have a perforation will require intravenous antibiotics, nasogastric or nasoduodenal suction, and bowel rest for 1 week. Early surgical consultation ensures prompt intervention when necessary, and delay in such an intervention leads to poor outcomes. Clip closure can be performed at the duodenal perforation site along with conservative management. Recently over-the-scope clips and purse-string sutures have also been used for closure of ERCP-associated perforation.[65] Covered self-expandable metal stents provide effective closure at sphincterotomy-associated perforation site. It must, however, be noted that despite endoscopic closure of the defect, if patients had a copious amount of enteral contents entering the peritoneal and retroperitoneal spaces, a surgical washout is indicated to prevent the formation of infected collections that are challenging to treat. Duodenal perforations occur when the descending duodenum stretches and in the setting of prior abdominal surgeries or malignancy; therefore, adequate care must be used to reduce the stretching maneuvers during ERCP. Other strategies to reduce the risk of ERCP-associated perforations include ensuring proper orientation of sphincterotomy, avoiding an extended length or zipper-cut sphincterotomy, use of balloon dilation in conjunction with sphincterotomy, and the use of CO_2 gas instead of air.

ENDOSCOPIC RETROGRADE CHOLANGIOPANCREATOGRAPHY INSTRUMENT–RELATED COMPLICATIONS

Spyglass cholangioscopy allows improved visualization of the bile duct, facilitating targeted biopsies and endotherapy such as electrohydraulic lithotripsy (EHL), and this led to widespread utilization in the clinical practice of biliary endoscopy. However, direct mechanical injury from spyglass cholangioscopy or spy biopsies, EHL-related bile duct injury was noted to occur in up to 2.1% of the procedures, and therefore, adequate care must be taken to ensure visualization when performing such procedures.[66] Prophylactic antibiotics should also be considered during such interventions as discussed previously due to the use of high-pressure injections into the bile duct.

Migration of the stents proximally into the bile duct was noted to occur in 3.5% of the biliary endoscopy procedure (**Fig. 4**).[67] Risk factors for proximal migration of the stents include benign strictures, use of short and straight stents, severe bile duct dilation, and distal biliary obstruction. The proximally migrated stents can be retrieved by

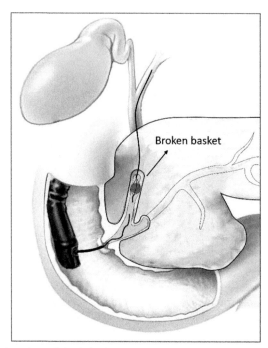

Fig. 4. Proximal migration of the bile duct stent.

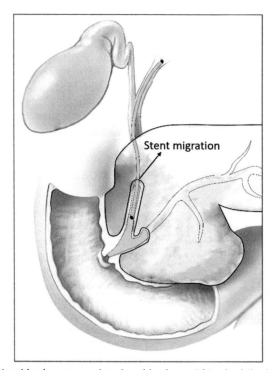

Fig. 5. Stone retrieval basket strangulated and broken within the bile duct.

using Soehendra stent retriever or a balloon catheter or by using fluoroscopy-guided forceps, snare, or a basket.

Mechanical lithotripsy and stone retrieval baskets with improved breaking strengths made it possible to treat large bile duct stones with biliary endoscopy. However, the baskets can often strangulate and break within the bile duct (**Fig. 5**); this especially occurs in the setting of large stones and small papillary incisions, and fluoroscopy-guided removal stools can be used as a rescue technique to remove the broken basket.[68]

SUMMARY

ERCP-based biliary endoscopy procedures are vital in the management of biliary disorders. However, serious complications can occur with such interventions, and endoscopists must be aware of the potential complications and techniques to prevent and manage such complications if they occur. Appropriate documentation of such complications is necessary to facilitate the endoscopy units to track such complications for quality improvement and identify techniques to prevent such complications.

CLINICS CARE POINTS

- PEP is the most common complication of ERCP; recognize the patient's procedure-related risk factors to determine the level of prophylaxis needed.
- PD injury with repeat passages of the guidewire significantly increases the risk of PEP, and therefore, a PD stent can be considered in this situation.
- Periprocedural IVF reduces PEP risk, and a combination of IVF and rectal NSAIDs is potentially more advantageous due to the cumulative additive benefit.
- Limit contrast use during biliary ERCP and avoid incomplete drainage.
- Consider balloon dilation over stent placement in patients with PSC.
- Use periprocedural antibiotics and antibiotic prophylaxis as indicated to reduce the risk of cholangitis after ERCP.
- Limit the injection of contrast into the gall bladder during ERCP.
- Consider early cholecystectomy after biliary endoscopy for stone therapy.
- Recognize patients at increased risk of ERCP-associated bleeding and modify or limit sphincterotomy techniques with the use of balloon sphincteroplasty.
- Endoscopic techniques with injection, hemostat clip, or stent therapy are effective in controlling and preventing ERCP-associated bleeding.
- Retroperitoneal air may be noted on imaging after ERCP sphincterotomy among asymptomatic patients, which does not warrant intervention.
- Conservative approach and endoscopic closure methods including clip, suture, and a covered metal stent can be used in selected cases of ERCP-associated perforation, but a free wall perforation warrants prompt surgical intervention.

DISCLOSURE

The authors have no disclosures relevant to this publication.

REFERENCES

1. Healthcare Cost and Utilization Project 2020. URL Available at: https://hcupnet. ahrq.gov/. Accessed on May 1, 2020.

2. Mutneja HR, Vohra I, Go A, et al. Temporal trends and mortality of post-ERCP pancreatitis in the United States: a nationwide analysis. Endoscopy 2021;53(4): 357–66.

3. Kochar B, Akshintala VS, Afghani E, et al. Incidence, severity, and mortality of post-ERCP pancreatitis: a systematic review by using randomized, controlled trials. Gastrointest Endosc 2015;81:143–149 e9.

4. Dumonceau JM, Kapral C, Aabakken L, et al. ERCP-related adverse events: European Society of Gastrointestinal Endoscopy (ESGE) Guideline. Endoscopy 2020;52:127–49.

5. Cotton PB. Analysis of 59 ERCP lawsuits; mainly about indications. Gastrointest Endosc 2006;63:378–82.

6. Vandervoort J, Soetikno RM, Tham TC, et al. Risk factors for complications after performance of ERCP. Gastrointest Endosc 2002;56:652–6.

7. Cheng CL, Sherman S, Watkins JL, et al. Risk factors for post-ERCP pancreatitis: a prospective multicenter study. Am J Gastroenterol 2006;101:139–47.

8. Rabenstein T, Schneider HT, Bulling D, et al. Analysis of the risk factors associated with endoscopic sphincterotomy techniques: preliminary results of a prospective study, with emphasis on the reduced risk of acute pancreatitis with low-dose anticoagulation treatment. Endoscopy 2000;32:10–9.

9. Christoforidis E, Goulimaris I, Kanellos I, et al. Post-ERCP pancreatitis and hyperamylasemia: patient-related and operative risk factors. Endoscopy 2002;34: 286–92.

10. Hookey LC, RioTinto R, Delhaye M, et al. Risk factors for pancreatitis after pancreatic sphincterotomy: a review of 572 cases. Endoscopy 2006;38:670–6.

11. Boender J, Nix GA, de Ridder MA, et al. Endoscopic papillotomy for common bile duct stones: factors influencing the complication rate. Endoscopy 1994;26: 209–16.

12. Christensen M, Matzen P, Schulze S, et al. Complications of ERCP: a prospective study. Gastrointest Endosc 2004;60:721–31.

13. Masci E, Toti G, Mariani A, et al. Complications of diagnostic and therapeutic ERCP: a prospective multicenter study. Am J Gastroenterol 2001;96:417–23.

14. Freeman ML, DiSario JA, Nelson DB, et al. Risk factors for post-ERCP pancreatitis: a prospective, multicenter study. Gastrointest Endosc 2001;54:425–34.

15. Freeman ML. Complications of endoscopic sphincterotomy. Endoscopy 1998;30: A216–20.

16. Chen JJ, Wang XM, Liu XQ, et al. Risk factors for post-ERCP pancreatitis: a systematic review of clinical trials with a large sample size in the past 10 years. Eur J Med Res 2014;19:26.

17. Ding X, Zhang F, Wang Y. Risk factors for post-ERCP pancreatitis: A systematic review and meta-analysis. Surgeon 2015;13:218–29.

18. Yasuda I, Isayama H, Bhatia V. Current situation of endoscopic biliary cannulation and salvage techniques for difficult cases: Current strategies in Japan. Dig Endosc 2016;28(Suppl 1):62–9.

19. Tse F, Yuan Y, Moayyedi P, et al. Guide wire-assisted cannulation for the prevention of post-ERCP pancreatitis: a systematic review and meta-analysis. Endoscopy 2013;45:605–18.

20. Tse F, Yuan Y, Bukhari M, et al. Pancreatic duct guidewire placement for biliary cannulation for the prevention of post-endoscopic retrograde cholangiopancreatography (ERCP) pancreatitis. Cochrane Database Syst Rev 2016;CD010571.

21. Kamal A, Akshintala VS, Talukdar R, et al. A Randomized Trial of Topical Epinephrine and Rectal Indomethacin for Preventing Post-Endoscopic Retrograde

Cholangiopancreatography Pancreatitis in High-Risk Patients. Am J Gastroenterol 2019;114:339–47.

22. Friedland S, Soetikno RM, Vandervoort J, et al. Bedside scoring system to predict the risk of developing pancreatitis following ERCP. Endoscopy 2002;34:483–8.

23. Park CH, Park SW, Yang MJ, et al. Pre- and post-procedure risk prediction models for post-endoscopic retrograde cholangiopancreatography pancreatitis. Surg Endosc 2021.

24. Chiba M, Kato M, Kinoshita Y, et al. The milestone for preventing post-ERCP pancreatitis using novel simplified predictive scoring system: a propensity score analysis. Surg Endosc 2020.

25. Rodrigues-Pinto E, Morais R, Sousa-Pinto B, et al. Development of an Online App to Predict Post-Endoscopic Retrograde Cholangiopancreatography Adverse Events Using a Single-Center Retrospective Cohort. Dig Dis 2021;39:283–93.

26. Development and validation of a risk stratification score for post-endoscopic retrograde cholangiopancreatography (ERCP) pancreatitis Kamal A., Akshintala V.S., Elmunzer B.J., Lehman G.A., Andriulli A., Talukdar R., Goenka M.K., Kochhar R., Faghih M., Kumbhari V., Ngamruengphong S., Khashab M.A., Kalloo A.N., Duvvur N.R., Singh V. Gastrointestinal Endoscopy 2018 87:6 Supplement 1 (AB573-).

27. Rex DK, Schoenfeld PS, Cohen J, et al. Quality indicators for colonoscopy. Gastrointest Endosc 2015;81:31–53.

28. Akshintala VS, Sperna Weiland CJ, Bhullar FA, et al. Non-steroidal anti-inflammatory drugs, intravenous fluids, pancreatic stents, or their combinations for the prevention of post-endoscopic retrograde cholangiopancreatography pancreatitis: a systematic review and network meta-analysis. Lancet Gastroenterol Hepatol 2021;6:733–42.

29. Akshintala VS, Tang B, Kamal A, et al. Risk estimation, machine learning based ercp decision-making tool for suspected choledocholithiasis. Gastrointest Endosc 2019;89:AB246–7.

30. Akshintala VS, Hutfless SM, Colantuoni E, et al. Systematic review with network meta-analysis: pharmacological prophylaxis against post-ERCP pancreatitis. Aliment Pharmacol Ther 2013;38:1325–37.

31. Serrano JPR, de Moura DTH, Bernardo WM, et al. Nonsteroidal anti-inflammatory drugs versus placebo for post-endoscopic retrograde cholangiopancreatography pancreatitis: a systematic review and meta-analysis. Endosc Int Open 2019;7:E477–86.

32. Choi JH, Kim HJ, Lee BU, et al. Vigorous Periprocedural Hydration With Lactated Ringer's Solution Reduces the Risk of Pancreatitis After Retrograde Cholangiopancreatography in Hospitalized Patients. Clin Gastroenterol Hepatol 2017;15: 86–92 e1.

33. Park CH, Paik WH, Park ET, et al. Aggressive intravenous hydration with lactated Ringer's solution for prevention of post-ERCP pancreatitis: a prospective randomized multicenter clinical trial. Endoscopy 2018;50:378–85.

34. Sugimoto M, Takagi T, Suzuki R, et al. Pancreatic stents for the prevention of post-endoscopic retrograde cholangiopancreatography pancreatitis should be inserted up to the pancreatic body or tail. World J Gastroenterol 2018;24:2392–9.

35. Dumonceau JM, Andriulli A, Elmunzer BJ, et al. Prophylaxis of post-ERCP pancreatitis: European Society of Gastrointestinal Endoscopy (ESGE) Guideline - updated June 2014. Endoscopy 2014;46:799–815.

36. Committee ASoP, Chandrasekhara V, Khashab MA, et al. Adverse events associated with ERCP. Gastrointest Endosc 2017;85:32–47.

37. Elmunzer BJ, Scheiman JM, Lehman GA, et al. A randomized trial of rectal indomethacin to prevent post-ERCP pancreatitis. N Engl J Med 2012;366:1414–22.

38. Avila P, Holmes I, Kouanda A, et al. Practice patterns of post-ERCP pancreatitis prophylaxis techniques in the United States: a survey of advanced endoscopists. Gastrointest Endosc 2020;91:568–73.e2.

39. Elmunzer BJ, Hernandez I, Gellad WF. The Skyrocketing Cost of Rectal Indomethacin. JAMA Intern Med 2020.

40. Radadiya D, Devani K, Arora S, et al. Peri-Procedural Aggressive Hydration for Post Endoscopic Retrograde Cholangiopancreatography (ERCP) Pancreatitis Prophylaxsis: Meta-analysis of Randomized Controlled Trials. Pancreatology 2019;19:819–27.

41. Sperna Weiland CJ, Smeets X, Kievit W, et al. Aggressive fluid hydration plus non-steroidal anti-inflammatory drugs versus non-steroidal anti-inflammatory drugs alone for post-endoscopic retrograde cholangiopancreatography pancreatitis (FLUYT): a multicentre, open-label, randomised, controlled trial. Lancet Gastroenterol Hepatol 2021;6:350–8.

42. Afghani E, Akshintala VS, Khashab MA, et al. 5-Fr vs. 3-Fr pancreatic stents for the prevention of post-ERCP pancreatitis in high-risk patients: a systematic review and network meta-analysis. Endoscopy 2014;46:573–80.

43. Choksi NS, Fogel EL, Cote GA, et al. The risk of post-ERCP pancreatitis and the protective effect of rectal indomethacin in cases of attempted but unsuccessful prophylactic pancreatic stent placement. Gastrointest Endosc 2015;81:150–5.

44. Elmunzer BJ, Serrano J, Chak A, et al. Rectal indomethacin alone versus indomethacin and prophylactic pancreatic stent placement for preventing pancreatitis after ERCP: study protocol for a randomized controlled trial. Trials 2016; 17:120.

45. Andriulli A, Loperfido S, Napolitano G, et al. Incidence rates of post-ERCP complications: a systematic survey of prospective studies. Am J Gastroenterol 2007; 102:1781–8.

46. Aumeran C, Poincloux L, Souweine B, et al. Multidrug-resistant Klebsiella pneumoniae outbreak after endoscopic retrograde cholangiopancreatography. Endoscopy 2010;42:895–9.

47. Navaneethan U, Gutierrez NG, Jegadeesan R, et al. Delay in performing ERCP and adverse events increase the 30-day readmission risk in patients with acute cholangitis. Gastrointest Endosc 2013;78:81–90.

48. Thosani N, Zubarik RS, Kochar R, et al. Prospective evaluation of bacteremia rates and infectious complications among patients undergoing single-operator choledochoscopy during ERCP. Endoscopy 2016;48:424–31.

49. Aabakken L, Karlsen TH, Albert J, et al. Role of endoscopy in primary sclerosing cholangitis: European Society of Gastrointestinal Endoscopy (ESGE) and European Association for the Study of the Liver (EASL) Clinical Guideline. Endoscopy 2017;49:588–608.

50. Kaya M, Petersen BT, Angulo P, et al. Balloon dilation compared to stenting of dominant strictures in primary sclerosing cholangitis. Am J Gastroenterol 2001; 96:1059–66.

51. ASoP Committee, Khashab MA, Chithadi KV, et al. Antibiotic prophylaxis for GI endoscopy. Gastrointest Endosc 2015;81:81–9.

52. Almadi MA, Barkun AN, Martel M. No benefit of covered vs uncovered self-expandable metal stents in patients with malignant distal biliary obstruction: a meta-analysis. Clin Gastroenterol Hepatol 2013;11:27–37 e1.

53. Saleem A, Leggett CL, Murad MH, et al. Meta-analysis of randomized trials comparing the patency of covered and uncovered self-expandable metal stents for palliation of distal malignant bile duct obstruction. Gastrointest Endosc 2011; 74:321–7.e1-3.
54. Xu J, Yang C. Cholecystectomy outcomes after endoscopic sphincterotomy in patients with choledocholithiasis: a meta-analysis. BMC Gastroenterol 2020; 20:229.
55. Gholson CF, Favrot D, Vickers B, et al. Delayed hemorrhage following endoscopic retrograde sphincterotomy for choledocholithiasis. Dig Dis Sci 1996;41:831–4.
56. Kim HJ, Kim MH, Kim DI, et al. Endoscopic hemostasis in sphincterotomy-induced hemorrhage: its efficacy and safety. Endoscopy 1999;31:431–6.
57. ASoP Committee, Acosta RD, Abraham NS, et al. The management of antithrombotic agents for patients undergoing GI endoscopy. Gastrointest Endosc 2016; 83:3–16.
58. Ratani RS, Mills TN, Ainley CC, et al. Electrophysical factors influencing endoscopic sphincterotomy. Gastrointest Endosc 1999;49:43–52.
59. Matsushita M, Takakuwa H, Shimeno N, et al. Prophylactic injection of hypertonic saline-epinephrine oral to the papilla for prevention of postsphincterotomy bleeding. J Clin Gastroenterol 2010;44:e167–70.
60. Baron TH, Norton ID, Herman L. Endoscopic hemoclip placement for post-sphincterotomy bleeding. Gastrointest Endosc 2000;52:662.
61. Shah JN, Marson F, Binmoeller KF. Temporary self-expandable metal stent placement for treatment of post-sphincterotomy bleeding. Gastrointest Endosc 2010; 72:1274–8.
62. Stapfer M, Selby RR, Stain SC, et al. Management of duodenal perforation after endoscopic retrograde cholangiopancreatography and sphincterotomy. Ann Surg 2000;232:191–8.
63. Lin LF, Siauw CP, Ho KS, et al. ERCP in post-Billroth II gastrectomy patients: emphasis on technique. Am J Gastroenterol 1999;94:144–8.
64. de Vries JH, Duijm LE, Dekker W, et al. CT before and after ERCP: detection of pancreatic pseudotumor, asymptomatic retroperitoneal perforation, and duodenal diverticulum. Gastrointest Endosc 1997;45:231–5.
65. Li Q, Ji J, Wang F, et al. ERCP-induced duodenal perforation successfully treated with endoscopic purse-string suture: a case report. Oncotarget 2015;6: 17847–50.
66. Ang TL, Kwek ABE. Safety and efficacy of SpyGlass cholangiopancreatoscopy in routine clinical practice in a regional Singapore hospital. Singapore Med J 2019; 60:538–44.
67. Kawaguchi Y, Ogawa M, Kawashima Y, et al. Risk factors for proximal migration of biliary tube stents. World J Gastroenterol 2014;20:1318–24.
68. Schneider MU, Matek W, Bauer R, et al. Mechanical lithotripsy of bile duct stones in 209 patients–effect of technical advances. Endoscopy 1988;20:248–53.

Multidisciplinary Approach to Indeterminate Biliary Strictures

Zaheer Nabi, MD, DNB,
D. Nageshwar Reddy, MD, DM, DSc, FAMS, FRCP, FASGE, MWGO, MASGE, FJGES*

KEYWORDS

- Indeterminate biliary stricture • ERCP • EUS • Cholangioscopy • Cytology
- Cholangiocarcinoma • FISH

KEY POINTS

- The evaluation of indeterminate biliary strictures requires a multidisciplinary approach.
- Cholangioscopy and endoscopic ultrasound have emerged as the frontrunners for the evaluation of biliary strictures that remain indeterminate after cross-sectional imaging and biliary cytology or biopsy.
- Upfront utilization of these modalities may be considered due to low diagnostic yield of biliary brush cytology and biopsy.
- Other diagnostic modalities including intraductal ultrasound, fluorescent in situ hybridization, and optical coherence tomography improve the diagnostic yield but do not provide with tissue diagnosis.
- In near future, next-generation sequencing is likely to play an important role in the evaluation of biliary strictures.

 Video content accompanies this article at http://www.giendo.theclinics.com.

INTRODUCTION

Indeterminate biliary strictures (IDBS) have been classically defined as those in which cross-sectional imaging (computed tomography and MRI) and endoscopic retrograde cholangiopancreatography (ERCP) with cytologic brushing or biopsy are nondiagnostic.[1] Majority (~70%) of the biliary strictures are malignant, with cholangiocarcinomas (CCA) and pancreatic cancers being the most common causes. However, up to one-fourth of the suspected malignant biliary strictures (MBS) ultimately turn out to be

Asian Institute of Gastroenterology & AIG Hospitals, Mind Space Road, Gachibowli, Hyderabad 500 032 India
* Corresponding author.
E-mail address: aigindia@yahoo.co.in

Gastrointest Endoscopy Clin N Am 32 (2022) 411–425
https://doi.org/10.1016/j.giec.2022.01.004

benign; this highlights the proportion of cases that remain undiagnosed after evaluation (imaging and endoscopic) and low sensitivity of the most widely used techniques for the determination of biliary strictures, that is, cross-sectional imaging and ERCP with brush cytology (BC) or forceps biopsy (FB). An accurate diagnosis is required not only for timely diagnosis of MBS and providing with a chance for curative resection but also for avoiding major surgery in cases with benign biliary strictures (BBS). The diagnostic dilemma and relative inefficacy of the conventional sampling techniques in differentiating BBS and MBS has propelled the development of newer modalities for the evaluation of IDBS. With the widespread availability of newer imaging and sampling techniques the indetermination of biliary strictures has reduced, albeit not completely eliminated. In the current era, the initial evaluation of biliary strictures incorporates one or more adjunctive modalities in addition to ERCP-assisted BC or FB.

The following section discusses the common causes of biliary strictures, clinical evaluation, limitations of the conventional techniques, role of newer modalities, and overall approach in cases with IDBS.

Biliary Strictures: Causes

The common causes of MBS include pancreatic adenocarcinoma, CCA, gall bladder cancers, and ampullary cancers. Relatively uncommon causes include lymphoma, metastases, and hepatocellular carcinoma. MBS not only differ with respect to their pathologies but also bear differences in terms of location and approach required for tissue sampling. Pancreatic adenocarcinomas usually result in distal strictures due to infiltration or extrinsic compression of bile duct by mass in head of pancreas. Low yield of ERCP sampling (BC/FB) in these cases is explained by intense desmoplastic reaction leading to relative acellularity.[2] Similarly, strictures due to extrinsic compression and encasement of biliary tract due to other causes are likely to pose diagnostic challenges when assessed using ERCP-based sampling techniques. Therefore, endosonography (EUS) may be a better adjunctive modality to assess and sample these strictures. On the other hand, CCA can involve any portion of the biliary tract and tend to grow from within. Therefore, direct visualization from within and targeted biopsies under cholangioscopic guidance are likely to improve the diagnostic yield.

Endoscopic Retrograde Cholangiopancreatography–Based Tissue Sampling

Brush cytology, biopsy, and bile aspiration: optimizing outcomes

The most commonly used ERCP sampling techniques, BC and FB, have very low sensitivity and negative predictive value. In a systematic review and meta-analysis, the pooled sensitivity of brush cytology, intraductal biopsies, and combined modalities were 45% (95% confidence interval [CI], 40%–50%), 48.1% (95% CI, 42.8%–53.4%), and 59.4% (95% CI, 53.7%– 64.8%), respectively.[3] The accuracy of BC and FB is especially lower for flat type MBS, nonbile duct cancer, and short (<30 mm) length of stricture.[4] However, technical ease, universal availability, and perfect specificity have kept these ancillary sampling techniques in business.

Several modifications in the ERCP-based sampling techniques have been evaluated to improve the diagnostic yield in cases with biliary strictures, which include triple sampling (bile aspiration + BC + FB), stricture dilatation before brushing/biopsy, modified biopsy forceps (slim type, long type, bent tip), wire grasping technique of biopsy, and rapid on-site evaluation (ROSE).[5–10] Balloon dilatation before sampling may expose submucosal tumor tissue and allow better accommodation of biopsy forceps especially in cases with tight biliary stenoses. Although balloon dilatation improved the sensitivity (41% to 71%) of biopsy in one study, the results were conflicting with regard to yield of brush cytology in 2 studies.[11–13] Overall, none of these amendments in the

ERCP sampling techniques have consistently augmented the diagnostic accuracy in biliary strictures. Therefore, adjunctive diagnostic modalities are considered upfront for the characterization of biliary strictures to avoid diagnostic delays.

Fluorescent In Situ Hybridization

Fluorescent in situ hybridization (FISH) uses chromosome-specific DNA probes (chromosome 3, 7, 17) to identify cells with mutations or abnormal number of chromosomes. Multiple studies have confirmed the utility of FISH in IDBS. The sensitivity of FISH is higher (60%–90%) with similar specificity (>90%) to ERCP-BC.[14–17] Levy and colleagues evaluated the role of FISH in 86 patients with IDBS.[14] In 21 patients with negative cytology and final diagnosis of malignant stricture, FISH was able to predict malignancy in 62% cases.[14]

The advantage of FISH is that the sample can be obtained easily using ERCP, high specificity (>90%), and improved sensitivity over brushing alone. The drawbacks of FISH include modest sensitivity, high additional cost, limited availability, need of expertise, and that interpretation is prone to subjective errors.[18] Polysomy may be detected in benign, inflammatory strictures such as primary sclerosing cholangitis (PSC). Therefore, caution is advised while interpreting the results of FISH in these cases.

The sensitivity of FISH can be potentially improved by using a different set of FISH probes. Fritcher confirmed higher sensitivity with similar specificity with the use of a new set of FISH probes (1q21, 7p12, 8q24, and 9p21) when compared with the conventional FISH probes (UroVysion) (sensitivity 65% vs 46%; specificity 93% vs 91%).[17] Similarly, serial FISHing in patients with PSC can reduce the frequency of false positives due to inflammation. Detection of polysomy on serial FISH analysis imparts a high risk for developing CCA in patients with PSC (36.4% vs 6.3%).[19]

Concluding remarks: FISH is a promise unfulfilled mainly due to low sensitivity. Therefore, the diagnosis of MBS cannot be ruled out based on a negative result. Novel DNA probes seem promising but need evaluation in future studies.

Cholangioscopy

Cholangioscopy systems currently available include single operator cholangioscopes (SOC) and direct per-oral cholangioscopes. The digital SOC system (SpyGlass, Boston Scientific Corp, Massachusetts, USA) provides better image quality as compared with previously available fiber optic versions. Cholangioscopic evaluation of IDBS is based on visual impression and targeted biopsies (Videos 1 and 2).[20] On visual impression, characteristics of MBS include tumor vessels, papillary projection, nodular or polypoid mass, and infiltrative lesions (**Fig. 1**).[21] Although, visual impression

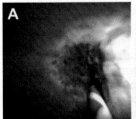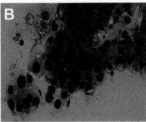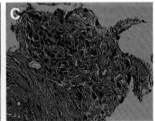

Fig. 1. Cholangioscopy with targeted biopsy in a case with indeterminate biliary stricture. (*A*) Cholangioscopic image revealing mucosal irregularity and tumor vessels. (*B*) Rapid on-site evaluation in the same case revealed pleomorphic cells that suggest malignancy. (*C*) Histopathology confirmed the diagnosis of cholangiocarcinoma.

on cholangioscopy is more sensitive when compared with guided biopsy, lower specificity limits the use of visual impression alone for diagnostic purposes. In a multicenter randomized trial by Gerges and colleagues, the sensitivity of visual impression (96% vs 67%), SOC guided biopsies (68% vs 21%), and overall accuracy (87.1% vs 66%) was significantly higher in the cholangioscopy group versus ERCP-BC.[22] Kulpatcharapong and colleagues performed a systematic review and meta-analysis (13 studies, 876 patients) pertaining to the diagnostic performance of digital and video cholangioscopes in patients with suspected MBS.[23] Cholangioscopic visual impression provided significantly higher sensitivity (93% vs 82%) but lower specificity (86% vs 98%) than cholangioscopic-guided biopsy.[23] Besides lower specificity, poor interobserver agreement is another issue with cholangioscopic visual impression in biliary strictures. In a recent study by the European cholangioscopy group, there was significant interobserver variation for the appraisal of IDBS.[24] In addition, the sensitivity as well as the specificity for blinded (74% and 47%) and unblinded (73% and 63%) SOC video appraisal were low. Similarly, low interobserver agreement for visual impression has been confirmed by other investigators using different sets of criteria for evaluation of IDBS.[25] The implications of findings from recent studies are 2-fold. First, it may not be appropriate to conclude the diagnosis based on visual impression alone and directed biopsies should be taken whenever feasible. Second, there is a need for more formal training and refinements in the visual criteria to improve interobserver variation.

Concluding remark: cholangioscopy has emerged as one of the first-line modalities for the evaluation of IDBS. It can be performed either during the index ERCP or after indeterminate results with initial ERCP-BC/FB. Visual impression alone has lower specificity and should be accompanied by targeted biopsies during cholangioscopy.

Optimizing the Outcomes of Cholangioscopy

Several factors have been shown to negatively affect the diagnostic yield of cholangioscopy in cases with IDBS, which include distal location of the strictures, operator's experience less than 25 cases, severe hyperbilirubinemia, and presence of a biliary stent.[26] Of these, operator's experience and biliary stenting are modifiable factors. Another potential strategy to improve the diagnostic yield of SOC is ROSE of touch imprint cytology (ROSE-TIC) or taking 3 biopsies for offsite evaluation.[27,28] Interobserver agreement can be improved by optimizing the objective parameters used for visual impression. Kahaleh and colleagues proposed a new cholangioscopic classification system (Mendoza criteria).[29] The interobserver agreement was better (16% higher) as compared with previous criteria and the overall diagnostic accuracy was 77%. Validation of these new criteria and confirmation of low interobserver variability is required before incorporating them into clinical practice. With the emerging role of artificial intelligence, the accuracy of SOC may improve and overcome interobserver variation while interpreting the images.[30]

Endosonography

EUS has emerged as an important tool for establishing diagnosis in cases with IDBS. EUS is superior to cross-sectional imaging for demonstrating small masses in bile duct and regional lymph nodes (**Fig. 2**). In a retrospective cohort study from Mayo clinic including 157 patients with CCA, lymph node detection was higher with EUS when compared with cross-sectional imaging (86% vs 47%; $P < .001$).[31] The detection of malignant regional lymph nodes bears a diagnostic, prognostic as well as therapeutic relevance in cases with MBS. The other advantage of EUS is avoidance of ERCP and associated complications in cases where biliary drainage is not indicated.

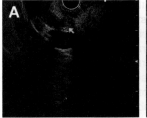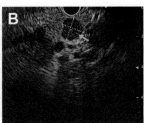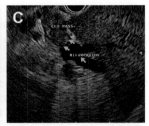

Fig. 2. Endosonography (EUS) in cases with indeterminate biliary strictures. (*A*) EUS image revealing hypoechoic thickening of distal bile duct (*green arrow*). EUS-guided sampling from the same confirmed the diagnosis of distal cholangiocarcinoma. (*B*) EUS image showing hypoechoic lymph node in periportal region in a case with hilar stricture. (*C*) EUS image revealing hypoechoic mass at the level of common hepatic duct (*green arrow*).

Several studies have confirmed the utility of EUS in IDBS. In a recent meta-analysis including 1123 patients with CCA (32 studies), the pooled diagnostic sensitivity with EUS-FNA was significantly better than ERCP-BC (73.6% vs 56.0%).[32] The diagnostic yield of EUS-FNA seems to be incremental over ERCP-BC/FB. In a multicenter study from Korea including 263 patients, the overall diagnostic sensitivity and accuracy were significantly higher for EUS/ERCP combination (85.8% and 87.1%) as compared with either modality alone (EUS-FNA 73.6% and 76.1%; ERCP 56.5% and 60.5%).[33]

The accuracy of EUS may be lower in proximal or hilar strictures as compared with distal biliary strictures. In a prospective study including 81 patients with CCA, the sensitivity of EUS-FNA was significantly higher in distal as compared with proximal CCA (81% vs 59%, respectively; $P = .04$).[34] In another large, retrospective study, the accuracy rate of EUS was significantly higher for distal biliary strictures (79% vs 57%, $P < .0001$).[35] Overall, the sensitivity of EUS-FNA in proximal or hilar strictures in different studies ranges from 50% to 89%.[36–39] Besides hilar location, the diagnostic performance of EUS-FNA may be suboptimal in cases with PSC and in the presence of biliary stent.[39] In a prospective study (n = 97), the sensitivity of EUS-FNA in the presence of a stent in patients with hilar and distal biliary strictures was 56% and 65%, respectively.[39] Several small studies have advised caution while performing EUS-FNA from hilar strictures due to the risk of needle tract seeding and peritoneal dissemination.[40–43] Transperitoneal (percutaneous or EUS guided) sampling of biliary strictures is considered as a contraindication for liver transplant at many centers.[44]

Concluding remark: EUS is widely available and provides with a good diagnostic yield (sensitivity>70%) especially in cases with distal biliary strictures. EUS should be considered as one of the primary modalities for the evaluation of IDBS along with cholangioscopy. Whenever feasible, EUS should be performed before the placement of a biliary stent. EUS may be preferred over cholangioscopy in distally located IDBS.

Intraductal Ultrasound

Intraductal ultrasound (IDUS) uses a small (6 Fr), high-frequency (12–20 MHz) probe that can be introduced through the working channel of duodenoscope. On IDUS, normal bile duct wall appears as a 3-layered structure, that is, hyperechoic mucosal layer, hypoechoic muscle layer, and hyperechoic outer connective tissue layer. A disruption of normal layer pattern suggests malignancy. Other features that suggest malignancy on IDUS include irregular and eccentric thickening, stricture dimensions (length>20 mm, thickness 7 mm), presence of mass infiltrating into surrounding tissue, and enlarged lymph nodes.[45,46] IDUS also provides useful information regarding longitudinal extent of tumor, identification of regional lymph nodes, and invasion into surrounding structures such as pancreatic parenchyma, portal vein, and right hepatic artery.[47]

Chen and colleagues evaluated 193 patients (97 malignant, 96 benign) with biliary strictures with IDUS.[48] The sensitivity, specificity, and accuracy rate of IDUS was 97%, 79%, and 88%, respectively. The diagnostic accuracy of IDUS was higher for proximal obstruction than that of distal bile duct obstruction (98% vs 83%, $P = .006$). The positive predictive value of biliary wall thickness greater than 7 mm without extrinsic compression and length greater than or equal to 20 mm was 100% and 93%, respectively.[48] In another large study including 264 patients, the sensitivity, specificity, and accuracy rates of IDUS were 93.2%, 89.5%, and 91.4%, respectively.[49] The sensitivity was better in cases with CCA (97.6%) followed by pancreatic carcinoma (93.8%), gallbladder cancer (88.9%), and ampullary cancer (80.8%).[49] IDUS seems to be better than ERCP-BC/FB for the characterization of IDBS.[50] The addition of IDUS to BC can provide accurate differentiation between benign and MBS in 80% to 90% cases.[14,51,52]

The pitfalls of IDUS include inability to perform tissue sampling, limited depth of field, suboptimal staging accuracy, and difficulty in estimating the longitudinal extent of tumor in the presence of inflammation.[53]

Concluding remark: in the current era, the place of IDUS in the diagnostic algorithm of IDBS remains to be defined. IDUS may be used in selected cases where the biliary stricture remains indeterminate after evaluation with EUS and cholangioscopy. However, the utility of IDUS in this setting requires evaluation in future studies.

Confocal Laser Endomicroscopy

Confocal laser endomicroscopy (CLE) provides microscopic details of the tissue structures in real time during endoscopy. Probe-based CLE (pCLE) can be passed through a cholangioscope or therapeutic channel of duodenoscope for use in pancreatobiliary tract.[54] The commercially available pCLE probe (Cellvizio CholangioFlex probe, Maunakea Tech, Paris, France) has an external diameter of 0.94 mm, field of view of 325 μm, a lateral resolution of 3.5 μm, and an optical slice thickness of 30 μm.[54] Imaging with pCLE requires prior administration of intravenous contrast injection, that is, 2.5 mL of 10% fluorescein sodium.

Meining and colleagues evaluated the role of pCLE and proposed a classification system (Miami Classification) for pancreatobiliary strictures.[54,55] The characteristics of malignant strictures included thick white bands (>20 μm), or thick dark bands (>40 μm), or dark clumps or epithelial structures.[55] With pCLE, the nature of biliary strictures could be determined with a high sensitivity (88%–97%). However, low specificity (33%–36%) was a concern especially in cases with a history of biliary stenting.[54–56] Caillol and colleagues proposed a new classification system (Paris classification) to improve the specificity of pCLE.[56] The investigators identified 4 criteria specific to benign inflammatory strictures, which included vascular congestion, dark granular patterns with scales, increased interglandular space, and thickened reticular structure. Taunk and colleagues confirmed the better specificity of Paris classification system in those with prior biliary stenting (73% vs 36%).[57] Slivka and colleagues also confirmed the utility of new pCLE classification system in IDBS in a prospective, multicenter study (sensitivity 89%, specificity 71%, accuracy 82%).[58]

Overall, pCLE is a safe procedure, and minor adverse events related to intravenous fluorescein dye include transient yellowish skin discoloration, hypotension, injection site erythema, and rash. High sensitivity and negative predictive value with pCLE means that a negative test virtually rules out malignancy in a given case with biliary stricture. However, interobserver variability and modest specificity limit the use of pCLE as a sole imaging modality to confirm malignancy in cases with IDBS.[59] The other technical limitation is that the pCLE probe should make a perpendicular contact with the bile duct wall for optimum image quality; this may result in differential sensitivity of pCLE in relation to the location of strictures.[60]

Concluding remark: the specificity of CLE-based evaluation seems to be lower as compared with cholangioscopic visual impression and targeted biopsies. Limited availability, lack of validated diagnostic criteria, and interobserver variations are other concerns. Therefore, the present utility of CLE over and above the commonly available modalities (EUS and cholangioscopy) is uncertain.

Optical Coherence Tomography

Optical coherence tomography (OCT) is performed using slim probes passed through the working channel of duodenoscopes. OCT provides high-resolution cross-sectional images of the biliary tract and enables scanning a large area in short duration. On OCT, normal bile duct has a differentiated 3-layer architecture: a thin and regular hyporeflective layer (single layer of epithelial cells), a larger intermediate hyperreflective layer (connective-fibromuscular layer), and an outer hyporeflective layer (connective tissue with muscular strips).[44] The layered pattern is disturbed in malignancies, and the tumor vessels are represented by large hyporeflective areas.

Arvanitakis and colleagues evaluated the role of intraductal OCT in 35 patients with confirmed malignant (19 cases) or benign (16 cases) strictures.[61] The OCT probe (PENTAX Corporation Tokyo, Japan/Lightlab Imaging Ltd. Boston, USA) used in this study has an outer diameter of 0.75 mm, a penetration depth of ~ 1 mm, and a resolution of ~ 10 μm. The criteria for diagnosing malignancy included a disorganized and subverted layer structure and large hypo- or nonreflective areas that suggest tumor vessels. Both the criteria were fulfilled by 53% of MBS, whereas at least one criterion was met by 79% of MBS. The use of OCT increased the sensitivity of ERCP-BC/FB from 63% to 84%. In a prospective study including 86 patients, Tyberg and colleagues evaluated the role of OCT using a new imaging system (NVision Volumetric Laser Endomicroscopy Imaging System [NinePoint Bedford, MA]).[62] The presence of hyperglandular mucosa, hyperreflective surface, and scalloping significantly increased the odds of malignancy by 6, 4.7, and 7.9 times, respectively.[62] Although, OCT seems appealing, a substantial proportion of benign strictures may fulfill at least one criterion for malignant strictures, thereby reducing its specificity.[61]

Concluding remark: although, OCT seems to be a promising imaging technique, there are limited data on its utility, lack of formal criteria to distinguish benign and malignant strictures, and interobserver variability in interpreting images. The currently available probes have not been designed for use over guidewire. Therefore, it may be difficult to traverse and image tight stenoses. Because of limited depth of field, OCT may be of limited utility in extraductal malignancies such as pancreatic cancer or metastatic biliary compression.

Next-Generation Sequencing

Next-generation sequencing (NGS) includes a highly sensitive assay for analyzing multiple genes that are commonly mutated, amplified, and/or deleted in malignant neoplasms involving biliary tract.[18] NGS can be performed using specimens obtained during ERCP.

In a prospective study, the sensitivity and specificity of NGS for MBS was 73% and 100%, respectively.[18] NGS improved the sensitivity of ERCP-BC and FB from 35% to

Table 1
Current modalities used for evaluation of biliary strictures

	Sensitivity	Specificity	Advantages	Drawbacks	Scope of Improvement
ERCP Brush cytology	26%–72%	100%[b]	Universally available, cheap, highly specific	Low sensitivity	ROSE
ERCP-Forceps biopsy	15%–100%	100%	Improves diagnostic yield of brushing	Multiple biopsies required	Newly designed forceps may improve yield
Bile aspiration	6%–32%	100%	Easy, can be performed during index ERCP	Very low sensitivity, uncertain utility	Scraping before aspiration may improve yield
Cholangioscopy (visual)	83%–90%	89%–96%	Widely available, high sensitivity	Lower specificity	Training, improved classification system
Cholangioscopy (biopsy)	80%–85%	100%	Highly specific	Lower sensitivity, difficult in distal strictures	Modified biopsy forceps
FISH	34%–89%	90%–100%	Improves sensitivity of ERCP-brushing	High cost, lower specificity in PSC, limited availability	Newer probes may improve sensitivity
Intraductal ultrasound	80%–90%	80%–92%	T-staging, detects invasion of adjacent structures[a]	Sampling not feasible, fragile probe, limited field of vision	IDUS-directed biopsies
pCLE	83%–97%	33%–36% 77%–81%[c]	Safe, high sensitivity	Interobserver agreement, low specificity, IV dye	Validation of diagnostic criteria
Endosonography	75%–94%	100%	Best imaging for RLN identification, good sensitivity, ERCP may be avoided in some cases	Less sensitive in proximal strictures, risk of transperitoneal seeding	Ideal needle to sample biliary lesions
Next generation sequencing	73%–96%	69%–100%	Good sensitivity and specificity	Limited data	Target amplification/enrichment techniques

Abbreviations: IV, intravenous; RLN, regional lymph node.
[a] Portal vein, right hepatic artery, and pancreatic parenchyma.
[b] Specificity drops if suspicious lesions on pathology considered as malignant.
[c] Better specificity with newer criteria (Paris).

77% and 52% to 83%, respectively. The sensitivity improved remarkably in patients with PSC (NGS 83% vs ERCP-BC/FB 8%). An additional advantage of NGS was identification of therapeutically relevant genomic alterations in 20 (8%) patients.[18] The prognostic significance of NGS in biliary tract malignancies was also suggested in another study where mutations in CDKN2A and TP53 were associated with poor prognosis and predicted response with gemcitabine- and platinum-based chemotherapy.[63] NGS may offer better sensitivity over FISH when added to cytology, especially in cases with high-risk strictures associated with PSC (NGS 85% vs FISH 76%).[64,65]

Concluding remark: NGS seems a promising technique for evaluation of IDBS. In future, the sensitivity of NGS is likely to improve further with target amplification/enrichment techniques and analysis of additional genes.

Putting It All Together

The evaluation of IDBS is determined by the relative diagnostic accuracies as well as availability of different modalities (**Table 1**). The current modalities can be broadly divided into those that work on visual impression (imaging: IDUS, CLE, OCT), tissue acquisition (ERCP-BC/FB, EUS-FNA), or both (EUS and cholangioscopy). The modalities based on visual impression have reasonable sensitivity but suffer with the issue of interobserver variability and suboptimal specificity especially in the presence of inflammation. Therefore, modalities that allow tissue diagnosis are deemed necessary in cases with IDBS. Per-oral cholangioscopy and EUS-FNA have emerged as major diagnostic modalities in cases with IDBS. Both of these modalities allow characterization of the stricture as well as acquisition of tissue for confirmation of diagnosis. The use of EUS-FNA and cholangioscopy may be individualized based on the available expertise and characteristics of stricture (proximal vs distal or extrinsic vs intrinsic). The utility of a tailored approach toward IDBS was demonstrated in a recent prospective study where cholangioscopy and EUS-FNA were performed for proximal and distal biliary strictures, respectively.[66] In this study, the overall diagnostic accuracy for ERCP-FB with cholangioscopy-biopsy and EUS-FNA was 98.3% and 98.4% for proximal strictures and distal strictures, respectively. When performed, EUS and cholangioscopy should be preferably performed before biliary stenting (**Fig. 3**).

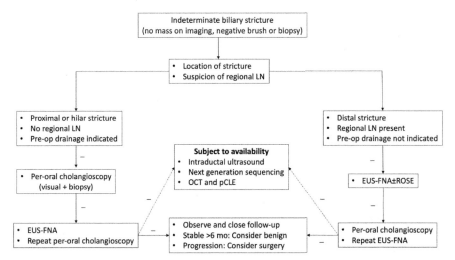

Fig. 3. Algorithmic approach for the evaluation of indeterminate biliary strictures.

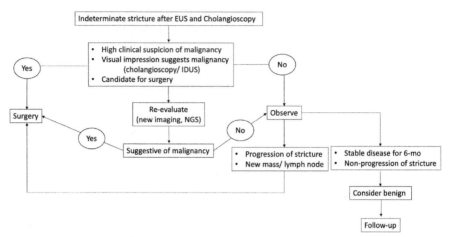

Fig. 4. Algorithmic approach for the evaluation of biliary strictures after negative results with adjunctive techniques.

Indeterminate Tissue Diagnosis: Beyond Endosonography and Cholangioscopy

The diagnostic dilemma may persist in a proportion of IDBS even after use of adjunctive modalities described earlier. EUS and cholangioscopy are widely available and often used upfront in cases with biliary strictures. Biliary strictures with indeterminate nature after use of these modalities represent IDBS in true sense in the current era. The approach in such cases should be individualized based on the likelihood of malignancy in a given case. The factors that may be considered with regard to further management include the clinical features, availability of advanced modalities for further evaluation, and candidacy for surgery. In selected patients, close follow-up, serial imaging, and assessment of clinical symptoms may unveil the diagnosis. Although there is no strict cut-off, stable disease and nonprogression of strictures beyond 6 months usually indicate benign disease. Longer follow-up (>12 months) may be warranted in those with dominant strictures associated with PSC. On the other hand, surgery may be considered especially if at least one of the adjunct modalities strongly suggests malignancy (eg, IDUS, visual impression on cholangioscopy, pCLE). The involvement of patients in the process of shared decision-making is paramount, and the pros and cons of available options (surgery, reevaluation, or surveillance) should be detailed (**Fig. 4**).

CLINICS CARE POINTS

- The diagnostic yield of biliary brush cytology and biopsy is sufficiently low, warranting the upfront utilization of additional diagnostic modalities.
- EUS is superior to cross-sectional imaging for identification of regional lymph nodes. It also allows sampling from the stricture as well as lymph nodes.
- EUS is preferred in distal strictures in view of technical difficulty and risk of needle tract seeding involved in proximal biliary strictures.
- Cholangioscopy and targeted biopsy should be preferred to visual impression alone due to interobserver variability with the latter.

DISCLOSURES

Both the authors (D.N. Reddy and Z. Nabi) have nothing to disclose.

SUPPLEMENTARY DATA

Supplementary data related to this article can be found online at https://doi.org/10.1016/j.giec.2022.01.004.

REFERENCES

1. Bowlus CL, Olson KA, Gershwin ME. Evaluation of indeterminate biliary strictures. Nat Rev Gastroenterol Hepatol 2016;13:28–37.

2. Naitoh I, Nakazawa T, Kato A, et al. Predictive factors for positive diagnosis of malignant biliary strictures by transpapillary brush cytology and forceps biopsy. J Dig Dis 2016;17:44–51.

3. Navaneethan U, Njei B, Lourdusamy V, et al. Comparative effectiveness of biliary brush cytology and intraductal biopsy for detection of malignant biliary strictures: a systematic review and meta-analysis. Gastrointest Endosc 2015;81:168–76.

4. Nishikawa T, Tsuyuguchi T, Sakai Y, et al. Factors affecting the accuracy of endoscopic transpapillary sampling methods for bile duct cancer. Dig Endosc 2014;26:276–81.

5. Archibugi L, Mariani A, Ciambriello B, et al. High sensitivity of ROSE-supported ERCP-guided brushing for biliary strictures. Endosc Int Open 2021;9:E363–70.

6. Fior-Gozlan M, Giovannini D, Rabeyrin M, et al. Monocentric study of bile aspiration associated with biliary brushing performed during endoscopic retrograde cholangiopancreatography in 239 patients with symptomatic biliary stricture. Cancer Cytopathol 2016;124:330–9.

7. Curcio G, Traina M, Mocciaro F, et al. Intraductal aspiration: a promising new tissue-sampling technique for the diagnosis of suspected malignant biliary strictures. Gastrointest Endosc 2012;75:798–804.

8. Yamamoto K, Tsuchiya T, Itoi T, et al. Evaluation of novel slim biopsy forceps for diagnosis of biliary strictures: Single-institutional study of consecutive 360 cases (with video). World J Gastroenterol 2017;23:6429–36.

9. Lee SJ, Lee YS, Lee MG, et al. Triple-tissue sampling during endoscopic retrograde cholangiopancreatography increases the overall diagnostic sensitivity for cholangiocarcinoma. Gut Liver 2014;8:669–73.

10. Fogel EL, deBellis M, McHenry L, et al. Effectiveness of a new long cytology brush in the evaluation of malignant biliary obstruction: a prospective study. Gastrointest Endosc 2006;63:71–7.

11. de Bellis M, Fogel EL, Sherman S, et al. Influence of stricture dilation and repeat brushing on the cancer detection rate of brush cytology in the evaluation of malignant biliary obstruction. Gastrointest Endosc 2003;58:176–82.

12. Farrell RJ, Jain AK, Brandwein SL, et al. The combination of stricture dilation, endoscopic needle aspiration, and biliary brushings significantly improves diagnostic yield from malignant bile duct strictures. Gastrointest Endosc 2001;54:587–94.

13. Porner D, Kaczmarek DJ, Heling D, et al. Transpapillary tissue sampling of biliary strictures: balloon dilatation prior to forceps biopsy improves sensitivity and accuracy. Sci Rep 2020;10:17423.

14. Levy MJ, Baron TH, Clayton AC, et al. Prospective evaluation of advanced molecular markers and imaging techniques in patients with indeterminate bile duct strictures. Am J Gastroenterol 2008;103:1263–73.

15. Fritcher EG, Kipp BR, Halling KC, et al. A multivariable model using advanced cytologic methods for the evaluation of indeterminate pancreatobiliary strictures. Gastroenterology 2009;136:2180–6.

16. Gonda TA, Glick MP, Sethi A, et al. Polysomy and p16 deletion by fluorescence in situ hybridization in the diagnosis of indeterminate biliary strictures. Gastrointest Endosc 2012;75:74–9.

17. Barr Fritcher EG, Voss JS, Brankley SM, et al. An Optimized Set of Fluorescence In Situ Hybridization Probes for Detection of Pancreatobiliary Tract Cancer in Cytology Brush Samples. Gastroenterology 2015;149:1813–1824 e1.

18. Singhi AD, Nikiforova MN, Chennat J, et al. Integrating next-generation sequencing to endoscopic retrograde cholangiopancreatography (ERCP)-obtained biliary specimens improves the detection and management of patients with malignant bile duct strictures. Gut 2020;69:52–61.

19. Quinn KP, Tabibian JH, Lindor KD. Clinical implications of serial versus isolated biliary fluorescence in situ hybridization (FISH) polysomy in primary sclerosing cholangitis. Scand J Gastroenterol 2017;52:377–81.

20. Ramchandani M, Reddy DN, Gupta R, et al. Role of single-operator peroral cholangioscopy in the diagnosis of indeterminate biliary lesions: a single-center, prospective study. Gastrointest Endosc 2011;74:511–9.

21. Kulpatcharapong S, Pittayanon R, Stephen JK, et al. Diagnostic performance of different cholangioscopes in patients with biliary strictures: a systematic review. Endoscopy 2020;52:174–85.

22. Gerges C, Beyna T, Tang RSY, et al. Digital single-operator peroral cholangioscopy-guided biopsy sampling versus ERCP-guided brushing for indeterminate biliary strictures: a prospective, randomized, multicenter trial (with video). Gastrointest Endosc 2020;91:1105–13.

23. Kulpatcharapong S, Pittayanon R, Kerr SJ, et al. Diagnostic performance of digital and video cholangioscopes in patients with suspected malignant biliary strictures: a systematic review and meta-analysis. Surg Endosc 2021. https://doi.org/10.1007/s00464-021-08571-2. In press.

24. Stassen PMC, Goodchild G, de Jonge PJF, et al. Diagnostic accuracy and interobserver agreement of digital single-operator cholangioscopy for indeterminate biliary strictures. Gastrointest Endosc 2021;94:1059–68.

25. Kahaleh M, Raijman I, Gaidhane M, et al. Digital Cholangioscopic Interpretation: When North Meets the South. Dig Dis Sci 2021. https://doi.org/10.1007/s10620-021-06961-z. In press.

26. Jang S, Stevens T, Kou L, et al. Efficacy of digital single-operator cholangioscopy and factors affecting its accuracy in the evaluation of indeterminate biliary stricture. Gastrointest Endosc 2020;91:385–393 e1.

27. Bang JY, Navaneethan U, Hasan M, et al. Optimizing Outcomes of Single-Operator Cholangioscopy-Guided Biopsies Based on a Randomized Trial. Clin Gastroenterol Hepatol 2020;18:441–448 e1.

28. Varadarajulu S, Bang JY, Hasan MK, et al. Improving the diagnostic yield of single-operator cholangioscopy-guided biopsy of indeterminate biliary strictures: ROSE to the rescue? (with video). Gastrointest Endosc 2016;84:681–7.

29. Kahaleh M, Gaidhane M, Shahid HM, et al. Digital single-operator cholangioscopy interobserver study using a new classification: the Mendoza Classification

(with video). Gastrointest Endosc 2022;95(2):319–26. https://doi.org/10.1016/j.gie.2021.08.015.

30. Saraiva MM, Ribeiro T, Ferreira JPS, et al. Artificial intelligence for automatic diagnosis of biliary stricture malignancy status in single-operator cholangioscopy: a pilot study. Gastrointest Endosc 2022;95(2):339–48. https://doi.org/10.1016/j.gie.2021.08.027.

31. Malikowski T, Levy MJ, Gleeson FC, et al. Endoscopic Ultrasound/Fine Needle Aspiration Is Effective for Lymph Node Staging in Patients With Cholangiocarcinoma. Hepatology 2020;72:940–8.

32. Yoon SB, Moon SH, Ko SW, et al. Brush Cytology, Forceps Biopsy, or Endoscopic Ultrasound-Guided Sampling for Diagnosis of Bile Duct Cancer: A Meta-Analysis. Dig Dis Sci 2021. https://doi.org/10.1007/s10620-021-07138-4. In press.

33. Jo JH, Cho CM, Jun JH, et al. Same-session endoscopic ultrasound-guided fine needle aspiration and endoscopic retrograde cholangiopancreatography-based tissue sampling in suspected malignant biliary obstruction: A multicenter experience. J Gastroenterol Hepatol 2019;34:799–805.

34. Mohamadnejad M, DeWitt JM, Sherman S, et al. Role of EUS for preoperative evaluation of cholangiocarcinoma: a large single-center experience. Gastrointest Endosc 2011;73:71–8.

35. Heinzow HS, Kammerer S, Rammes C, et al. Comparative analysis of ERCP, IDUS, EUS and CT in predicting malignant bile duct strictures. World J Gastroenterol 2014;20:10495–503.

36. Fritscher-Ravens A, Broering DC, Knoefel WT, et al. EUS-guided fine-needle aspiration of suspected hilar cholangiocarcinoma in potentially operable patients with negative brush cytology. Am J Gastroenterol 2004;99:45–51.

37. DeWitt J, Misra VL, Leblanc JK, et al. EUS-guided FNA of proximal biliary strictures after negative ERCP brush cytology results. Gastrointest Endosc 2006;64:325–33.

38. Nayar MK, Manas DM, Wadehra V, et al. Role of EUS/EUS-guided FNA in the management of proximal biliary strictures. Hepatogastroenterology 2011;58:1862–5.

39. Raine T, Thomas JP, Brais R, et al. Test performance and predictors of accuracy of endoscopic ultrasound-guided fine-needle aspiration for diagnosing biliary strictures or masses. Endosc Int Open 2020;8:E1537–44.

40. Kim SH, Woo YS, Lee KH, et al. Preoperative EUS-guided FNA: effects on peritoneal recurrence and survival in patients with pancreatic cancer. Gastrointest Endosc 2018;88:926–34.

41. El Chafic AH, Dewitt J, Leblanc JK, et al. Impact of preoperative endoscopic ultrasound-guided fine needle aspiration on postoperative recurrence and survival in cholangiocarcinoma patients. Endoscopy 2013;45:883–9.

42. Heimbach JK, Sanchez W, Rosen CB, et al. Trans-peritoneal fine needle aspiration biopsy of hilar cholangiocarcinoma is associated with disease dissemination. HPB (Oxford) 2011;13:356–60.

43. Yane K, Kuwatani M, Yoshida M, et al. Non-negligible rate of needle tract seeding after endoscopic ultrasound-guided fine-needle aspiration for patients undergoing distal pancreatectomy for pancreatic cancer. Dig Endosc 2020;32:801–11.

44. Testoni PA, Mariani A, Mangiavillano B, et al. Main pancreatic duct, common bile duct and sphincter of Oddi structure visualized by optical coherence tomography: An ex vivo study compared with histology. Dig Liver Dis 2006;38:409–14.

45. Del Vecchio Blanco G, Mossa M, Troncone E, et al. Tips and tricks for the diagnosis and management of biliary stenosis-state of the art review. World J Gastrointest Endosc 2021;13:473–90.

46. Krishna NB, Saripalli S, Safdar R, et al. Intraductal US in evaluation of biliary strictures without a mass lesion on CT scan or magnetic resonance imaging: significance of focal wall thickening and extrinsic compression at the stricture site. Gastrointest Endosc 2007;66:90–6.

47. Sun B, Hu B. The role of intraductal ultrasonography in pancreatobiliary diseases. Endosc Ultrasound 2016;5:291–9.

48. Chen L, Lu Y, Wu JC, et al. Diagnostic Utility of Endoscopic Retrograde Cholangiography/Intraductal Ultrasound (ERC/IDUS) in Distinguishing Malignant from Benign Bile Duct Obstruction. Dig Dis Sci 2016;61:610–7.

49. Meister T, Heinzow HS, Woestmeyer C, et al. Intraductal ultrasound substantiates diagnostics of bile duct strictures of uncertain etiology. World J Gastroenterol 2013;19:874–81.

50. Vazquez-Sequeiros E, Baron TH, Clain JE, et al. Evaluation of indeterminate bile duct strictures by intraductal US. Gastrointest Endosc 2002;56:372–9.

51. Domagk D, Wessling J, Reimer P, et al. Endoscopic retrograde cholangiopancreatography, intraductal ultrasonography, and magnetic resonance cholangiopancreatography in bile duct strictures: a prospective comparison of imaging diagnostics with histopathological correlation. Am J Gastroenterol 2004;99:1684–9.

52. Stavropoulos S, Larghi A, Verna E, et al. Intraductal ultrasound for the evaluation of patients with biliary strictures and no abdominal mass on computed tomography. Endoscopy 2005;37:715–21.

53. Farrell RJ, Agarwal B, Brandwein SL, et al. Intraductal US is a useful adjunct to ERCP for distinguishing malignant from benign biliary strictures. Gastrointest Endosc 2002;56:681–7.

54. Meining A, Chen YK, Pleskow D, et al. Direct visualization of indeterminate pancreaticobiliary strictures with probe-based confocal laser endomicroscopy: a multicenter experience. Gastrointest Endosc 2011;74:961–8.

55. Meining A, Shah RJ, Slivka A, et al. Classification of probe-based confocal laser endomicroscopy findings in pancreaticobiliary strictures. Endoscopy 2012;44:251–7.

56. Caillol F, Filoche B, Gaidhane M, et al. Refined probe-based confocal laser endomicroscopy classification for biliary strictures: the Paris Classification. Dig Dis Sci 2013;58:1784–9.

57. Taunk P, Singh S, Lichtenstein D, et al. Improved classification of indeterminate biliary strictures by probe-based confocal laser endomicroscopy using the Paris Criteria following biliary stenting. J Gastroenterol Hepatol 2017;32:1778–83.

58. Slivka A, Gan I, Jamidar P, et al. Validation of the diagnostic accuracy of probe-based confocal laser endomicroscopy for the characterization of indeterminate biliary strictures: results of a prospective multicenter international study. Gastrointest Endosc 2015;81:282–90.

59. Talreja JP, Sethi A, Jamidar PA, et al. Interpretation of probe-based confocal laser endomicroscopy of indeterminate biliary strictures: is there any interobserver agreement? Dig Dis Sci 2012;57:3299–302.

60. Han S, Kahaleh M, Sharaiha RZ, et al. Probe-based confocal laser endomicroscopy in the evaluation of dominant strictures in patients with primary sclerosing cholangitis: results of a U.S. multicenter prospective trial. Gastrointest Endosc 2021;94:569–576 e1.

61. Arvanitakis M, Hookey L, Tessier G, et al. Intraductal optical coherence tomography during endoscopic retrograde cholangiopancreatography for investigation of biliary strictures. Endoscopy 2009;41:696–701.
62. Tyberg A, Raijman I, Novikov AA, et al. Optical coherence tomography of the pancreatic and bile ducts: are we ready for prime time? Endosc Int Open 2020;8:E644–9.
63. Ahn DH, Javle M, Ahn CW, et al. Next-generation sequencing survey of biliary tract cancer reveals the association between tumor somatic variants and chemotherapy resistance. Cancer 2016;122:3657–66.
64. Dudley JC, Zheng Z, McDonald T, et al. Next-Generation Sequencing and Fluorescence in Situ Hybridization Have Comparable Performance Characteristics in the Analysis of Pancreaticobiliary Brushings for Malignancy. J Mol Diagn 2016;18: 124–30.
65. Scheid JF, Rosenbaum MW, Przybyszewski EM, et al. Next-generation sequencing in the evaluation of biliary strictures in patients with primary sclerosing cholangitis. Cancer Cytopathol 2021. https://doi.org/10.1002/cncy.22528. In press.
66. Lee YN, Moon JH, Choi HJ, et al. Tissue acquisition for diagnosis of biliary strictures using peroral cholangioscopy or endoscopic ultrasound-guided fine-needle aspiration. Endoscopy 2019;51:50–9.

Role of ERCP in Malignant Hilar Biliary Obstruction

Tae Hoon Lee, MD, PhD[a], Jong Ho Moon, MD, FASGE, FJGES[b],*,
Sherman Stuart, MD, MASGE[c]

KEYWORDS

- Malignant Hilar Obstruction • Drainage • Endoscopy

KEY POINTS

- Malignant hilar biliary obstruction (MHO), an aggressive perihilar biliary obstruction caused by cholangiocarcinoma, gallbladder cancer, or other metastatic malignancies, has a poor prognosis. Surgical resection is the only curative treatment method for biliary malignancies. However, most of the patients with MHO cannot undergo surgeries on presentation because of an advanced inoperable state or a poor performance state due to old age or comorbid diseases.
- Palliative biliary drainage is mandatory to improve symptomatic jaundice and quality of life. Among drainage methods, endoscopic biliary drainage is the current standard for the palliation of unresectable advanced MHO.
- The development of stents and various accessories and advances in endoscopic techniques including endoscopic ultrasonography have facilitated primary endoscopic intervention in difficult high-grade hilar strictures. However, some issues are still under debate, such as palliation methods, appropriate stents, the number of stents, deployment methods, and additional local ablation therapies.

INTRODUCTION

Curative management of malignant hilar biliary obstruction (MHO) remains a challenge because of difficulty in its early diagnosis and its advanced state at diagnosis. Cholangiocarcinoma is known to be prevalent in Eastern and Southeastern Asia whereby infection by *Opisthorchis viverrini* or *Clonorchis sinensis* (liver flukes, flatworms) is

[a] Division of Gastroenterology and Hepatology, Department of Internal Medicine, SoonChunHyang University Cheonan Hospital, SoonChunHyang University School of Medicine, Cheonan, 31, Sooncheonhyang 6-gil, Dongnam-gu, Cheonan-si, Chungcheongnam-do, 31151, Republic of Korea; [b] Division of Gastroenterology and Hepatology, Department of Internal Medicine, SoonChunHyang University Bucheon Hospital, SoonChunHyang University School of Medicine, 170 Jomaru-Ro, Bucheon 14584, Republic of Korea; [c] Department of Medicine, Division of Gastroenterology/Hepatology, Indiana University School of Medicine, Indiana University Health-University Hospital, 550 North University Boulevard, Suite 1634, Indianapolis, IN 46202, USA
* Corresponding author.
E-mail addresses: jhmoon@schmc.ac.kr; jhmoonsch@gmail.com

Gastrointest Endoscopy Clin N Am 32 (2022) 427–453
https://doi.org/10.1016/j.giec.2022.01.003

Abbreviations	
MHO	malignant hilar biliary obstruction
HCCA	hilar cholangiocarcinoma
MDCT	multidetector computed tomography
MRI	magnetic resonance image
MRCP	magnetic resonance cholangiopancreatography
IHDs	intrahepatic ducts
PTBD	percutaneous transhepatic biliary drainage
PBD	preoperative biliary drainage
FLR	future liver remnant
RCT	randomized controlled trials
SEMS	self-expandable metal stent
CBD	common bile duct
SIS	stent-in-stent
SBS	stent-by-stent
EUS-BD	endoscopic ultrasound-guided biliary drainage
RBO	recurrent biliary obstruction
PDT	photodynamic therapy
RFA	radiofrequency ablation

known to be a high risk factor for cholangiocarcinomas.[1,2] In Western countries, primary sclerosing cholangitis is the most common predisposing condition, especially for hilar cholangiocarcinoma (HCCA).[3] HCCA, traditionally known as a Klatskin tumor, accounts for more than 50% of all cholangiocarcinomas. It is the main cause of MHO.[1,4–6] Gallbladder cancers, hepatocellular carcinomas, lymphomas, and metastatic malignancies can also result in perihilar obstruction.

Pathologically and morphologically, HCCA shows a characteristic spreading feature of longitudinal extension along the bile duct with the transmural invasion of bile ducts and radial extension into periductal tissues and adjacent structures. Especially, the most common sclerosing (scirrhous) type is characterized by an intense desmoplastic reaction.[7] Because of these pathologic and morphologic characteristics, imaging diagnosis of these microscopic spreading is limited currently, making it difficult to define resectability clearly despite numerous advanced image modalities. Although surgical resection undoubtedly remains the standard treatment of MHO, most of the patients are diagnosed at an advanced stage at the initial presentation with a poor survival outcome.

Therefore, primary palliative biliary drainage is necessary till end-of-life regardless of whether or not surgical resection is performed. It may improve their quality of life by ameliorating pruritus, general weakness, and poor appetite. However, compared with drainage of extrahepatic distal obstruction, primary palliative biliary drainage has different technical and clinical feasibilities. Although there are various palliation strategies for advanced MHO, they remain under debate. The aim of this review is to define the current role of endoscopy in the palliation of MHO according to its application in various clinical settings.

FACTORS TO CONSIDER BEFORE PERFORMING DRAINAGE OF MALIGNANT HILAR BILIARY OBSTRUCTION
Biliary Anatomy for Endoscopic Drainage

Multidetector computed tomography (MDCT) and magnetic resonance image (MRI)/ magnetic resonance cholangiopancreatography (MRCP) are the best imaging modalities for presumptive diagnosis, staging, and evaluating resectability of MHO as well as for determining the best route of drainage.[8] For effective biliary drainage, it is necessary to understand the anatomy and optimal amounts of liver volume to drain before selecting the procedure and establishing an appropriate drainage strategy.

The normal anatomy of intrahepatic ducts (IHDs) should be considered to obtain effective drainage. The Bismuth classification is widely used by radiologists and endoscopists because it describes the extent of the tumor into the IHD, which can have a practical impact on drainage strategy.[9] The left hepatic duct is usually 3 cm long before dividing into ducts for segments 2, 3, and 4, while the right hepatic duct is about 1 cm in length before dividing early into 2 sectorial ducts (anterior for segments 5 and 8; posterior for segments 6 and 7).[10] Therefore, as HCCA advances, right lobe sectors are involved and obstructed earlier than left lobe ones. When the 2 right sectorial ducts (anterior and posterior) are separated such as in Bismuth type IIIA, multiple stents are required to obtain complete drainage of these 2 ducts.

Optimal amount of liver volume to drain

Approximately 55% to 60%, 30% to 35%, and 10% of the liver volume are excreted through the right hepatic duct, the left hepatic duct, and the caudate lobe, respectively. Ameliorating symptoms and improving quality of life and survival by prolonging stent patency without increasing adverse events are clinical goals of biliary drainage. It has been recommended to drain at least 25% of the total liver volume for adequate biliary drainage in biliary obstruction.[11] However, more than 50% drainage of total liver volume has been suggested recently.[2] Factor analysis for predicting drainage effectiveness during endoscopic stenting for MHO has shown that drainage greater than 50% is associated with prolonged survival than drainage less than 50% (119 days vs. 59 days, $P = .005$).[12] Especially for high-grade strictures such as Bismuth type III or IV, a major factor related to drainage efficiency is to drain more than 50% of the liver volume.[12] Therefore, if a single stent cannot drain more than 50% of estimated liver volume, multiple liver segments should be drained by an endoscopic or a percutaneous approach. Adequate drainage of liver volume is physiologically ideal.

Level of experience

Endoscopic stenting for perihilar obstruction is known to have a difficulty level of 3 (a total of 4 levels: 1–4), meaning that its risk of technical failure is relatively high.[13] In such cases, complications might seriously affect the survival rate. Compared with the drainage of distal biliary obstruction, a more advanced level of experience is needed for effective hilar drainage.[14,15] Especially, high-grade hilar stricture may need more experience of the endoscopist because technical failure can increase the rate of adverse events. Therefore, some guidelines recommend a percutaneous approach for multiple drainages in advanced MHO.[2,16] However, with the advance of techniques, endoscopic palliation shows outstanding results now. The American Society for Gastrointestinal Endoscopy (ASGE) guideline 2021 suggests that endoscopic or percutaneous transhepatic biliary drainage (PTBD) should be based on patient preferences, disease characteristics, and local expertise.[17]

PREOPERATIVE BILIARY DRAINAGE OF MALIGNANT HILAR BILIARY OBSTRUCTION

There is a slight difference in opinion about preoperative biliary drainage (PBD) for resectable MHO according to the results of previous studies. The indication for PBD should be conducted by balancing risks and benefits for each patient. In resectable MHO, PBD is not routinely performed. There is a consensus that PBD is indicated in patients with cholangitis, hyperbilirubinemia-induced malnutrition, hepatic insufficiency or renal insufficiency, patients needing neo-adjuvant therapy, severely symptomatic patients, and those with delays in surgery.[8] In addition, expected future liver remnant (FLR) volume should be considered. If the FLR volume is predicted to be less than 30% after surgery, the risk of postoperative liver failure and death is high. Quantification of FLR volume is essential to indicate whether PBD should be performed.[18,19] When the FLR volume is less than 30%, portal vein embolization is required to obtain hypertrophy of the remnant liver. In this setting, PBD seems to reduce the risk for hepatic insufficiency. Thus, it should be definitely performed.[20]

However, no randomized controlled trials (RCT) have been reported to clarify the safety of major hepatectomy without PBD for cholestatic patients with HCCA. Several retrospective studies have shown that PBD can increase the risk of postsurgical infections without any effect on survival.[21–23] Scheufele *and colleagues*[24] have demonstrated that PBD can induce a shift of biliary microbiome with an increase of aggressive and resistant bacteria. Meta-analysis studies have revealed that preoperative PTBD is associated with lower risk of cholangitis, particularly in patients with Bismuth-Corlette type II, III, and IV compared with endoscopic drainage. Preoperative PTBD showed a lower risk of drainage-related complications and higher success rates of palliative relief of cholestasis than endoscopic drainage.[25–27] Two meta-analysis studies have reported that procedure-related morbidity in the ERCP group is similar to or higher than PTBD group.[28,29] However, another meta-analysis has shown higher morbidity in the PTBD group.[30] Hameed *and colleagues*[28] have reported a relatively lower 5-year survival rate in the PTBD group (30% vs 46%). Importantly, Takahashi Y *and colleagues.*[31] have shown more common peritoneal metastasis in PTBD drainage (5.2%). Hirano *and colleagues*[32] have also performed an adjusted analysis on factors influencing peritoneal recurrence. After controlling for age and tumor stage, they found that preoperative PTBD was the only independent factor predictive of the development of peritoneal recurrence (OR: 6.9; 95% CI: 1.9–25.7; $P = .004$). The ASGE guideline also suggests against routine use of PTBD as first-line therapy compared with endoscopic biliary drainage in patients with MHO undergoing PBD.[17]

Therefore, PBD should be performed in indicated patients as described above and the lower FLR (<30%). Although endoscopic drainage has lower technical success rates with higher rates of pancreatitis or cholangitis and the occasional need for conversion to PTBD, endoscopic drainage is more preferred by patients and physicians because it can avoid external drainage. Also, if endoscopic drainage is performed by experienced endoscopists, serious adverse events might not be different from those in PTBD. A major concern with preoperative PTBD is its association with higher rates of peritoneal metastasis, higher postprocedure mortality, and worse survival than endoscopic drainage. However, well-designed RCTs are needed to obtain high-level evidence.

ENDOSCOPIC PALLIATION
Primary role of ERCP Compared with Percutaneous Drainage

Asia-Pacific consensus and the recent European Society of Gastrointestinal Endoscopy (ESGE) guideline prefer a percutaneous approach than an endoscopic approach for bilateral or multi-segmental drainage in high-grade hilar strictures such as bismuth type II or more for drainage of more than 50% of liver volume.[2,33] PTBD is still superior to endoscopic drainage in advanced MHO based on reported studies. PTBD shows higher technical feasibility and enables a selective lobar approach for drainage of selective bile ducts than an endoscopic approach. Previous retrospective studies have shown that technical success rate and durability are higher in PTBD than in endoscopic drainage with comparable complication rates.[34–36] A meta-analysis and systematic review has revealed that PTBD is superior to endoscopic drainage in patients with advanced unresectable MHO.[37]

However, PTBD also has some limitations. First, PTBD is very inconvenient to patients because of pain and discomfort at the puncture site. In addition, patients have to keep an external catheter for a long time, which diminishes their quality of life. Second, external loss of bile out of the body with external drainage is not physiologic. Third, although PTBD is a relatively safe and effective tailored method when it is performed by experts, it is technically difficult when IHD is not fully expanded or when multiple liver metastasis, ascites, or blood clotting disorders are present. Also, for multiple stenting, multiple percutaneous punctures are needed. Usually, 2 interval steps are needed for the placement of internal stents.

Therefore, endoscopic palliation is actually more frequently performed as a primary intervention in terms of convenience and quality of life for patients. Recent studies using self-expandable metal stent (SEMS) via endoscopy have shown higher technical and clinical success rates with promising stent patency without increasing adverse events even in multiple or bilateral drainage.[38–50] The development of various metal stents and accessories such as guidewires and the technical advances of endoscopists skills have facilitated a primary endoscopic approach as a preferred method even in advanced MHO.

The 2021 ASGE guideline suggests that the final decision of the palliative drainage method should be based on patient preferences, disease characteristics, and local expertise for patients with unresectable MHO.[51] PTBD and endoscopic drainage should be selected according to surrounding circumferences including patients, physicians, and hospitals. These 2 methods each have their pros and cons.

Plastic and Metal Stents

Plastic stents are most commonly used for endoscopic biliary drainage regardless of the level of biliary stricture. A plastic stent is easy to exchange, remove, and add on for effective drainage. It does not impair subsequent therapies such as local ablation therapies or surgery either. Thus, the plastic stent is also indicated for PBD. Finally, stent size can be adapted to the common bile duct (CBD) diameter which is not dilated in most MHO cases. However, a relatively higher rate of stent malfunction occurs due to the smaller diameter requiring frequent stent exchange during the survival period, which may decrease quality of life and increase the cost.

In contrast to plastic stents, metal stents with relatively larger diameters provide more prolonged stent patency. In addition, an open wire mesh of a metal stent does not occlude side branches of IHDs or cystic ducts. Technically, in severe or tight strictures, longer plastic stent insertion using a pushing catheter may be difficult due to less pushability. However, an SEMS is preloaded in a delivery catheter via a thin delivery system (5.4–8.5 Fr according to the manufactures), which facilitates easy passage across tight biliary strictures with better pushability.[52–55] Therefore, SEMSs have been used for the prolongation of stent patency with lower rate of reintervention without increasing complications during the survival period. Clinical studies comparing SEMS and plastic stents in MHO have shown a higher success rate of SEMS technically and clinically with the prolongation of stent patency by reducing the number of reinterventions, resulting in its cost-effectiveness.[56–59]

The 2013 Asia-Pacific consensus and the 2018 ESGE guideline have suggested metal stents in patients with high-grade MHO with a predicted survival longer than 3 months. SEMS was superior to plastic stenting for palliation with respect to outcomes and cost-effectiveness.[2,16] The 2021 ASGE guideline also suggests SEMS rather than plastic stent in patients with a short life expectancy (<3 months) and those who place a high value on avoiding repeated interventions.[17]

Despite these benefits of SEMS, stent occlusion by tumor ingrowth and/or overgrowth still occurs in 20% to 50% of cases, which is unavoidable when the survival period is longer. Embedded stents are very hard to remove after the malfunction of stents. Stent revision is also very difficult compared with plastic stents.[38,52,53,60] To overcome these shortfalls, covered SEMS can be used because they are easy to remove or exchange without becoming embedded. However, it is difficult to deploy multiple covered SEMSs to hilar lesions due to limited narrow space. In addition, occlusion of side branches of IHDs might result in liver abscess or cholangitis. For multiple (more than 2) drainages, the actual diameter of the stent will be decreased, which might decrease the original benefit of covered SEMS to prolong the patency of stent. In addition, biofilm formation cannot be prevented, resulting in sludge or stones. Therefore, inserting covered SEMS in advanced MHO is not generally recommended.

Unilateral Versus Bilateral Drainage

Unilateral (single) drainage: Evidence supporting the efficacy of unilateral drainage in advanced MHO is that it is enough for the perihilar palliation whether a right or left duct drainage is performed. Polydorou *and colleagues*[61] have reported that there is no significant difference in successful drainage, complications, number of endoprosthesis changes, or survival between drainage to the right bile duct and drainage to the left bile duct. Regarding drainage volume of liver, it has been known that only 25% of the liver volume requires drainage to have adequate palliation of obstructive cholestasis and to improve biochemical parameters.[11]

Previous studies have reported that bilateral drainage can result in relatively higher rate of adverse events without the prolongation of stent patency, which is the main reason why bilateral drainage is not recommended routinely.[62–65] Unilateral drainage with either a metal or plastic stent has a higher technical success rate, a lower incidence of complications, and a higher successful drainage rate than bilateral stenting.[61–65] De Palma *and colleagues*[62,63] have shown that unilateral drainage using a metal stent is safe and effective in a large majority of patients with unresectable MHO. In their results, compared with bilateral SEMS, unilateral SEMS had a significantly higher technical success rate (88.6% in unilateral vs. 76.9% in bilateral, $P = .041$) and a significantly lower rate of adverse events (18.9% vs. 26.9%, $P = .026$).[63] The authors concluded that inserting more than one stent could not be justified as a routine procedure in patients with MHO. Regarding adverse events, Iwano *and colleagues*[65] have shown that unilateral drainage is associated with a lower incidence of liver abscess without any significant difference in stent patency rate or complication-free survival than bilateral drainage. Recent studies using a percutaneous approach have also shown no significant difference between unilateral and bilateral drainages (**Table 1**).[66,67]

Bilateral (multiple) drainage: Recent factor analysis studies predicting drainage effectiveness after endoscopic stenting of MHO have shown that drainage greater than 50% is associated with prolonged survival than drainage less than 50% (119 days vs. 59 days, $P = .005$).[12] Therefore, bilateral or multiple stenting for drainage greater than 50% might be warranted to achieve clinical efficacy in high-degree MHO. The Asia-Pacific consensus also suggests that the goal of palliative stenting is to perform drainage greater than 50% of liver volume in Bismuth type II to IV.[2] If a single stent cannot drain more than 50% of liver volume, bilateral or multisegmental drainage is recommended. It will be particularly helpful when both hepatic lobes are diseased or opacified, or when a nondominant or atrophic lobe has been inadvertently stented

Table 1
Unilateral versus bilateral drainage using SEMS in MHO

% (No.)	Design	SEMS, No.	Technical Success	Clinical Success	Adverse Events	Re-intervention	Stent Patency, day[a]	Survival, day[a]
Endoscopic method								
Naitoh et al,[73] 2009	Retrospective	Uni:17 Bi:29 P-value	100 (17) 90 (26)	94 (16) 90 (25)	65 (11) 64 (17)	59 (10) 23 (6) 0.02	210 488 0.009	166 205 0.559
Iwano et al,[65] 2011	Retrospective	Uni: 65 Bi. 17 P-value	95.2 (60/63) 89.5 (17/19)	n/a	36.9 (24) 41.2 (7)	26.2 (17) 29.4 (5)	133 125 0.322	170 184 0.490
Liberato & Canena[56] 2012	Retrospective (plastic + metal)	Uni:35 Bi.42 P-value	98.8 (total)	97.9 (total)	Early 2 Late 24.4 (total)	24.4 (total)	Longer patency in bilateral	n/a
Mukai et al,[57] 2013	RCT (plastic + metal)	Uni. 14 Bi. 16 P-value	100 (total)	n/a	n/a	29 (4) 50 (8)	363 295 0.347	219.5 (total)
Lee et al,[74] 2017	RCT	Uni. 66 Bi. 67 P-value	100 (66) 95.5 (64) 0.244	84.9 (56) 95.3 (61) 0.047	27.3 (18) 6.3 (4) 0.001 (early)	57.6 (38) 42.2 (27) 0.079	139 252 <0.01	178 270 0.053
Percutaneous method								
Teng et al,[66] 2019	Retrospective	Uni. 58 Bi. 52 P-value	93.1 (54) 90.4 (47) 0.864	96.4 (53) 97.9 (46) 1.00	9/55 7/47 0.839	9/55 4/47 0.236	185 198 0.999	189 199 0.867
Chang et al,[67] 2017	Retrospective	Uni. 33 Bi. SBS 30 P-value	93.9 (31) 90 (27) 0.912	93.5 (29) 96.3 (26) 0.637	4 7 0.207	16.1 (5) 11.1 (3) 0.58	368 387 0.685	200 198 0.751

SEMS, self-expandable metal stent; Uni., unilateral; Bi., bilateral; RCT, randomized controlled trial.
n/a; not available.
Data are expressed as % (patient number).
[a] Median.

without achieving drainage. The 2021 ASGE guideline also suggests the placement of bilateral stents instead of a single unilateral stent in MHO.[17]

Regarding adverse events, when bilateral drainage fails after contrast injection passes the hilar stricture and into atrophied and/or unintended multiple hepatic segments, post-ERCP cholangitis and abscess are problematic as they are associated with a lower survival rate.[68] The incidence of cholangitis in patients with MHO is significantly higher than that in those with a distal obstruction.[69] However, unintended contrast injection can be avoided or reduced by using MRI/MRCP or three-dimensional CT imaging. Based on advanced image analysis, targeted and planned endoscopic drainages can reduce unintentional contrast injection, which can result in postprocedure adverse events such as cholangitis and abscess.[69–72] Therefore, proper procedure based on prior image analysis and performance by experienced endoscopists is highly recommended to reduce adverse events, which can result in the prolongation of stent patency and higher complication-free survival.

As Chang *and colleagues*[68] first showed that bilateral SEMS might improve stent patency and survival by ensuring adequate drainage in MHO, several studies revealed the benefit of bilateral SEMS in stent patency, survival, and reintervention rate.[56,73,74] The first RCT comparing unilateral and bilateral drainage using SEMS in advanced MHO has shown the superiority of bilateral drainage in term of stent patency (adjusted HR: 0.30, 95% CI: 0.17–0.52; $P < .001$) and reintervention rate.[74] Adverse event rates with unilateral stents were not different from those of bilateral stents. A meta-analysis and systematic review have shown that unilateral plastic drainage is comparable to bilateral plastic drainage in terms of overall adverse events and 30-day mortality in patients with MHO. Bilateral metal stenting seems to have lower odds of overall complications than unilateral metallic stenting. Bilateral SEMS were superior in palliating jaundice. However, 30-day mortality showed no difference between unilateral and bilateral drainages by SEMS.[75]

Therefore, although previous initial reports supporting benefits of unilateral drainage suggested that multiple biliary drainages could not be justified as a routine procedure in patients with MHO, for effective and physiologic drainage $\geq 50\%$ of liver volume, multiple drainages using SEMS or plastic stents is now recommended as primary palliation in advanced MHO.

Endoscopic Multisectoral Drainage using Metal Stents

Self-expandable metal stents for bilateral stenting

Numerous types of SEMS are now available for the palliation of MHO. Basically, wire structure and materials are similar. They are usually made of stainless steel or nickel shape-retaining titanium (Nitinol). According to the stent's cell structure, it can be divided into a small closed-cell or large open-cell type. Large open-cell type stents (Zilver stent, Wilson-Cook Medical Inc., Winston-Salem, NC, USA; JOSTENT SelfX stent, Abbott Vascular Devices, Redwood City, Calif., USA; Niti-S Y-type or Niti-S large cell D-type, Taewoong Medical Inc., Seoul, Korea) can be easily dilated by ballooning or a second stent. They then remain in a dilated state. Such stents may facilitate primary insertion or reintervention when stent malfunction develops. However, this type of stent might be suboptimal for stent patency due to vulnerability of tumor ingrowth and relatively decreased radial force on the central portion in severe strictures. Small closed-cell design stents (WallFlex, Boston Scientific Co., Natick, MA, USA; Bonastent, Standard SciTech Inc., Seoul, Korea; Hanarostent; M.I. Tech Co., Seoul, Korea) have relatively smaller sized cells which may overcome the weakness of the central portion of stent caused by the extent of stricture or tumor burden. On the other hand, this benefit of a closed or small-cell design makes it technically difficult for primary second stent insertion and stent revision, especially when it is placed as a stent-in-stent (SIS) configuration. As a mixed form of small closed-cell type, cross-wired type (M-Hilar stent, Standard SciTech Inc., Seoul, Korea) **(Fig. 1)** has the conventional hook and a cross-wired structure on the proximal and distal portions. However, on the 25-mm-long central portion, it only has a cross-wired structure to facilitate the placement of the contralateral stent across it. However, comparative results regarding technical feasibility and functionality according to the type of stents have not been reported yet.

An open-cell or cross-wired type is adequate for SIS deployment and a closed-cell type is adequate for stent-by-stent (SBS) deployment. Thus, appropriate deployment methods and stents should be selected according to technical difficulty, experience of endoscopists, whether a second procedure is considered, and stent availability.

Endoscopic bilateral stent-in-stent versus stent-by-stent (side-by-side) deployment

Bilateral or multiple deployment methods of SEMS are divided into SIS and SBS techniques. Reported studies for each method have shown various technical and clinical feasibilities ranging from 73.3% to 100% for experts using SIS and SBS techniques.[35–39,41–50,52–57,76–78] There are still debates about which method is better for effective drainage in MHO. In a retrospective comparison, Naitoh and colleagues[47] showed that rates of early and late adverse events including cholangitis, cholecystitis, and liver abscess were higher in the SBS group than in the SIS group (44% vs. 13%, respectively; $P = .016$). Despite more frequent adverse events in the SBS group, the cumulative stent patency tended to be prolonged in the SBS group than in the SIS group. On the other hand, another small-sized study revealed that there was no significant difference in adverse events, stent patency, or survival between SBS and SIS groups.[79] The first RCT of SIS and SBS deployment by Lee and colleagues[78] has revealed that there is no significant difference in technical feasibility, adverse events, or stent patency duration. Technical feasibility of SIS deployed by experts was not different from that of the SBS method. Stent patency rates at 3 months and 6 months after the successful deployment of bilateral SEMS tended to be higher in the SIS group without showing a statistically significant difference **(Table 2)**. A recent meta-analysis study has revealed that SIS is technically superior to SBS without any other differences.[80] However, among 5 enrolled studies, there was only one RCT. Thus, more comparative studies are needed to support these results.

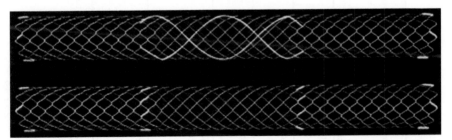

Fig. 1. Cross-wired type M-Hilar stent. The 1st stent had 2 spiral radiopaque markings (X mark) on the central portion and 4-spot markings on each end. It had the conventional hook and cross-wired structure on the proximal and distal portions. However, on the 25-mm-long central portion, this stent had only the cross-wired structure. The 2nd stent was of the same design, except that it had 4 spot radiopaque markings on each end of the central portion to differentiate it from the 1st stent.

Table 2
Comparative studies for endoscopic SIS versus SBS deployment in MHO

% (No.)	Design	Stent, No.	Sex (male), No.	Age, Mean (SD)	Technical Success	Clinical Success	Early Adverse Events	Late Adverse Events	Total Adverse Events	Occlusion Rate	Stent Patency, day[a]	Survival, day[a]
Naitoh et al,[47] 2012	Retrospective	SIS, 24	14	69.5 (11)	89 (25)	96 (24/25)	11 (3/28)	32 (8/25)	44 (11/25)	20 (5/25)	155	198
		SBS, 28	11									
		P-value	0.137	0.105	0.148	0.51	0.366	0.074	0.016	0.091	0.388	0.952
Kim et al,[79] 2012	Retrospective	SIS, 22	17	65.0 (3.1)	100 (22)	81.8 (18)	22.7 (5/22)	50 (11/22)	72.7 (16/22)	59.1 (13/22)	134	225
		SBS, 19	11	64.2 (2.8)	100 (19)	78.9 (15)	31.6 (6/19)	36.8 (7/19)	68.4 (13/19)	47.4 (9/19)	118	146
		P-value	0.313	0.637	n/s	1	0.725	0.531	0.538	0.538	0.074	0.266
Law et al,[77] 2013	Retrospective	SIS, 7	Total 19	68	100 (7)	n/a	Total 4/0		Total 4/0	42.9 (3/7)	Total 86	n/a
		SBS, 17		68	100 (17)					52.9 (9/17)		
		P-value		0.99	n/s					0.31		
Lee et al,[78] 2018	Randomized study	SIS, 34	15	74.5 (10.04)	100 (34)	94.1 (32/34)	11.8 (4/34)	17.6 (6/34)	23.5 (8/34)	44.1 (15/34)	253	209
		SBS, 35	21	72.5 (11.05)	91.4 (32)	90.6 (29/32)	11.4 (4/35)	22.9 (8/35)	28.6 (10/35)	34.3 (12/35)	262	221
		P-value	0.187	0.438	0.081	0.668	0.965	0.591	0.633	0.403	0.865	0.197
Ishigaki et al,[54] 2020	Retrospective	SIS, 40	22	72	100 (40)	93 (37)	23 (9)	10 (4)	32.5 (13)	48 (19)	169	238
		SBS, 24	13	74	96 (23)	96 (23)	46 (11)	12 (3)	58.3 (14)	43 (11)	205	381
		P-value	0.99	0.90	0.99	0.99	0.09	0.99	n/a	0.99	0.67	0.07

SIS, stent-in-stent; SBS, stent-by-stent; n/a, not available; n/s, not significant; SD, standard deviation.
Data are shown as % (patient number).
a Median.

Stent-by-stent (SBS) deployment: SBS deployment is a sequential or simultaneous parallel placement of 2 or more SEMS into both IHDs or multi-sectoral branches.[50,81] Following selective insertion of guidewires into intended multi-sectoral branches of the bile duct, 2 or more SEMS are then sequentially inserted parallel over the inserted guidewires using the "side-by-side" method. The distal end of both stents should be placed at the same level within CBD or across the ampulla of Vater (**Fig. 2**). Simultaneous SBS placement is also possible using a smaller 6F stent delivery system (Zilver 635, Cook Medical, Winston-Salem, NC, USA; Epic, Boston Scientific, Natick, MA, USA).

The advantage of the SBS technique is its technical feasibility. Compared with SIS deployment, bilateral SBS deployment is relatively easier after the insertion of 2 guidewires as mentioned in the technique. Also, revision of stents is technically easier when stents have crossed the major papilla. Selective guidewire insertion and stent revision are also relatively easy through the deployed 2 stents in the duodenum. Although this position of stents might be vulnerable to duodenal reflux, few studies have examined the effect of stent position on patients' outcomes in MHO. In malignant bile duct obstruction, the placement of 10-Fr Teflon stents above or across the sphincter of Oddi showed no difference in stent function.[82]

Regarding limitations, technically after the deployment of the first SEMS, inserting the second delivery system can be difficult due to the resistance or impaction of the second delivery catheter against the previously deployed SEMS. However, insertion following delivery catheter preloading on the guidewire may speed the procedure, and pneumatic balloon dilatation before the deployment of the first stent enables sequential SBS deployment in severe obstruction. Other technical issues include potential entanglement of the 2 guidewires, difficulty of precise deployment of both ends of stents when they are placed within the CBD to facilitate endoscopic revision when stents are occluded.[3] Second, when 2 SEMSs with large diameters are deployed in parallel in a normal CBD, they may compress the adjacent portal vein at the CBD level.[83] Usually, the bile duct below the obstruction level is not dilated. Finally, stents with relatively smaller diameters due to the diameter of CBD may decrease stent patency and preclude the full expansion of 2 stents in nondilated CBD.

Stent-in-stent (SIS) deployment: SIS is named its final configuration of bilateral stents. Following sequential insertion and deployment of the second SEMS over a guidewire into the contralateral duct through the central portion of the first stent, a configuration of a Y-shape bilateral SEMS is obtained (**Fig. 3**).[52,53] Usually, distal ends of stents are placed above the level of papilla. To preserve the function of the

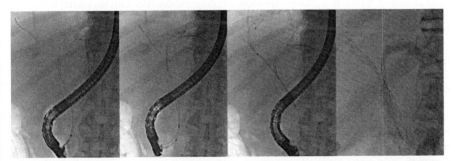

Fig. 2. Endoscopic bilateral stent-by-stent (SBS) deployment showing a parallel configuration of 2 metal stents into both IHDs. Each stent is positioned at the same level within CBD, above the level of the major papilla.

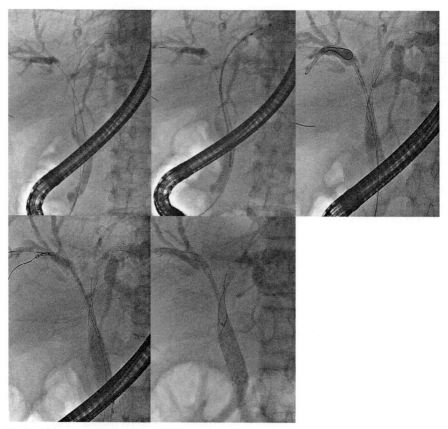

Fig. 3. Endoscopic bilateral stent-in-stent (SIS) showing a Y-shaped configuration after the deployment of 2 stents into both IHDs due to the second stent passing through the first deployed metal stent. Distal margins of each stent are also positioned within CBD.

sphincter of Oddi as much as possible and to prevent duodenal reflux, a large endoscopic sphincterotomy should not be performed routinely. For successful bilateral SIS, open-celled or cross-wired type is useful for second stenting.

The strength of SIS is its final configuration in a Y-shape according to the normal bile duct anatomy, which is a more physiologic configuration. SIS with less axial force can fit the bile duct configuration well with less pressure to proximal and distal sides of the bile duct wall or surrounding vascular structures.[84] Second, SIS may minimize duodenal reflux which can facilitate cholangitis or biofilm formation because the distal end of the stent in the SIS method is usually placed above the level of papilla. Duodenal reflux and deposition of organic material or bacteria can result in sludge or stone formation in the stent. Third, multi-sectoral drainage through the SIS method is possible as a primary insertion or revisionary method.[42,85,86] Despite these benefits, the main issue of SIS is that it is a technically difficult procedure involving guidewire manipulation for negotiating multiple ducts, primary 2nd stent insertion, and revision after stent malfunction. In particular, when stent malfunction occurs due to tumor ingrowth, bilaterally crossed wire mesh may prohibit the reinsertion of a guidewire or stent regardless of a plastic or a metal stent. Also, it is unavailable in several countries.

Based on reported literature, SIS and SBS deployment methods each have pros and cons, suggesting that these 2 methods are complimentary techniques rather than competitive techniques. According to technical difficulty, bile duct dilatation, and level of experience, the primarily intended method can be changed to one or the other.

Triple branched stenting

Multi-sectoral drainage has been suggested as a reasonable option to avoid cholangitis in the course of chemotherapy and to preserve the functional volume of the liver as much as possible, even in patients who are anicteric with a high-grade MHO.[42] Theoretically, triple drainage of the right anterior, right posterior, and left-sided bile ducts may be ideal when treating a high-grade MHO. Placement of more than 3 plastic stents is technically feasible, whereas it is less likely with metal stents. Triple stenting using SEMS can be performed by SIS, SBS, or combined deployment methods. SBS is possible if multiple guidewire insertion into IHDs is possible. However, inserting more than 3 SEMSs with SBS deployment can overextend the normal extrahepatic bile duct and increase the risk of pancreatitis. Triple stenting by the SIS method can also be performed in the same manner. Kawamoto *and colleagues*[42,86] have reported that triple stenting using the SIS method has a high technical success rate (100%) with occlusion rates of stents of 33% ~ 37%. Compared with bilateral drainage, its technical feasibility and adverse events were not different.

Additional insertion of a third metal stent into a bilateral SIS configuration as a revisionary method is also technically feasible and efficacious when technically successful bilateral SIS deployment has failed clinically (**Fig. 4**). Stent dysfunction during follow-up developed in 35.7% (5/14) of patients who underwent functionally successful placement of a third metal stent.[85]

These reported studies for triple stenting were performed by experts in advanced centers and the numbers of enrolled patients were small. In addition, they were not comparative studies. However, primary or revisionary method of triple stenting might be promising in selected patients for the prolongation of stent patency or the decrease of adverse events during the follow-up period. More large-sized studies are needed to confirm the efficacy of triple stenting.

Endoscopic Ultrasound-Guided Biliary Drainage in MHO

Endoscopic ultrasound-guided biliary drainage (EUS-BD) is now being increasingly used even in palliative drainage of MHO when conventional ERCP is unsuccessful

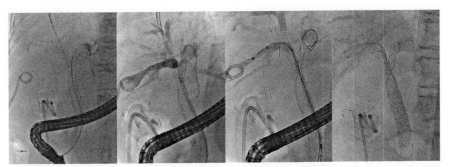

Fig. 4. Endoscopic triple branched stenting of SEMS following successful bilateral SIS deployment. As a revisionary method, following the insertion of a guidewire through the bilateral SEMS, a third metal stent was inserted into the right posterior segment. Final configuration showed triple branched SIS deployment.

or difficult due to surgically altered anatomy.[87,88] Still, primary EUS-BD for unresectable MHO is limited. It is not widely practiced due to limited data from some specialized centers or experts. However, when conventional ERCP is impossible or failed due to gastric outlet obstruction or surgically altered anatomy, EUS-BD can be used as a rescue method as an alternative to PTBD. Contraindications are similar to those of PTBD such as uncontrolled or severe coagulopathy, massive ascites, intervening vessels, and unstable state for endoscopy. EUS-guided hepaticogastrostomy (EUS-HGS), hepaticoduodenostomy, and bridging method are also availabe.[89,90] In the bridging method, the left IHD is accessed through the hilar stricture from the right IHD and stomach. An uncovered bridging SEMS is placed across the hilar stricture, followed by another covered or partially covered SEMS placement from the left IHD to the stomach, as seen in EUS-HGS.

Reintervention after Stent Malfunction

Reported recurrent biliary obstruction (RBO) rates after the placement of bilateral SEMS in MHO range from 3% to 45%.[53] RBO cannot be avoided during the survival period due to progression of tumor or stent-related adverse events. Primary endoscopic reintervention is usually effective and less invasive. Percutaneous or EUS-guided interventions are alternatives when primary endoscopic intervention using ERCP fails. Intended technical success of PTBD is usually higher than endoscopic success. Recently, EUS-BD has also been used as a reintervention in failed ERCP. However, it has too many limitations for primary use.[89]

Regarding the primary endoscopic method, plastic stents or fully covered SEMSs are technically easy for exchange and revision after the malfunction of stents. Therefore, considering reintervention, primary uses of these types of stents are likely to be more popular and easier than bare-metal stents. In general, stent revision of deployed metal stents is more difficult than the primary deployment of SEMS. In cases of primary deployment of multiple SEMS, reinsertion of metal stent or plastic stent through the previously deployed stent should be considered. Bilateral SBS deployment across the papilla is relatively easy for revision regardless of the type of stent. However, SIS or SBS deployment within the CBD level is relatively difficult to access bilaterally. A recent systematic review of 10 retrospective studies has revealed that placing a plastic stent as a reintervention is as effective as a second SEMS in malignant biliary obstruction.[91] Risks of reocclusion and patency duration after second stents were similar between plastic stents and SEMS. However, that systematic review included mostly distal biliary obstruction cases.[91] More large-scaled prospective studies for hilar lesions are needed to validate these findings. A relatively small number of patients with advanced MHO, a relatively short survival time, and follow-up loss after the placement of stents might preclude effective evaluation of studies.

LOCAL ABLATION THERAPIES

Besides traditional chemotherapy and radiotherapy, endoscopic local ablation therapies such as photodynamic therapy and radiofrequency ablation (RFA) are also promising local ablation therapies to prolong the patency of stent and survival.[92–94]

Photodynamic Therapy (PDT)

Photodynamic therapy (PDT) can result in a local tumor ablation effect after the photosensitization of a neoplastic tissue. A photosensitizer drug (commonly a hematoporphyrin derivative) is activated in the target tumor tissue by means of a laser with a specific wavelength. The production of oxygen free radicals can lead to the destruction of cellular and lysosomal membranes and damage of microvasculature, thus inducing tumor necrosis.[95–97] PDT offers the possibility of tumor "remodeling," which can enhance or prolong the decompressive effect (**Fig. 5**).[95] Based on this theory, the ability of PDT to destroy cancer cells and lessen cholestasis may prolong stent patency by diminishing the need for further procedures, such as stent reintervention, which may result in improved quality of life for patients with advanced MHO. Therefore, endoscopic drainage in combination with intraluminal PDT might be the best palliative option to prolong stent patency or survival by reducing tumor burden in appropriately selected patients. Even in patients with advanced MHO, it has been shown that PDT can improve survival and quality of life, out-performing biliary stenting alone in both uncontrolled and RCTs (**Table 3**).[97–104] An RCT by Ortner and colleagues[98] has demonstrated that PDT can lead to improved survival and Karnofsky performance status when compared with biliary stenting only in patients with unresectable cholangiocarcinoma. Zoepf and colleagues[99] have also shown an increased survival duration in patients treated with both PDT and stents than in those treated with biliary stenting alone. A trend suggestive of a longer patency duration for biliary stents was observed in patients with HCCA receiving PDT (compared with those receiving stents alone).[105] Moreover, PDT plus stenting seems to be associated with survival outcomes as good as those for operable patients who have R1 resections.[102] Furthermore, this combination treatment is associated with lower rates of adverse events than stenting alone.[102] However, as these findings are generally from retrospective and noncontrolled studies, conclusions based on these data must be made with caution. In a prospective cohort study comparing radical surgical

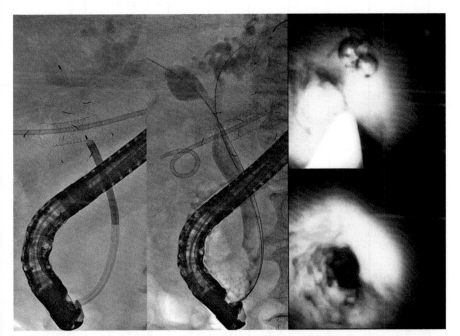

Fig. 5. Endoscopic PDT. PDT was performed via Spyglass system (Boston Scientific, Natick, MA, USA) assistance. Fluoroscopy showed that the Spyglass system assisted PDT. Following PDT, recanalization was noted after 1 week. Guidewire was then inserted bilaterally for the insertion of biliary stents.

Table 3
Comparative studies using PDT with stent and stent only in MHO

N (%)	Study		Group	PDT Session (Range)	Stent	Adverse Events Early/Late	Survival (day) median
Ortner et al,[98] 2003	RCT	HCCA B II ~ IV	PDT 20 Stent 19	2.4 (1–5)	10F plastic	7 (35) 7 (37)	493 98 (P < .0001)
Zoepf et al,[99] 2005	RCT	HCCA B II, IV	PDT 16 Stent 16	1~2	Plastic	4[a] 1[a]	21m 7m (P < .0109)
Dumoulin et al,[100] 2003	Retrospective	HCCA B III, IV	PDT 24 Stent 20	n/a	Plastic, Metal	Cholangitis 2(0–5) per patient/0 in control	9.9 m 5.6 m (not significant)
Kahaleh et al,[101] 2008	Retrospective	HCCA B I ~ IV	PDT 19 Stent 29	1.6 (1~3)	7~10F plastic	7[b] 10[b]	16.2 m 7.4 m (P = .003)
Witzigman et al,[102] 2006	Prospective	HCCA B I ~ IV	PDT 68 Stent 56	2 (1–6)	9, 11.5 F plastic	46 (67.6) 37 (66.1)	12m 6.4 m (P < .01)
Quyn et al,[103] 2009	Cohort	HCCA B II ~ IV	PDT 23 Palliative 17	1 Endoscopic or Percutaneous	10F plastic or metal	7/23, 4/23	425 169 (P < .0001)
Cheon et al,[104] 2012	Retrospective	HCCA B II ~ IV	PDT 72 Stent 71	n/a	n/a	n/a	9.8 m 7.3 m (P = .029)

RCT, randomized controlled trial; HCCA, hilar cholangiocarcinoma; PDT, photodynamic therapy.
n/a, not available.
[a] Severe infectious complications.
[b] Cholangitis.

resection, PDT, and biliary stenting in patients with advanced HCCA, mean and median survival were both significantly better in radical resection and PDT groups than in the biliary stent alone group.[103] The combination of chemotherapy and PDT for cholangiocarcinoma might be promising because the nature of chemotherapy is systemic while that of PDT is regional.

In summary, reported studies have suggested a benefit of PDT in patients with HCCA. However, these encouraging results are often obtained in comparison with patients who have received suboptimal biliary drainage. Thus, they could be misinterpreted as positive outcomes in support of PDT. Additional large-scale RCTs are needed to clarify this. Second, in advanced MHO, diffuse longitudinal tumor spreading is difficult to estimate the exact length of local ablation, and phototoxicity is also a troublesome complication. Third, it remains unknown whether radiotherapy, chemotherapy, PDT, or a combination of these therapies can provide superior outcomes.

Radiofrequency Ablation

RFA is a different type of local ablation therapy such as PDT. It does not need a photosensitizer. Thus, it has no phototoxicity. Its procedure method is also very simple (**Fig. 6**). The cost for treatment is relatively lower than that of PDT. Although no sufficient data exist to prove the equivalence or superiority to PDT in MHO, RFA is now widely used. It shows similar results to PDT. It might be an effective therapeutic alternative of PDT for the palliative treatment of malignant biliary obstruction (**Table 4**).[106–110] However, the effective and safe treatment mode of RFA for advanced MHO is still debatable. In Bismuth type I and type II MHO, which are difficult to perform surgical resection, the group with stent and RFA showed longer survival and stent patency than the stent-only group.[93] However, the effect for high-grade advanced

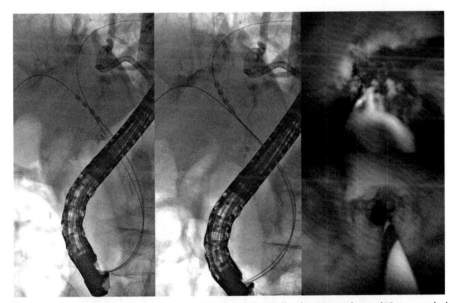

Fig. 6. Endoscopic RFA. After placing guidewires bilaterally, the RFA catheter (18 mm probe) was advanced to both IHDs over the guidewire sequentially and bilateral strictures were ablated, respectively. Cholangioscopic view shows resolution of obstruction at 1 month after RFA.

Table 4
Efficacy of RFA for MHO

	No.	Technical Success	RFA Session (Range)	Stent	Complication Early/late	Recurrent Biliary Obstruction	Patency (day)	Survival (day)
Inoue et al,[107] 2020	41	95.1% (39/41)	[a]39	SBS, SEMS	2.4%/7.7%	38.5% (15/39)	230	n/a
Bokemeyer et al,[108] 2019	32 (21 hilar)	100%	[a]54 (1–2)	Plastic 85.2%, SEMS 14.8%	18.5% (10/54)	n/a	n/a	342/221 (control; P = .046)
Tal et al,[109] 2014	12	100%	[a]19 (1–5)	Plastic	Late bleeding 3 Cholangitis 4	n/a	n/a	6.4 m
Kim et al,[110] 2019	11	100%	[c]4 (2–8)	Plastic, SEMS	Early; pancreatitis (1) fever only (5)	27.3% (3)	30-d stent patency, 100%	191
Schmidt et al,[106] 2016	14	100%	31	Plastic, SEMS	28% (4); cholangitis, liver abscess, sepsis	premature stent replacements (<3 m), 29% (4)	n/a	n/a

[c]Temperature-controlled ID-RFA catheter (ELRA; STARmed, Goyang, Korea) and RF generator (VIVA Combo; STARmed)
SEMS, self-expandable metal stent; n/a, not available.
[a] Habib EndoHPB Biopolar Radiofrequency Catheter (Boston Scientific, Marlborough, USA; EMcision UK, London, United Kingdom).

MHO such as Bismuth type III and IV still needs more research results. Cholangitis, hepatic abscesses, and deaths due to severe bleeding during RFA in MHO have been reported in previous studies.[106–110] Therefore, more large-sized comparative studies are needed to determine the appropriate mode of therapy, especially in high-grade MHO. Recent RCT of intraductal RFA demonstrated that a temperature-controlled RFA with a power of 7 W and temperature of 80°C for 60 to 120 seconds was safe for advanced MHO.[110,111] The RFA catheter was advanced over the guidewire and performed for both IHDs. The electrode length of the RFA catheter is selected according to the stricture length. To ablate strictures in full-length, serial overlapped ablations can be allowed.

A meta-analysis study has analyzed a group that has undergone PDT, RFA, or stent alone. It found that the group with a stent alone for extrahepatic cholangiocarcinoma showed a lower survival rate (PDT 11.9 months, RFA 8.1 months, and stent 6.7 months) and a middle 30-day mortality (PDT 3.3%, RFA 7%, and stent 4.9%). The PDT group seemed to demonstrate better results than RFA or simple stent implantation.[112] Although these studies were not exclusively targeting high-grade MHO, they suggested that PDT and RFA might be effective as a local tumor treatment. The 2021 ASGE guideline also mentions that RFA and PDT through SEMS can be considered as a topical treatment at research institutes or tertiary-referral hospitals or higher.[17]

Therefore, concurrently administering local endoscopic treatment along with active chemotherapy is expected to contribute to improved stent patency, reduced complications, and improved survival rate than stenting alone.

SUMMARY

In surgically inoperable or unsuitable patients, endoscopic palliation can be chosen as a primary drainage method even in advanced MHO. For more effective drainage of liver volume, multisegmental drainage is more helpful than single drainage physiologically and can be conducted because technical limitations are now much ameliorated due to the development of various stents, accessories, and delivery systems. SEMS is recommended in terms of patency duration, reintervention rate, and cost-effectiveness in patients who cannot receive surgical resection. However, according to the possibility of surgery after chemotherapy or combined radiotherapy or add-on therapies such as PDT and RFA, regular exchange of plastic stents or conversion to SEMS after stent malfunction can be chosen for a better treatment strategy. Regarding bilateral or multi-sectoral deployment of SEMS, both SIS and SBS techniques have their pros and cons in technical aspects and clinical outcomes. Deployment methods should be selected according to the level of experience, technical difficulties. anatomic status, and consideration of second reintervention. Finally, as a local treatment, traditional PDT and RFA can be added to reduce the tumor burden of MHO to prolong stent patency and/or survival. However, more large-scaled studies are needed to validate their efficacy in advanced MHO. The final goal of endoscopic palliation of inoperable MHO is to increase the quality of life by the prolongation of stent patency and survival. Therefore, according to patient status, adequate endoscopic palliation with or without local therapies as well as chemoradiation therapies should be provided.

CLINICS CARE POINTS

- Endoscopic palliative drainage for patients with unresectable MHO has recently become the preferred procedure, but it is complementary rather than competitive compared with PTBD. It should be based on patient preferences, disease characteristics, and experts.

- For effective and physiologic drainage ≥ 50% of liver volume, multiple drainages using SEMS or plastic stents is recommended as primary palliation in advanced MHO. Usually, SEMS provides more prolonged stent patency and cost-effectiveness. However, the selection of plastic or metal stent is based on life expectancy, cost-effectiveness, and future therapeutic plan.

- Bilateral SIS and SBS deployment methods are technically and clinically feasible. According to technical difficulty, bile duct dilatation, and level of experience, the primary intended method can be changed to one or the other.

- Combined local ablation therapies such as PDT or RFA can be promising as a local treatment option to prolong the patency of stent or survival.

CONFLICTS OF INTEREST

The authors have nothing to disclose.

ACKNOWLEDGMENTS

This work was supported by Soonchunhyang University Research Fund.

REFERENCES

1. Shin HR, Oh JK, Masuyer E, et al. Epidemiology of cholangiocarcinoma: an update focusing on risk factors. Cancer Sci 2010;101(3):579–85.
2. Rerknimitr R, Angsuwatcharakon P, Ratanachu-ek T, et al. Asia-Pacific consensus recommendations for endoscopic and interventional management of hilar cholangiocarcinoma. J Gastroenterol Hepatol 2013;28(4):593–607.
3. Welzel TM, Graubard BI, El-Serag HB, et al. Risk factors for intrahepatic and extrahepatic cholangiocarcinoma in the United States: a population-based case-control study. Clin Gastroenterol Hepatol 2007;5(10):1221–8.
4. Blechacz B, Komuta M, Roskams T, et al. Clinical diagnosis and staging of cholangiocarcinoma. Nat Rev Gastroenterol Hepatol 2011;8(9):512–22.
5. Deoliveira ML, Schulick RD, Nimura Y, et al. New staging system and a registry for perihilar cholangiocarcinoma. Hepatol 2011;53(4):1363–71.
6. Yusoff AR, Siti ZM, Muzammil AR, et al. Cholangiocarcinoma: a 10-year experience of a single tertiary centre in the multi ethnicity-Malaysia. Med J Malaysia 2012;67(1):45–51.
7. Weinbren K, Mutum SS. Pathological aspects of cholangiocarcinoma. The Journal of pathology 1983;139(2):217–38.
8. Mansour JC, Aloia TA, Crane CH, et al. Hilar cholangiocarcinoma: expert consensus statement. HPB 2015;17(8):691–9.
9. Bismuth H, Nakache R, Diamond T. Management strategies in resection for hilar cholangiocarcinoma. Annals of surgery 1992;215(1):31–8.
10. Tibble JA, Cairns SR. Role of endoscopic endoprostheses in proximal malignant biliary obstruction. J hepato-biliary-pancreatic Surg 2001;8(2):118–23.
11. Dowsett JF, Vaira D, Hatfield AR, et al. Endoscopic biliary therapy using the combined percutaneous and endoscopic technique. Gastroenterology 1989; 96(4):1180–6.
12. Vienne A, Hobeika E, Gouya H, et al. Prediction of drainage effectiveness during endoscopic stenting of malignant hilar strictures: the role of liver volume assessment. Gastrointest Endosc 2010;72(4):728–35.

13. Cotton PB, Eisen G, Romagnuolo J, et al. Grading the complexity of endoscopic procedures: results of an ASGE working party. Gastrointest Endosc 2011;73(5): 868–74.
14. Ekkelenkamp VE, de Man RA, Ter Borg F, et al. Prospective evaluation of ERCP performance: results of a nationwide quality registry. Endosc 2015;47(6):503–7.
15. Keswani RN, Qumseya BJ, O'Dwyer LC, et al. Association Between Endoscopist and Center Endoscopic Retrograde Cholangiopancreatography Volume With Procedure Success and Adverse Outcomes: A Systematic Review and Meta-analysis. Clin Gastroenterol Hepatol 2017;15(12):1866–75.e3.
16. Dumonceau JM, Tringali A, Papanikolaou IS, et al. Endoscopic biliary stenting: indications, choice of stents, and results: European Society of Gastrointestinal Endoscopy (ESGE) Clinical Guideline - Updated October 2017. Endoscopy 2018;50(9):910–30.
17. Qumseya BJ, Jamil LH, Elmunzer BJ, et al. ASGE guideline on the role of endoscopy in the management of malignant hilar obstruction. Gastrointest Endosc 2021. https://doi.org/10.1016/j.gie.2020.12.035.
18. Wiggers JK, Groot Koerkamp B, Cieslak KP, et al. Postoperative Mortality after Liver Resection for Perihilar Cholangiocarcinoma: Development of a Risk Score and Importance of Biliary Drainage of the Future Liver Remnant. J Am Coll Surg 2016;223(2):321–31.e1.
19. Olthof PB, Wiggers JK, Groot Koerkamp B, et al. Postoperative Liver Failure Risk Score: Identifying Patients with Resectable Perihilar Cholangiocarcinoma Who Can Benefit from Portal Vein Embolization. J Am Coll Surg 2017;225(3):387–94.
20. Kennedy TJ, Yopp A, Qin Y, et al. Role of preoperative biliary drainage of liver remnant prior to extended liver resection for hilar cholangiocarcinoma. HPB 2009;11(5):445–51.
21. Farges O, Regimbeau JM, Fuks D, et al. Multicentre European study of preoperative biliary drainage for hilar cholangiocarcinoma. The British journal of surgery 2013;100(2):274–83.
22. Ferrero A, Lo Tesoriere R, Viganò L, et al. Preoperative biliary drainage increases infectious complications after hepatectomy for proximal bile duct tumor obstruction. World Journal Surgery 2009;33(2):318–25.
23. Hochwald SN, Burke EC, Jarnagin WR, et al. Association of preoperative biliary stenting with increased postoperative infectious complications in proximal cholangiocarcinoma. Archives of surgery (Chicago, Ill : 1960) 1999;134(3):261–6.
24. Scheufele F, Aichinger L, Jäger C, et al. Effect of preoperative biliary drainage on bacterial flora in bile of patients with periampullary cancer. *The British journal of surgery* 2017;104(2):e182–8.
25. Tang Z, Yang Y, Meng W, et al. Best option for preoperative biliary drainage in Klatskin tumor: A systematic review and meta-analysis. Medicine 2017;96(43): e8372.
26. Chen GF, Yu WD, Wang JR, et al. The methods of preoperative biliary drainage for resectable hilar cholangiocarcinoma patients: A protocol for systematic review and meta analysis. Medicine 2020;99(21):e20237.
27. Celotti A, Solaini L, Montori G, et al. Preoperative biliary drainage in hilar cholangiocarcinoma: Systematic review and meta-analysis. Eur J Surg Oncol : J Eur Soc Surg Oncol Br Assoc Surg Oncol 2017;43(9):1628–35.
28. Hameed A, Pang T, Chiou J, et al. Percutaneous vs. endoscopic pre-operative biliary drainage in hilar cholangiocarcinoma - a systematic review and meta-analysis. HPB : official J Int Hepato Pancreato Biliary Assoc 2016;18(5):400–10.

29. Al Mahjoub A, Menahem B, Fohlen A, et al. Preoperative Biliary Drainage in Patients with Resectable Perihilar Cholangiocarcinoma: Is Percutaneous Transhepatic Biliary Drainage Safer and More Effective than Endoscopic Biliary Drainage? A Meta-Analysis. J Vasc Interv Radiol 2017;28(4):576–82.

30. Kishi Y, Shimada K, Nara S, et al. The type of preoperative biliary drainage predicts short-term outcome after major hepatectomy. Langenbecks Arch Surg 2016;401(4):503–11.

31. Takahashi Y, Nagino M, Nishio H, et al. Percutaneous transhepatic biliary drainage catheter tract recurrence in cholangiocarcinoma. Br J Surg 2010; 97(12):1860–6.

32. Hirano S, Tanaka E, Tsuchikawa T, et al. Oncological benefit of preoperative endoscopic biliary drainage in patients with hilar cholangiocarcinoma. J hepato-biliary-pancreatic Sci 2014;21(8):533–40.

33. Aghaie Meybodi M, Shakoor D, Nanavati J, et al. Unilateral versus bilateral endoscopic stenting in patients with unresectable malignant hilar obstruction: a systematic review and meta-analysis. Endosc Int open 2020;8(3):E281–90.

34. Jang SI, Hwang JH, Lee KH, et al. Percutaneous biliary approach as a successful rescue procedure after failed endoscopic therapy for drainage in advanced hilar tumors. J Gastroenterol Hepatol 2017;32(4):932–8.

35. Paik WH, Park YS, Hwang JH, et al. Palliative treatment with self-expandable metallic stents in patients with advanced type III or IV hilar cholangiocarcinoma: a percutaneous versus endoscopic approach. Gastrointest Endosc 2009;69(1): 55–62.

36. Lee SH, Park JK, Yoon WJ, et al. Optimal biliary drainage for inoperable Klatskin's tumor based on Bismuth type. World J Gastroenterol 2007;13(29): 3948–55.

37. Moole H, Dharmapuri S, Duvvuri A, et al. Endoscopic versus Percutaneous Biliary Drainage in Palliation of Advanced Malignant Hilar Obstruction: A Meta-Analysis and Systematic Review. Can J Gastroenterol Hepatol 2016;4726078. https://doi.org/10.1155/2016/4726078.

38. Chahal P, Baron TH. Expandable metal stents for endoscopic bilateral stent-within-stent placement for malignant hilar biliary obstruction. Gastrointest Endosc 2010;71(1):195–9.

39. Hwang JC, Kim JH, Lim SG, et al. Y-shaped endoscopic bilateral metal stent placement for malignant hilar biliary obstruction: prospective long-term study. Scand J Gastroenterol 2011;46(3):326–32.

40. Ishiwatari H, Hayashi T, Ono M, et al. Newly designed plastic stent for endoscopic placement above the sphincter of Oddi in patients with malignant hilar biliary obstruction. Dig Endosc 2013;25(Suppl 2):94–9.

41. Kato H, Tsutsumi K, Harada R, et al. Endoscopic bilateral deployment of multiple metallic stents for malignant hilar biliary strictures. Dig Endosc 2013;25(Suppl 2):75–80.

42. Kawamoto H, Tsutsumi K, Fujii M, et al. Endoscopic 3-branched partial stent-in-stent deployment of metallic stents in high-grade malignant hilar biliary stricture (with videos). Gastrointest Endosc 2007;66(5):1030–7.

43. Kogure H, Isayama H, Nakai Y, et al. Newly designed large cell Niti-S stent for malignant hilar biliary obstruction: a pilot study. Surg Endosc 2011;25(2):463–7.

44. Lee JH, Kang DH, Kim JY, et al. Endoscopic bilateral metal stent placement for advanced hilar cholangiocarcinoma: a pilot study of a newly designed Y stent. Gastrointest Endosc 2007;66(2):364–9.

45. Lee TH, Moon JH, Kim JH, et al. Primary and revision efficacy of cross-wired metallic stents for endoscopic bilateral stent-in-stent placement in malignant hilar biliary strictures. Endoscopy 2013;45(2):106–13.

46. Lee TH, Park do H, Lee SS, et al. Technical feasibility and revision efficacy of the sequential deployment of endoscopic bilateral side-by-side metal stents for malignant hilar biliary strictures: a multicenter prospective study. Dig Dis Sci 2013; 58(2):547–55.

47. Naitoh I, Hayashi K, Nakazawa T, et al. Side-by-side versus stent-in-stent deployment in bilateral endoscopic metal stenting for malignant hilar biliary obstruction. Dig Dis Sci 2012;57(12):3279–85.

48. Park do H, Lee SS, Moon JH, et al. Newly designed stent for endoscopic bilateral stent-in-stent placement of metallic stents in patients with malignant hilar biliary strictures: multicenter prospective feasibility study (with videos). Gastrointest Endosc 2009;69(7):1357–60.

49. Kim JY, Kang DH, Kim HW, et al. Usefulness of slimmer and open-cell-design stents for endoscopic bilateral stenting and endoscopic revision in patients with hilar cholangiocarcinoma (with video). Gastrointest Endosc 2009;70(6): 1109–15.

50. Dumas R, Demuth N, Buckley M, et al. Endoscopic bilateral metal stent placement for malignant hilar stenoses: identification of optimal technique. Gastrointestinal endoscopy 2000;51(3):334–8.

51. Bismuth H, Castaing D, Traynor O. Resection or palliation: priority of surgery in the treatment of hilar cancer. World journal of surgery 1988;12(1):39–47.

52. Kim JH. Endoscopic stent placement in the palliation of malignant biliary obstruction. Clin Endosc 2011;44(2):76–86.

53. Lee TH. Technical tips and issues of biliary stenting, focusing on malignant hilar obstruction. Clin Endosc 2013;46(3):260–6.

54. Ishigaki K, Hamada T, Nakai Y, et al. Retrospective Comparative Study of Side-by-Side and Stent-in-Stent Metal Stent Placement for Hilar Malignant Biliary Obstruction. Dig Dis Sci 2020;65(12):3710–8.

55. Kawakami H, Itoi T, Kuwatani M, et al. Technical tips and troubleshooting of endoscopic biliary drainage for unresectable malignant hilar biliary obstruction. J hepato-biliary-pancreatic Sci 2015;22(4):E12–21.

56. Liberato MJ, Canena JM. Endoscopic stenting for hilar cholangiocarcinoma: efficacy of unilateral and bilateral placement of plastic and metal stents in a retrospective review of 480 patients. BMC Gastroenterol 2012;12:103.

57. Mukai T, Yasuda I, Nakashima M, et al. Metallic stents are more efficacious than plastic stents in unresectable malignant hilar biliary strictures: a randomized controlled trial. Journal of hepato-biliary-pancreatic sciences 2013;20(2): 214–22.

58. Aljiffry M, Abdulelah A, Walsh M, et al. Evidence-based approach to cholangiocarcinoma: a systematic review of the current literature. J Am Coll Surg 2009; 208(1):134–47.

59. Sangchan A, Kongkasame W, Pugkhem A, et al. Efficacy of metal and plastic stents in unresectable complex hilar cholangiocarcinoma: a randomized controlled trial. Gastrointest Endosc 2012;76(1):93–9.

60. Polydorou AA, Cairns SR, Dowsett JF, et al. Palliation of proximal malignant biliary obstruction by endoscopic endoprosthesis insertion. Gut 1991;32(6): 685–9.

61. Polydorou AA, Chisholm EM, Romanos AA, et al. A comparison of right versus left hepatic duct endoprosthesis insertion in malignant hilar biliary obstruction. Endosc 1989;21(6):266–71.

62. De Palma GD, Galloro G, Siciliano S, et al. Unilateral versus bilateral endoscopic hepatic duct drainage in patients with malignant hilar biliary obstruction: results of a prospective, randomized, and controlled study. Gastrointest Endosc 2001; 53(6):547–53.

63. De Palma GD, Pezzullo A, Rega M, et al. Unilateral placement of metallic stents for malignant hilar obstruction: a prospective study. Gastrointest Endosc 2003; 58(1):50–3.

64. Sherman S. Endoscopic drainage of malignant hilar obstruction: is one biliary stent enough or should we work to place two? Gastrointest Endosc 2001; 53(6):681–4.

65. Iwano H, Ryozawa S, Ishigaki N, et al. Unilateral versus bilateral drainage using self-expandable metallic stent for unresectable hilar biliary obstruction. Dig Endosc 2011;23(1):43–8.

66. Teng F, Xian YT, Lin J, et al. Comparison of Unilateral With Bilateral Metal Stenting for Malignant Hilar Biliary Obstruction. Surgical laparoscopy, endoscopy & percutaneous techniques 2019;29(1):43–8.

67. Chang G, Xia FF, Li HF, et al. Unilateral versus bilateral stent insertion for malignant hilar biliary obstruction. Abdominal Radiology (New York) 2017;42(11): 2745–51.

68. Chang WH, Kortan P, Haber GB. Outcome in patients with bifurcation tumors who undergo unilateral versus bilateral hepatic duct drainage. Gastrointest Endosc 1998;47(5):354–62.

69. Nomura T, Shirai Y, Hatakeyama K. Cholangitis after endoscopic biliary drainage for hilar lesions. Hepatogastroenterology 1997;44(17):1267–70.

70. Khan SA, Davidson BR, Goldin R, et al. Guidelines for the diagnosis and treatment of cholangiocarcinoma: consensus document. Gut 2002;51(Suppl 6): VI1–9.

71. Freeman ML, Overby C. Selective MRCP and CT-targeted drainage of malignant hilar biliary obstruction with self-expanding metallic stents. Gastrointest Endosc 2003;58(1):41–9.

72. Hintze RE, Abou-Rebyeh H, Adler A, et al. Magnetic resonance cholangiopancreatography-guided unilateral endoscopic stent placement for Klatskin tumors. Gastrointest Endosc 2001;53(1):40–6.

73. Naitoh I, Ohara H, Nakazawa T, et al. Unilateral versus bilateral endoscopic metal stenting for malignant hilar biliary obstruction. J Gastroenterol Hepatol 2009;24(4):552–7.

74. Lee TH, Kim TH, Moon JH, et al. Bilateral versus unilateral placement of metal stents for inoperable high-grade malignant hilar biliary strictures: a multicenter, prospective, randomized study (with video). Gastrointest Endosc 2017;86(5): 817–27.

75. Puli SR, Kalva N, Pamulaparthy SR, et al. Bilateral and unilateral stenting for malignant hilar obstruction: a systematic review and meta-analysis. Indian Journal Gastroenterology 2013;32(6):355–62.

76. Chennat J, Waxman I. Initial performance profile of a new 6F self-expanding metal stent for palliation of malignant hilar biliary obstruction. Gastrointest Endosc 2010;72(3):632–6.

77. Law R, Baron TH. Bilateral metal stents for hilar biliary obstruction using a 6Fr delivery system: outcomes following bilateral and side-by-side stent deployment. Dig Dis Sci 2013;58(9):2667–72.

78. Lee TH, Moon JH, Choi JH, et al. Prospective comparison of endoscopic bilateral stent-in-stent versus stent-by-stent deployment for inoperable advanced malignant hilar biliary stricture. Gastrointest Endosc 2019;90(2):222–30.

79. Kim KM, Lee KH, Chung YH, et al. A comparison of bilateral stenting methods for malignant hilar biliary obstruction. Hepatogastroenterology 2012;59(114): 341–6.

80. Shim SR, Lee TH, Yang JK, et al. Endoscopic Bilateral Stent-in-Stent Versus Stent-by-Stent Deployment in Advanced Malignant Hilar Obstruction: A Meta-Analysis and Systematic Review. Dig Dis Sci 2021. https://doi.org/10.1007/s10620-021-06885-8.

81. Cheng JL, Bruno MJ, Bergman JJ, et al. Endoscopic palliation of patients with biliary obstruction caused by nonresectable hilar cholangiocarcinoma: efficacy of self-expandable metallic Wallstents. Gastrointest Endosc 2002;56(1):33–9.

82. Pedersen FM, Lassen AT, Schaffalitzky de Muckadell OB. Randomized trial of stent placed above and across the sphincter of Oddi in malignant bile duct obstruction. Gastrointest Endosc 1998;48(6):574–9.

83. Moon JH, Rerknimitr R, Kogure H, et al. Topic controversies in the endoscopic management of malignant hilar strictures using metal stent: side-by-side versus stent-in-stent techniques. Journal of hepato-biliary-pancreatic sciences 2015; 22(9):650–6.

84. Fukasawa M, Takano S, Shindo H, et al. Endoscopic biliary stenting for unresectable malignant hilar obstruction. Clin J Gastroenterol 2017;10(6):485–90.

85. Lee TH, Moon JH, Choi HJ, et al. Third metal stent for revision of malignant hilar biliary strictures. Endoscopy 2016;48(12):1129–33.

86. Kawamoto H, Tsutsumi K, Harada R, et al. Endoscopic deployment of multiple JOSTENT SelfX is effective and safe in treatment of malignant hilar biliary strictures. Clin Gastroenterol Hepatol 2008;6(4):401–8.

87. Lee TH, Choi JH, Park do H, et al. Similar Efficacies of Endoscopic Ultrasound-guided Transmural and Percutaneous Drainage for Malignant Distal Biliary Obstruction. Clin Gastroenterol Hepatol : official Clin Pract J Am Gastroenterological Assoc 2016;14(7):1011–9.e3.

88. Paik WH, Lee TH, Park DH, et al. EUS-Guided Biliary Drainage Versus ERCP for the Primary Palliation of Malignant Biliary Obstruction: A Multicenter Randomized Clinical Trial. Am J Gastroenterol 2018;113(7):987–97.

89. Nakai Y, Kogure H, Isayama H, et al. Endoscopic Ultrasound-Guided Biliary Drainage for Unresectable Hilar Malignant Biliary Obstruction. Clin Endosc 2019;52(3):220–5.

90. Nakai Y, Isayama H, Yamamoto N, et al. Indications for endoscopic ultrasonography (EUS)-guided biliary intervention: Does EUS always come after failed endoscopic retrograde cholangiopancreatography? Dig Endosc 2017;29(2): 218–25.

91. Shah T, Desai S, Haque M, et al. Management of occluded metal stents in malignant biliary obstruction: similar outcomes with second metal stents compared to plastic stents. Dig Dis Sci 2012;57(11):2765–73.

92. Sharaiha RZ, Natov N, Glockenberg KS, et al. Comparison of metal stenting with radiofrequency ablation versus stenting alone for treating malignant biliary strictures: is there an added benefit? Dig Dis Sci 2014;59(12):3099–102.

93. Yang J, Wang J, Zhou H, et al. Efficacy and safety of endoscopic radiofrequency ablation for unresectable extrahepatic cholangiocarcinoma: a randomized trial. Endosc 2018;50(8):751–60.

94. Hong MJ, Cheon YK, Lee EJ, et al. Long-term outcome of photodynamic therapy with systemic chemotherapy compared to photodynamic therapy alone in patients with advanced hilar cholangiocarcinoma. Gut and liver 2014;8(3): 318–23.

95. Berr F, Tannapfel A, Lamesch P, et al. Neoadjuvant photodynamic therapy before curative resection of proximal bile duct carcinoma. J Hepatol 2000; 32(2):352–7.

96. Cheon YK. The role of photodynamic therapy for hilar cholangiocarcinoma. Korean J Intern Med 2010;25(4):345–52.

97. Cheon YK, Cho YD, Baek SH, et al. [Comparison of survival of advanced hilar cholangiocarcinoma after biliary drainage alone versus photodynamic therapy with external drainage]. Korean J Gastroenterol 2004;44(5):280–7.

98. Ortner ME, Caca K, Berr F, et al. Successful photodynamic therapy for nonresectable cholangiocarcinoma: a randomized prospective study. *Gastroenterol* Nov 2003;125(5):1355–63.

99. Zoepf T, Jakobs R, Arnold JC, et al. Palliation of nonresectable bile duct cancer: improved survival after photodynamic therapy. Am J Gastroenterol 2005; 100(11):2426–30.

100. Dumoulin FL, Gerhardt T, Fuchs S, et al. Phase II study of photodynamic therapy and metal stent as palliative treatment for nonresectable hilar cholangiocarcinoma. Gastrointest Endosc 2003;57(7):860–7.

101. Kahaleh M, Mishra R, Shami VM, et al. Unresectable cholangiocarcinoma: comparison of survival in biliary stenting alone versus stenting with photodynamic therapy. Clin Gastroenterol Hepatol 2008;6(3):290–7.

102. Witzigmann H, Berr F, Ringel U, et al. Surgical and palliative management and outcome in 184 patients with hilar cholangiocarcinoma: palliative photodynamic therapy plus stenting is comparable to r1/r2 resection. Ann Surg 2006;244(2): 230–9.

103. Quyn AJ, Ziyaie D, Polignano FM, et al. Photodynamic therapy is associated with an improvement in survival in patients with irresectable hilar cholangiocarcinoma. HPB 2009;11(7):570–7.

104. Cheon YK, Lee TY, Lee SM, et al. Longterm outcome of photodynamic therapy compared with biliary stenting alone in patients with advanced hilar cholangiocarcinoma. HPB 2012;14(3):185–93.

105. Gerhardt T, Rings D, Höblinger A, et al. Combination of bilateral metal stenting and trans-stent photodynamic therapy for palliative treatment of hilar cholangiocarcinoma. Z Gastroenterologie 2010;48(1):28–32.

106. Schmidt A, Bloechinger M, Weber A, et al. Short-term effects and adverse events of endoscopically applied radiofrequency ablation appear to be comparable with photodynamic therapy in hilar cholangiocarcinoma. United Eur Gastroenterol J 2016;4(4):570–9.

107. Inoue T, Ibusuki M, Kitano R, et al. Endobiliary radiofrequency ablation combined with bilateral metal stent placement for malignant hilar biliary obstruction. Endosc 2020;52(7):595–9.

108. Bokemeyer A, Matern P, Bettenworth D, et al. Endoscopic Radiofrequency Ablation Prolongs Survival of Patients with Unresectable Hilar Cholangiocellular Carcinoma - A Case-Control Study. Scientific Rep 2019;9(1):13685.

109. Tal AO, Vermehren J, Friedrich-Rust M, et al. Intraductal endoscopic radiofrequency ablation for the treatment of hilar non-resectable malignant bile duct obstruction. World J Gastrointest Endosc 2014;6(1):13–9.
110. Kim EJ, Cho JH, Kim YJ, et al. Intraductal temperature-controlled radiofrequency ablation in malignant hilar obstruction: a preliminary study in animals and initial human experience. Endosc Int open 2019;7(10):E1293–300.
111. Kang H, Han SY, Cho JH, et al. Efficacy and safety of temperature-controlled intraductal radiofrequency ablation in advanced malignant hilar biliary obstruction: A pilot multicenter randomized comparative trial. J hepato-biliary-pancreatic Sci 2021. https://doi.org/10.1002/jhbp.1082.
112. Mohan BP, Chandan S, Khan SR, et al. Photodynamic Therapy (PDT), Radiofrequency Ablation (RFA) With Biliary Stents in Palliative Treatment of Unresectable Extrahepatic Cholangiocarcinoma: A Systematic Review and Meta-analysis. J Clin Gastroenterol 2021.

Role of ERCP in Benign Biliary Strictures

Tommaso Schepis, MD[a], Ivo Boškoski, MD, PhD[a,b,*], Andrea Tringali, MD, PhD[a,b], Guido Costamagna, MD, FACG, FJGES[a,b]

KEYWORDS

- Benign biliary stricture • Endoscopy • ERCP

KEY POINTS

- Benign biliary strictures are a clinical challenge requiring a multidisciplinary evaluation.
- Endoscopy represents the first-line treatment in the management of benign biliary strictures.
- The endoscopic procedure to choose depends on etiologic factors, characteristics of the single patients, and local facilities.

INTRODUCTION

Biliary strictures can be broadly classified as benign and malignant (BBS and MBS). BBS can be associated with several causes resulting in local inflammation with secondary fibrosis and scarring. Postoperative and inflammatory strictures are the most common BBS causes. Laparoscopic cholecystectomy is the most common procedure associated with postoperative biliary stricture (POBS) with a higher incidence in laparoscopic if compared with open cholecystectomy (0.24%–0.42% vs 0.1%).[1,2] POBSs develop intraoperatively as a consequence of a partial or complete clipping of the biliary duct, a thermal injury during tissues dissection, a vascular damage with consequent ischemic injuries or postoperatively due to adhesions.[3] The presence of anatomic variants, local inflammation, and the poor surgeon's expertise are well-known risk factors for the development of POBS.[3] Liver transplantation (LT) is the second surgical procedure most commonly associated with POBS. The estimated

[a] Digestive Endoscopy Unit, Fondazione Policlinico Universitario Agostino Gemelli IRCCS, Rome, Italy; [b] Centre for Endoscopic Research Therapeutics and Training (CERTT), Università Cattolica Del Sacro Cuore di Roma, Italy
* Corresponding author. Digestive Endoscopy Unit, Fondazione Policlinico Universitario Agostino Gemelli IRCCS, Largo A. Gemelli, 8, Rome 00168, Italy.
E-mail address: ivo.boskoski@policlinicogemelli.it

Gastrointest Endoscopy Clin N Am 32 (2022) 455–475
https://doi.org/10.1016/j.giec.2022.01.006
1052-5157/22/© 2022 Elsevier Inc. All rights reserved.
giendo.theclinics.com

incidence of POBS after LT ranges from 5% to 15% in deceased donor LT and from 28% to 32% in living donor LT.[4] POBS occurring after LT can develop at the anastomosis (anastomotic biliary stricture) or elsewhere in the biliary tree (nonanastomotic biliary stricture).[5] Chronic pancreatitis is the most common inflammatory cause of BBS. Roughly 20% of patients with chronic pancreatitis develop BBS that generally occur in the distal part of the common biliary duct. Bilioenteric anastomosis, primary sclerosing cholangitis, immunoglobulin G4 (IgG4)-related cholangiopathy, infections, and traumas are other possible but rare causes of BBS (**Box 1**).

Classifications

The Bismuth classification is the most used classification for postsurgical BBS based on the location of the stricture. Type I strictures are located more than 2 cm distal to the confluence of the left and right hepatic ducts (**Fig. 1**); type II strictures are located less than 2 cm from the hepatic confluence (**Fig. 2**); type III strictures involve the hepatic confluence but do not affect its patency (**Fig. 3**); type IV strictures involve and interrupt the confluence (**Fig. 4**); type V strictures involve the aberrant right sectoral hepatic duct alone (**Fig. 5**) or with concomitant injury of the common hepatic duct (**Table 1**).[6] The Strasberg classification is another classification originally introduced for laparoscopic injuries of the biliary ducts. The Strasberg classification includes the following: type A, bile leak from cystic duct stump or minor biliary radical in gallbladder fossa; type B, occluded right posterior sectoral duct; type C, bile leak from

---

Box 1
Causes of benign biliary strictures

Postsurgical
- Cholecystectomy
- Liver transplantation
- Bilioenteric anastomosis
- Biliary reconstruction
- Post-ERCP: sphincterotomy or stent placement

Inflammatory
- Chronic pancreatitis
- Primary sclerosing cholangitis
- Immunoglobulin G4–related cholangiopathy
- Acquired immune deficiency syndrome cholangiopathy
- Vasculitis
- Choledocholithiasis
- Mirizzi syndrome
- Sarcoidosis

Infective
- Recurrent cholangitis
- Ascaris lumbricoides
- Clonorchis sinensis
- Opisthorchis viverrini
- Tuberculosis
- Histoplasmosis
- Human immunodeficiency virus cholangiopathy

Miscellaneous
- Ischemia
- Trauma
- Portal biliopathy
- Radiation injury

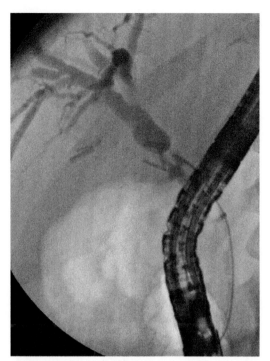

Fig. 1. Anastomotic biliary stricture after liver transplantation located greater than 2 cm distal to the main hepatic confluence (Bismuth I).

transected right posterior sectoral ducts; type D, bile leak from main bile duct without major tissue loss; and finally, the type E of the Strasberg classification is an analogue of the Bismuth classification (see **Table 1**).[7]

Clinical Presentation and Diagnosis

BBS clinical presentation varies, depending on the severity of the biliary obstruction, from subclinical mild elevation of liver function tests to a severe cholestatic syndrome. Jaundice, pruritus, dark urine, pale stools, and cholangitis are frequent signs and symptoms of BBS.[8] The clinical presentation also depends on the underlying cause. In patients presenting with a cholestatic syndrome the upper transabdominal ultrasound (US) is generally the first diagnostic imaging performed. US has a high sensitivity for detection of the biliary obstruction (95%) but it has a low accuracy in the determination of the extent of the stricture.[9] Moreover, US presents a low specificity in the differential diagnosis between BBS and MBS (30%–70%).[9] Computed tomography (CT) is commonly used as a second-level imaging examination in the assessment of suspect biliary obstruction. CT presents a higher sensitivity in the detection of biliary obstruction when compared with US.[10] The sensitivity of CT in the detection of biliary obstruction is greater than 90%, whereas the accuracy in determining the extent of the stricture is 75%.[11] CT can also be used to differentiate between BBS and MBS. Sundeep and colleagues in a prospective study reported that the sensitivity, specificity, positive predictive value, negative predictive value, and diagnostic accuracy of CT for predicting the nature of the stricture were 79.2%, 79.4%, 73.1%, 84.4%, and 79.3%, respectively (**Table 2**).[12] The presence of a mass, lymph node enlargement, hyperenhancement, long stricture, and higher proximal dilatation are

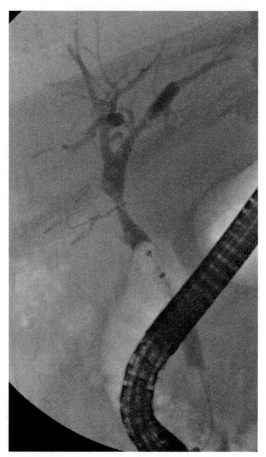

Fig. 2. Benign biliary stricture close (<2 cm) to the biliary confluence (Bismuth II).

some of the CT findings that predict the malignant nature of the stricture.[13,14] Magnetic resonance cholangiopancreatography (MRCP) is the most accurate imaging technique that provides a noninvasive detailed evaluation of biliary stricture and plays an important role in planning the subsequent endoscopic therapy. MRCP is increasingly used in the evaluation of biliary obstruction because of the lack of ionizing radiation, the ability to offer high-quality cholangiograms, and the ability to determine the location and extent of biliary strictures.[11] The reported sensitivity, specificity, positive predictive value, negative predictive value, and diagnostic accuracy of MRCP for predicting the nature of the stricture are 87.5%, 85.3%, 80.8%, 90.6%, and 82.7%, respectively (see **Table 2**).[12] The differential diagnosis between BBS and MBS can also be improved with the use of diffusion-weighted imaging.[15] Endoscopic US (EUS) is increasingly used for the evaluation of biliary obstruction. Despite standard imaging techniques, EUS not only provides a morphologic evaluation but also allows the performance of EUS-guided fine-needle aspiration (EUS-FNA) for a cytologic or histologic diagnosis to exclude the malignant nature of the biliary stricture. Jeffrey and colleagues reported that EUS-FNA of unexplained bile duct strictures presents high specificity and positive predictive value (close to 100%) but low sensitivity and negative predictive value (47% and 50%, respectively) (see **Table 2**).[16] In case the

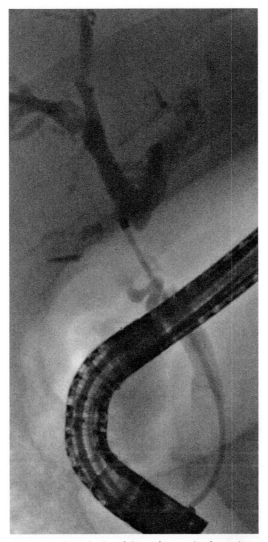

Fig. 3. Postcholecystectomy stenosis involving the main hepatic confluence but not affecting its patency (Bismuth III).

cause of the stricture is unclear, cholangioscopy can be performed to directly visualize the stricture and characterize it histologically (**Fig. 6**). Intraductal ultrasonography (IDUS) and confocal laser endomicroscopy (CLE) are recent options that can aid in differentiating between BBS and MBS. IDUS involves the insertion of a high-frequency US probe into the bile duct that provides high-resolution images of the ductal wall and periductal tissues.[17] The reported sensitivity, specificity, and accuracy of IDUS in differentiating malignant from benign strictures are 97.6%, 98%, and 92%, respectively.[18] CLE involves the intravenous injection of a contrast agent (generally fluorescein) and the subsequent insertion of a catheter probe through the working channel of the endoscope or through the FNA. CLE provides a real-time microscopic evaluation of the tissues contacted by the probe.[19] The reported sensitivity and

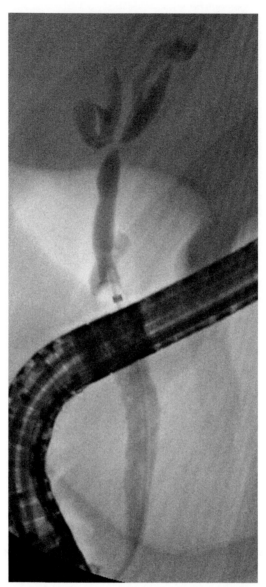

Fig. 4. Postsurgical stricture interrupting the hepatic confluence (Bismuth IV).

specificity of CLE in the detection of MBS are respectively 73% to 83% and 33% to 50%.[20] Nevertheless, IDUS and CLE are not systematically included in the diagnostic workup of BBS being technically demanding, expensive, and not widely available. Moreover, the interobserver agreement is extremely poor, especially for CLE.

The diagnostic algorithm for biliary strictures management is summarized in **Fig. 7**.

ENDOSCOPIC MANAGEMENT

Surgery, interventional radiology, and endoscopy are the techniques available for the management of BBS and to achieve biliary decompression. Endoscopic retrograde

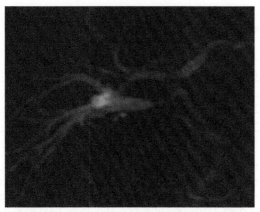

Fig. 5. MRCP showing transection of an aberrant right sectorial hepatic duct.

cholangiopancreatography (ERCP), since its introduction, has widely evolved representing nowadays the first-choice treatment in the management of several kinds of biliopancreatic diseases including BBS. The endoscopic techniques available for the treatment of BBS include balloon dilatation, plastic stent (PS) placement, fully covered metal stent placement, and magnetic compression anastomosis (MCA).

Endoscopic Balloon Dilatation

Endoscopic balloon dilatation implies bile duct cannulation, the insertion of a guide-wire across the stricture, and the advancement of the dilating balloon.[5] The balloon

---

Table 1
Benign biliary stricture classifications

Bismuth Classification	Strasberg Classification
Type I • Strictures located >2 cm distal to the confluence of the left and right hepatic ducts.	Type A • Bile leak from cystic duct stump or minor biliary radical in gallbladder fossa.
Type II • Strictures located <2 cm from the hepatic confluence.	Type B • Occluded right posterior sectoral duct.
Type III • Strictures involving the hepatic confluence but not affecting its patency.	Type C • Bile leak from divided right posterior sectoral ducts.
Type IV • Strictures involving and interrupting the hepatic confluence.	Type D • Bile leak from main bile duct without major tissue loss.
Type V • Strictures involving the aberrant right sectoral hepatic duct alone or with concomitant injury of the common hepatic duct.	Type E • E1: injury >2 cm from the hepatic confluence. • E2: injury <2 cm from the hepatic confluence. • E3: hilar stricture with the hepatic confluence preserved. • E4: hilar stricture with involvement of the hepatic confluence. • E5: combined common hepatic duct and aberrant right hepatic duct injury.

Table 2
Diagnostic tools for benign biliary strictures

	Sensitivity (%)	Specificity (%)	Positive Predictive Value (%)	Negative Predictive Value (%)
CT	79.2	79.4	73.1	84.4
MRCP	87.5	85.3	80.8	90.6
EUS-FNA	47	100	100	50

in then fully inflated under fluoroscopic guidance and is maintained across the stricture for 30 to 60 seconds[21] after disappearance of the waist. The dilating balloon size generally ranges between 4 and 8 mm, and it is chosen depending on the diameter of the upstream bile duct. Particular attention should be paid to in the early postoperative period (<30 days) after biliary anastomosis for higher risk of anastomotic dehiscence and biliary leaks.[22,23] The BBS dilatation can be followed by the placement of a biliary stent to avoid stricture recurrence. In fact, the main limitation of balloon dilatation alone is the occurrence of restenosis in up to 47% of cases.[24,25]

Plastic Stent Placement

PSs are the most used device for the endoscopic management of BBS. Several types of PS are available differing in their length, angulation, construction material, coating, and antimigration mechanism. The removability of PS is an essential characteristic for devices used for a benign disease, allowing the performance of a temporary treatment. Moreover, the caliber and the length of PS can be easily adapted to the biliary tree shape of the specific patient to obtain a tailored treatment. To achieve an adequate and progressive dilatation of the biliary stricture, a multistenting technique can be used with the insertion of an increasing number of PSs placed side by side.[26] Stent exchange is generally performed every 3 to 4 months for a total of 12 to 18 months (**Fig. 8**).[27] The major downside with PS is the need to undergo multiple ERCPs for stent exchange; however, the multistenting technique may reduce the need for frequent exchanges, as biliary drainage continues even after stent occlusion through the spaces between the stents.[28] Stent migration and stent occlusion are

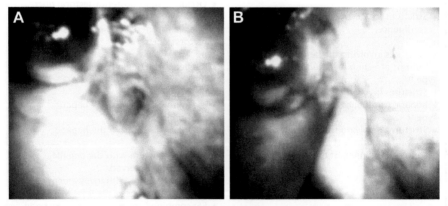

Fig. 6. Cholangioscopy shows a tight anastomotic biliary stricture after liver transplantation (*A*); a guidewire is placed through the stricture under direct cholangioscopy view (*B*).

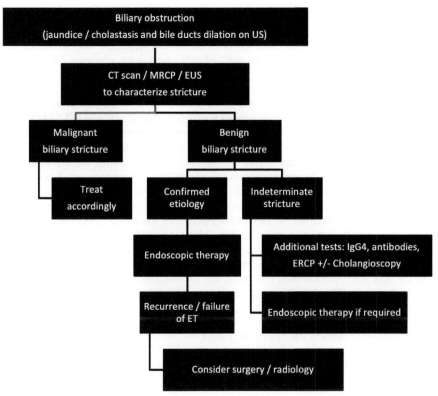

Fig. 7. Approach to benign biliary strictures.

other complications associated with PSs.[29,30] PS migration occurs in 5% to 10% of cases, with distal migration more common than proximal migration.[29] Stent migration occurs more commonly with a single stent.[31] Stent occlusion occurs in up to 30% of cases, and it is related to bacterial biofilm formation, biliary sludge, biliary reflux of dietary fibers, and clot formation.[30]

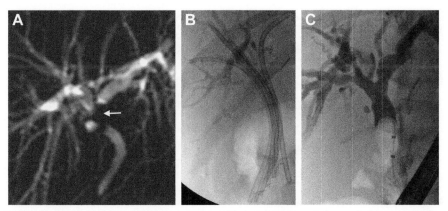

Fig. 8. Postcholecystectomy biliary stricture with interruption of the main hepatic confluence (*A*); after insertion of a maximum of 7 plastic stents (*B*) the stricture is resolved (*C*).

Fully Covered Self-Expandable Metal Stent Placement

Self-expandable metal stents (SEMSs) are an available alternative to PS in the management of biliary strictures. Three kinds of SEMS are available: uncovered-SEMS (U-SEMS), partially covered SEMS (PC-SEMS), and fully covered SEMS (FC-SEMS).[32] In U-SEMS the metallic mesh is in direct contact with the stricture tissues. The ingrowth of reactive tissue through the metallic mesh leads to the risk for stent occlusion and the irretrievability of the stent.[33] U-SEMSs are indeed indicated for palliative purpose in MBS and are not indicated for BBS.[34] PC-SEMS and FC-SEMS have been designed to allow the stent retrieval in order to perform a temporary treatment. PC-SEMS presents a plastic polymer only in the central portion of stent with uncovered proximal and distal ends.[35] This design reduces the risk for stent migration if compared with FC-SEMS and increases the capability of stent removal if compared with U-SEMS.[36] The use of PC-SEMS in BBS has been reported; however, the bare ends of these stents still present the risk for tissue ingrowth, and their retrieval is not always easily performed.[37,38] FC-SEMS presents the plastic polymer all around the metallic mesh, reducing the risk for tissue ingrowth and allowing an easier removal.[39] FC-SEMS are the first choice among SEMSs in the management of BBS. The advantages of FC-SEMS if compared with PS are the greater diameter, the need for less stent exchanges, the lower risk for stent occlusion, and consequently the longer patency (**Fig. 9**).[40] The main limitation of FC-SEMS is the high risk for migration ranging between 20% and 40% of cases.[41–43] Therefore, FC-SEMSs with antimigratory mechanisms including flared ends, anchoring fins, and anchoring flaps have been designed to reduce the risk of migration.[44]

Magnetic Compression Anastomosis

In case of severe biliary stricture impeding the passage of a guidewire through the complete biliary obstruction, the MCA has been reported as a minimal invasive alternative to surgery or percutaneous treatments.[45,46] MCA is a hybrid technique involving both interventional radiology and endoscopy. Two different magnets are placed in the proximal and distal side of the stricture.[47] One magnet is generally delivered percutaneously through a transhepatic biliary drainage (PTBD), and the second magnet is then delivered endoscopically during an ERCP session (**Fig. 10**).[48] Once delivered, the 2 magnets attract to each other until a complete approximation is achieved. The

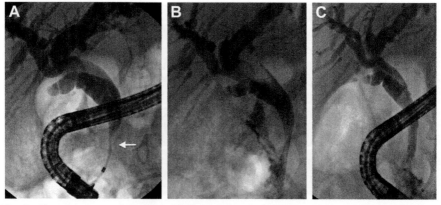

Fig. 9. Chronic pancreatitis–related biliary stricture (*A*), treated by insertion of a fully covered metal stent (*B*); stricture resolution after metal stent removal (*C*).

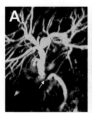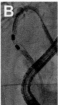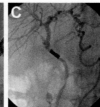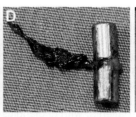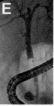

Fig. 10. Magnetic resonance cholangiography shows a complete stenosis of the anastomotic biliary stricture after liver transplantation (*A*); combined percutaneous and endoscopic insertion of 2 cylindrical magnets (*B*); magnets migration (*C*) and stricture resolution after insertion of 4 plastic stents (*D*); magnets with necrotic tissue in the middle (*E*).

magnets approximation determines the occurrence of ischemic necrosis of the compressed tissue, progressively leading to the formation of a fistula.[49] The magnets are then removed, and an endoscopic stent can be placed through the newly created fistula to increase the caliber of the stricture and consolidate the results.[47] The feasibility and safety of MCA have been reported in several experimental and clinical studies in patients with benign biliobiliary and bilioenteric strictures. The most common adverse event associated with MCA is cholangitis.[50] The reported success rate of MCA in the treatment of biliary strictures is 87.5%, and the reported recurrence rate is of 7.1%.[51]

ENDOSCOPIC APPROACH IN THE SPECIFIC CAUSES
Postcholecystectomy Biliary Strictures

Cholecystectomy is still today the first cause of BBS. The incidence of BBS after laparoscopic cholecystectomy is higher if compared with open cholecystectomy (0.23%–0.42% vs 0.1%).[21] The endoscopic approach is the standard of care in case of postcholecystectomy biliary stricture, and the multistenting treatment with periodic exchange of the PSs is generally considered the first choice.[26,27,52] The success rate of the multiple PS placement with a progressive increase in the number of PS and periodic exchanges (generally every 3 months for a period of 6–18 months) is reported to range between 80% and 100%.[5] The success rate differs depending on the location of the biliary stricture: BBS occurring in the distal part of the biliary duct presents the best outcomes with a success rate greater than 80%, whereas BBS occurring nearby the hepatic ductal confluence present a lower success rate (25%).[27] A long-term evaluation of 154 patients with POBS treated with the multistenting therapy was recently reported: a mean number of 4.3 stents were placed, and a mean of 4.2 ERCP per patient were performed.[53] They reported a success rate of 96.7% and a recurrence rate of 9.4% with a mean follow-up of 11 years. One of the most important risk factors for postcholecystectomy biliary injuries is the presence of anatomic variants of the biliary tree.[54] Overall, 12.3% to 24.1% of patients have an "aberrant duct" (the right posterior or the right anterior sectorial duct that join the common bile duct close to the cystic duct) that can lead to a wrong interpretation of the biliary tree anatomy during surgery, increasing the risk of biliary injuries.[55] The endoscopic multistenting therapy has been reported as an effective treatment of this subgroup of patients with a reported success rate depending on the specific type of aberrant duct injury: the duct patency in patients with Strasberg type C injury, Strasberg type E5, isolated aberrant duct stenosis, and Strasberg type B is achieved in 91%, 100%, 100%, and 16.6%, respectively.[56] The main downside to the multistenting approach is the need for multiple ERCP with PS exchanges. To overcome this limitation, the use of FC-SEMS has been reported. A prospective multinational study evaluated the efficacy of FC-SEMS in patients with BBS: the investigators performed a subgroup analysis of patients with postcholecystectomy BBS with a 5-year follow-up.[57] They reported a success rate of 72% with complete resolution of the biliary stricture. The endoscopic removal of the FC-SEMS was performed in 83.3% of cases, and in 3 patients the FC-SEMS spontaneously migrated without complications. The long-term follow-up (5 years) documented that 61% of patients remained stent-free. Procedure-related adverse events occurred in 38.9% of patients, with cholangitis representing the most common complication.

MPS (multiple plastic stent) still represents the first-line therapy for postcholecystectomy biliary strictures, especially if close to the main hepatic confluence.[31]

Postliver Transplant Biliary Strictures

LT is the second most common surgical procedure after cholecystectomy associated with BBS. Post-LT BBS can occur in the early postoperative course (<30 days) or later (>90 days) and can be classified as anastomotic strictures (ABS) (BBS occurring at the biliobiliary anastomosis) and nonanastomotic biliary strictures (NABS) (BBS occurring elsewhere in the biliary tree).[58] The use of T-tubes, Roux-en-Y anastomosis, ischemic injuries, acute hepatic artery thrombosis, infections, ABO mismatch, non–heart beating donors, and primary sclerosis cholangitis are considered risk factors for the development of post-LT BBS.[59–61] Endoscopy represents the first-line approach in patients with post-LT BBS, and percutaneous treatment, surgery and retransplantation are considered only in case of endoscopic therapy failure.[62]

ABSs present generally as short single strictures at the anastomosis site and result from the surgical technique, local tissue ischemia, or a fibrotic healing.[63] The overall success rate of endoscopy in the management of ABS is reported to be of 75%.[64] However, the endoscopic success rate varies depending on the time of presentation. ABS with early presentation (<30 days) is associated with better outcomes and a good response to endoscopic balloon dilatation followed by PS placement for a brief period of time (3–6 months).[65] ABS with later presentation (>90 days) generally need a longer time of stenting with more exchanges to avoid stricture recurrence.[5,66] The combination of endoscopic balloon dilatation and multiple PS placement has a success rate of 81% to 88%, significantly higher if compared with the balloon dilatation alone (success rate 37.5%).[23,67] The use of FC-SEMS for ABS has been described to reduce the need for stent exchanges and showed a high success rate (rage 92%–100%) but also a high rate of stent migration (>20%).[68,69] Min and colleagues performed a study with 75 patients with ABS and compared the efficacy of FC-SEMS, PS, and PTBD with a mean follow-up of 39 months.[70] The success rate, recurrence rate, and safety were comparable in the 3 groups of patients; however, FC-SEMSs were associated with fewer ERCP procedures and shorter time of treatment. The use of PC-SEMS has also been evaluated but its use is still today debated. Chaput and colleagues reported the use of PC-SEMS in 22 patients with ABSs and documented a sustained stricture resolution in 52.6% of patients with a high rate of stent migration or dislocation and technical difficulties in stent removal.[38] In cases of severe biliary stricture impeding the passage of a guidewire, MCA has been reported to be an innovative and effective procedure to treat post-LT BBS. Sung and colleagues reported the use of MCA in 39 patients, of which 29 were post-LT BBS.[47] A successful recanalization was obtained in 89% of patients with a median time from magnet approximation to recanalization of 52 days. One case of cholangitis was reported as the only adverse event. MPS is considered the most effective treatment of ABSs after LT.[31]

NABSs account for 10% to 25% of post-LT BBS and present generally as multiple and longer biliary strictures located at the hepatic confluence or at the intrahepatic biliary tree.[71] Graft ischemic injury, post-LT hepatic artery thrombosis, and donor-recipient ABO incompatibility are the main causes of NABS.[72] The endoscopic management of NABS is more challenging if compared with ABS. The reported long-term success rate of the endoscopic treatment ranges between 50% and 70%.[73] The success rate broadly depends on the strictures severity, number, and location. The extrahepatic single stricture presents better outcomes when compared with multiple intrahepatic BBS.[58] When the endoscopic approach fails, the patient may need a surgical or percutaneous approach. However, in patients resistant to conservative treatment, retransplantation may represent the only available treatment.[74]

Chronic Pancreatitis

BBS occurs in 3% to 23% of patients with chronic pancreatitis.[75] BBS occurs in the distal part of the common bile duct and is determined by the close anatomic relationship with the head of the pancreas. The occurrence of fibrosis secondary to repeated episodes of inflammation and scarring is the major etiologic factor determining the involvement of the biliary duct in chronic pancreatitis.[76] In patients with chronic pancreatitis presenting with a cholestatic syndrome, cross-sectional imaging to rule out the presence of malignancy is considered mandatory. Once the diagnosis of BBS has been established, biliary decompression is indicated in symptomatic patients and in case of persistent (>4 weeks) elevation of serum alkaline phosphatase and/or bilirubin.[77] The endoscopic approach is generally considered the first option in patients with BBS and chronic pancreatitis, reserving the surgical intervention for unresponsive patients and in the suspicion of malignancy.[77,78] Both the endoscopic placement of multiple PSs and the placement of a single FC-SEMS have been described in the management of chronic pancreatitis–related BBS.[32,79] Haapamäki and colleagues in a prospective, multicenter, randomized study compared the use of FC-SEMS and MPS in the management of 60 patients with BBS caused by chronic pancreatitis.[80] At 2-year follow-up, the success rate was 90% in the plastic stent group and 92% in the FC-SEMS group. No differences in terms of safety were reported. Similar results were described in a recent multicentric randomized controlled trial enrolling 164 patients (84 MPSs and 80 FC-SEMSs); the investigators reported a 19% FC-SEMS migration rate.[81]To overcome the risk for stent migration, the use of PC-SEMS has been described also in the context of chronic pancreatitis with a reported success rate of 90%; however, their use in clinical practice is still today debated for the potential difficulties in stent removal.[82]

FC-SEMSs are the first-line treatment of CP-related biliary strictures obtaining similar results compared with MPS with less procedures, being therefore cost-effective.[31]

Primary Sclerosing Cholangitis

Primary sclerosing cholangitis (PSC) is a rare, chronic cholestatic liver disease characterized by intrahepatic and/or extrahepatic strictures determined by chronic inflammation and consequent fibrosis of the biliary tree.[83] During the disease course, 50% of patients with PSC will develop a dominant stricture, defined as a narrowing of the common bile duct with a diameter less than or equal to 1.5 mm or in the right and left hepatic ducts with a diameter less than or equal to 1 mm.[84] Once dominant stricture is detected, it is mandatory to rule out the presence of malignancy, given the high risk for cholangiocarcinoma in patients with PSC (10%–15% over the lifetime).[85] The endoscopic treatment is indicated in cases of symptomatic dominant stricture (eg, jaundice, cholangitis, pruritus). Endoscopic balloon dilatation, often performed in multiple sessions, is considered the first-line treatment.[86] Kaya and colleagues in a retrospective study compared the efficacy and safety of balloon dilatation and PS placement.[87] They reported a similar success rate in terms of bilirubin decrease, but the stent group was associated with higher median number of procedures per patient, higher need for percutaneous intervention, and higher rate of complications (54% vs 15%). Balloon dilations are repeated at intervals of 1 to 4 weeks (average of 2–3 sessions) until a technical success is obtained. The balloon diameter is generally chosen depending on the bile duct diameter proximal and distal to the dominant stricture.[88] If balloon dilatation fails, a short-term stenting with PS is an available option. PS should be removed 1 to 2 weeks after the insertion considering that in patients with PSC stent occlusion seems to occur earlier.[86] No advantages in terms of efficacy were detected comparing short-term (1–2 week) and standard (8–12 weeks) stenting.[89,90] In any cases of biliary intervention, antibiotic prophylaxis is recommended to reduce the risk of cholangitis, bacteremia, and septicemia.[86,91]

Endoscopic resolution of PSC-related biliary strictures is rarely possible; repeated treatments during the course of the disease are usually needed due to stricture relapse or the onset of new stenosis secondary to the chronic nature of PSC.

Immunoglobulin G4–related Sclerosing Cholangitis

IgG4-related sclerosing cholangitis (IgG4-SC) is considered the biliary manifestation of the systemic IgG4-related disease, characterized by elevation of serum IgG4 levels and presence of IgG4-positive plasma cells, lymphocytes, fibrosis, and obliterative phlebitis in the bile duct wall.[92] IgG4-SC is commonly associated with autoimmune pancreatitis, and up to 20% of patients with autoimmune pancreatitis present also with IgG4-SC.[93] BBS is a clinical manifestation of IgG4-SC; the stricture can occur at any point of the biliary tree and can be associated with an inflammation of the biliary duct wall or an extraductal compression from an inflammatory or malignant mass in the head of the pancreas (association with autoimmune pancreatitis or pancreatic cancer). The endoscopic management with nasobiliary drainage or PS placement has been described in patients with symptomatic biliary stricture and IgG4-SC.[94] However, IgG4-SC presents a rapid response to steroid therapy that should be considered the first-line treatment of biliary obstruction.[95] Endoscopic biliary decompression can be considered the target therapy in cases of cholangitis, contraindication to steroid therapy, and uncertain diagnosis requiring brush cytology or biliary biopsy.[92]

SUMMARY

BBS represent a clinical challenge from the diagnosis to the definitive treatment. The exclusion of malignancy and the diagnosis of the underlying cause are the first crucial steps determining the choice of the best treatment of the single patient.[96] Endoscopy provides an efficient and minimally invasive therapy for the management of a wide range of BBS. Endoscopic balloon dilatation was the first treatment available and is considered still a valid endoscopic approach to biliary strictures. The introduction of endoscopic stents broadly increased the therapeutic efficacy of endoscopy. The multistenting approach is nowadays the most commonly used technique that involves the need for multiple ERCP sessions with PS exchanges every 3 to 6 months.[97] Although highly effective, the multistenting technique is a demanding approach needing for the patient compliance and organization of the endoscopy facilities in order to ensure the PS exchange up to the stricture resolution.[98] To overcome this limitation, SEMSs have been introduced in the daily clinical practice.[99] The advantages of SEMS are the larger diameter allowing a longer patency and the need for less frequent stent exchanges.[100] U-SEMSs do not have any role in the management of BBS and are reserved for MBS with palliative purpose. FC-SEMS and PC-SEMS have both been used in several types of BBS; however, PC-SEMSs are not still widely used in clinical practice for the evidence of common difficulties in stent removal. In case of severe biliary strictures not allowing the passage of a guidewire, a new technique called MCA has been described. Few reports have been published so far describing the role of MCA mainly in the management of post-LT ABS; however, the data available are promising and describe MCA as a safe and effective approach.[101] The efficacy of the endoscopic treatment strongly depends on the underling cause. Postcholecystectomy strictures and ABSs generally present a good response to the endoscopic management including both the multistenting technique and the placement of a single FC-SEMS. Conversely, NABSs and chronic pancreatitis-related strictures are more challenging with a lower success rate of the endoscopic approach. A multidisciplinary evaluation of the single clinical case with the involvement of the endoscopist, the interventional radiologist, and the surgeon is always recommended in order to choose the best treatment in the specific patient.

CLINICS CARE POINTS

- The definition of the cause of benign biliary strictures is determinant in the choice of the clinical treatment.
- Interventional radiology, surgery, and endoscopy are the available options for the management of benign biliary strictures.
- Endoscopy is considered the first-line treatment in the management of benign biliary stricture.
- Endoscopic balloon dilatation, plastic stent placement, fully covered metal stent placement, and MCA are the endoscopic techniques available.

DISCLOSURE

I. Boskoski is consultant for Apollo Endosurgery, Cook Medical, Boston Scientific, Nitinotes, and Endo Tools. Guido Costamagna is consultant for Olympus, Cook Medical, and Boston Scientific. Andrea Tringali and Tommaso Schepis have nothing to disclose.

REFERENCES

1. Adamsen S, Hansen OH, Funch-Jensen P, et al. Bile duct injury during laparoscopic cholecystectomy: a prospective nationwide series. J Am Coll Surg 1997; 184(6):571–8.
2. Barrett M, Asbun HJ, Chien HL, et al. Bile duct injury and morbidity following cholecystectomy: a need for improvement. Surg Endosc 2018;32(4):1683–8.
3. Cantù P, Mauro A, Cassinotti E, et al. Post-operative biliary strictures. Dig Liver Dis 2020;52(12):1421–7.
4. Sharma S, Gurakar A, Jabbour N. Biliary strictures following liver transplantation: past, present and preventive strategies. Liver Transpl 2008;14(6):759–69.
5. Visrodia KH, Tabibian JH, Baron TH. Endoscopic management of benign biliary strictures. World J Gastrointest Endosc 2015;7(11):1003–13.
6. Bismuth H. Postoperative strictures of the biliary tract. Edinburgh (UK): Churchill Livingstone; 1982.
7. Strasberg SM, Hertl M, Soper NJ. An analysis of the problem of biliary injury during laparoscopic cholecystectomy. J Am Coll Surg 1995;180(1):101–25.

8. Rustagi T, Jamidar PA. Endoscopic management of benign biliary strictures. Curr Gastroenterol Rep 2015;17(1):422.

9. Kapoor BS, Mauri G, Lorenz JM. Management of Biliary Strictures: State-of-the-Art Review. Radiology 2018;289(3):590–603.

10. Nesbit GM, Johnson CD, James EM, et al. Cholangiocarcinoma: diagnosis and evaluation of resectability by CT and sonography as procedures complementary to cholangiography. AJR Am J Roentgenol 1988;151(5):933–8.

11. Singh A, Gelrud A, Agarwal B. Biliary strictures: diagnostic considerations and approach. Gastroenterol Rep (Oxf) 2015;3(1):22–31.

12. Saluja SS, Sharma R, Pal S, et al. Differentiation between benign and malignant hilar obstructions using laboratory and radiological investigations: a prospective study. HPB (Oxford) 2007;9(5):373–82.

13. Han JK, Choi BI, Kim TK, et al. Hilar cholangiocarcinoma: thin-section spiral CT findings with cholangiographic correlation. Radiographics 1997;17(6):1475–85.

14. Choi SH, Han JK, Lee JM, et al. Differentiating malignant from benign common bile duct stricture with multiphasic helical CT. Radiology 2005;236(1):178–83.

15. Cui XY, Chen HW. Role of diffusion-weighted magnetic resonance imaging in the diagnosis of extrahepatic cholangiocarcinoma. World J Gastroenterol 2010; 16(25):3196–201.

16. Lee JH, Salem R, Aslanian H, et al. Endoscopic ultrasound and fine-needle aspiration of unexplained bile duct strictures. Am J Gastroenterol 2004;99(6): 1069–73.

17. Levy MJ, Vazquez-Sequeiros E, Wiersema MJ. Evaluation of the pancreaticobiliary ductal systems by intraductal US. Gastrointest Endosc 2002;55(3):397–408.

18. Meister T, Heinzow HS, Woestmeyer C, et al. Intraductal ultrasound substantiates diagnostics of bile duct strictures of uncertain etiology. World J Gastroenterol 2013;19(6):874–81.

19. Caillol F, Filoche B, Gaidhane M, et al. Refined probe-based confocal laser endomicroscopy classification for biliary strictures: the Paris Classification. Dig Dis Sci 2013;58(6):1784–9.

20. Chennat J, Konda VJ, Madrigal-Hoyos E, et al. Biliary confocal laser endomicroscopy real-time detection of cholangiocarcinoma. Dig Dis Sci 2011;56(12): 3701–6.

21. Tringali A. Endoscopic Management of Benign Biliary Strictures. J Gastroenterol Hepatol Res 2015. https://doi.org/10.17554/j.issn.2224-3992.2015.04.494.

22. Thuluvath PJ, Pfau PR, Kimmey MB, et al. Biliary complications after liver transplantation: the role of endoscopy. Endoscopy 2005;37(9):857–63.

23. Zoepf T, Maldonado-Lopez EJ, Hilgard P, et al. Balloon dilatation vs. balloon dilatation plus bile duct endoprostheses for treatment of anastomotic biliary strictures after liver transplantation. Liver Transpl 2006;12(1):88–94.

24. Foutch PG, Sivak MV Jr. Therapeutic endoscopic balloon dilatation of the extrahepatic biliary ducts. Am J Gastroenterol 1985;80(7):575–80.

25. Smith MT, Sherman S, Lehman GA. Endoscopic management of benign strictures of the biliary tree. Endoscopy 1995;27(3):253–66.

26. Costamagna G, Pandolfi M, Mutignani M, et al. Long-term results of endoscopic management of postoperative bile duct strictures with increasing numbers of stents. Gastrointest Endosc 2001;54(2):162–8.

27. Draganov P, Hoffman B, Marsh W, et al. Long-term outcome in patients with benign biliary strictures treated endoscopically with multiple stents. Gastrointest Endosc 2002;55(6):680–6.

28. Lawrence C, Romagnuolo J, Payne KM, et al. Low symptomatic premature stent occlusion of multiple plastic stents for benign biliary strictures: comparing standard and prolonged stent change intervals. Gastrointest Endosc 2010;72(3): 558–63.

29. Pfau PR, Pleskow DK, Banerjee S, et al, ASGE Technology Assessment Committee. Pancreatic and biliary stents. Gastrointest Endosc 2013;77(3):319–27 [Erratum apperars in Gastrointest Endosc 2013;78(1):193-5].

30. Kwon CI, Lehman GA. Mechanisms of biliary plastic stent occlusion and efforts at prevention. Clin Endosc 2016;49(2):139–46.

31. Arhan M, Odemiş B, Parlak E, et al. Migration of biliary plastic stents: experience of a tertiary center. Surg Endosc 2009;23(4):769–75.

32. Dumonceau JM, Tringali A, Papanikolaou IS, et al. Endoscopic biliary stenting: indications, choice of stents, and results: European Society of Gastrointestinal Endoscopy (ESGE) Clinical Guideline - Updated October 2017. Endoscopy 2018;50(9):910–30.

33. Isayama H, Nakai Y, Kogure H, et al. Biliary self-expandable metallic stent for unresectable malignant distal biliary obstruction: which is better: covered or uncovered? Dig Endosc 2013;25(Suppl 2):71–4.

34. Almadi MA, Barkun A, Martel M. Plastic vs. Self-Expandable Metal Stents for Palliation in Malignant Biliary Obstruction: A Series of Meta-Analyses. Am J Gastroenterol 2017;112(2):260–73.

35. Gómez-Oliva C, Guarner-Argente C, Concepción M, et al. Partially covered self-expanding metal stent for unresectable malignant extrahepatic biliary obstruction: results of a large prospective series. Surg Endosc 2012;26(1):222–9.

36. Jain D, Stein A, Hasan MK. Stepwise Algorithmic Approach to Endoscopic Removal of Biliary Partially Covered and Uncovered Self-Expanding Metal Stents. Clin Endosc 2021;54(4):608–12.

37. Cantù P, Hookey LC, Morales A, et al. The treatment of patients with symptomatic common bile duct stenosis secondary to chronic pancreatitis using partially covered metal stents: a pilot study. Endoscopy 2005;37(8):735–9.

38. Chaput U, Scatton O, Bichard P, et al. Temporary placement of partially covered self-expandable metal stents for anastomotic biliary strictures after liver transplantation: a prospective, multicenter study. Gastrointest Endosc 2010;72(6): 1167–74.

39. Sawas T, Al Halabi S, Parsi MA, et al. Self-expandable metal stents versus plastic stents for malignant biliary obstruction: a meta-analysis. Gastrointest Endosc 2015;82(2):256–67.e7.

40. Krishnamoorthi R, Jayaraj M, Kozarek R. Endoscopic Stents for the Biliary Tree and Pancreas. Curr Treat Options Gastroenterol 2017;15(3):397–415.

41. Mahajan A, Ho H, Sauer B, et al. Temporary placement of fully covered self-expandable metal stents in benign biliary strictures: midterm evaluation (with video). Gastrointest Endosc 2009;70(2):303–9.

42. Park JK, Moon JH, Choi HJ, et al. Anchoring of a fully covered self-expandable metal stent with a 5F double-pigtail plastic stent to prevent migration in the management of benign biliary strictures. Am J Gastroenterol 2011;106(10):1761–5.

43. Tarantino I, Mangiavillano B, Di Mitri R, et al. Fully covered self-expandable metallic stents in benign biliary strictures: a multicenter study on efficacy and safety. Endoscopy 2012;44(10):923–7.

44. Park DH, Lee SS, Lee TH, et al. Anchoring flap versus flared end, fully covered self-expandable metal stents to prevent migration in patients with benign biliary

strictures: a multicenter, prospective, comparative pilot study (with videos). Gastrointest Endosc 2011;73(1):64–70.

45. Jang SI, Rhee K, Kim H, et al. Recanalization of refractory benign biliary stricture using magnetic compression anastomosis. Endoscopy 2014;46(1):70–4.

46. Itoi T, Kasuya K, Sofuni A, et al. Magnetic compression anastomosis for biliary obstruction: review and experience at Tokyo Medical University Hospital. J Hepatobiliary Pancreat Sci 2011;18(3):357–65.

47. Jang SI, Lee KH, Yoon HJ, et al. Treatment of completely obstructed benign biliary strictures with magnetic compression anastomosis: follow-up results after recanalization. Gastrointest Endosc 2017;85(5):1057–66.

48. Takao S, Matsuo Y, Shinchi H, et al. Magnetic compression anastomosis for benign obstruction of the common bile duct. Endoscopy 2001;33(11):988–90.

49. Mimuro A, Tsuchida A, Yamanouchi E, et al. A novel technique of magnetic compression anastomosis for severe biliary stenosis. Gastrointest Endosc 2003;58(2):283–7.

50. Jang SI, Kim JH, Won JY, et al. Magnetic compression anastomosis is useful in biliary anastomotic strictures after living donor liver transplantation. Gastrointest Endosc 2011;74(5):1040–8.

51. Jang SI, Cho JH, Lee DK. Magnetic compression anastomosis for the treatment of post-transplant biliary stricture. Clin Endosc 2020;53(3):266–75.

52. Kuzela L, Oltman M, Sutka J, et al. Prospective follow-up of patients with bile duct strictures secondary to laparoscopic cholecystectomy, treated endoscopically with multiple stents. Hepatogastroenterology 2005;52(65):1357–61.

53. Costamagna G, Tringali A, Perri V, et al. Endotherapy of postcholecystectomy biliary strictures with multiple plastic stents: long-term results in a large cohort of patients. Gastrointest Endosc 2020;91(1):81–9.

54. Sharma V, Saraswat VA, Baijal SS, et al. Anatomic variations in intrahepatic bile ducts in a north Indian population. J Gastroenterol Hepatol 2008;23(7 Pt 2): e58–62.

55. Bageacu S, Abdelaal A, Ficarelli S, et al. Anatomy of the right liver lobe: a surgical analysis in 124 consecutive living donors. Clin Transplant 2011;25(4): E447–54.

56. Tringali A, Massinha P, Schepis T, et al. Long-term outcomes of endoscopic treatment of aberrant hepatic duct injuries after cholecystectomy. Gastrointest Endosc 2020;91(3):584–92.

57. Tringali A, Reddy DN, Ponchon T, et al. Treatment of post-cholecystectomy biliary strictures with fully-covered self-expanding metal stents - results after 5 years of follow-up. BMC Gastroenterol 2019;19(1):214.

58. Kochhar G, Parungao JM, Hanouneh IA, et al. Biliary complications following liver transplantation. World J Gastroenterol 2013;19(19):2841–6.

59. Greif F, Bronsther OL, Van Thiel DH, et al. The incidence, timing, and management of biliary tract complications after orthotopic liver transplantation. Ann Surg 1994;219(1):40–5.

60. Davidson BR, Rai R, Kurzawinski TR, et al. Prospective randomized trial of end-to-end versus side-to-side biliary reconstruction after orthotopic liver transplantation. Br J Surg 1999;86(4):447–52.

61. Pascher A, Neuhaus P. Biliary complications after deceased-donor orthotopic liver transplantation. J Hepatobiliary Pancreat Surg 2006;13(6):487–96.

62. Londoño MC, Balderramo D, Cárdenas A. Management of biliary complications after orthotopic liver transplantation: the role of endoscopy. World J Gastroenterol 2008;14(4):493–7.

63. Verdonk RC, Buis CI, Porte RJ, et al. Anastomotic biliary strictures after liver transplantation: causes and consequences. Liver Transpl 2006;12(5):726–35.
64. Park JS, Kim MH, Lee SK, et al. Efficacy of endoscopic and percutaneous treatments for biliary complications after cadaveric and living donor liver transplantation. Gastrointest Endosc 2003;57(1):78–85.
65. Graziadei IW, Schwaighofer H, Koch R, et al. Long-term outcome of endoscopic treatment of biliary strictures after liver transplantation. Liver Transpl 2006;12(5): 718–25.
66. Alazmi WM, Fogel EL, Watkins JL, et al. Recurrence rate of anastomotic biliary strictures in patients who have had previous successful endoscopic therapy for anastomotic narrowing after orthotopic liver transplantation. Endoscopy 2006; 38(6):571–4.
67. Pasha SF, Harrison ME, Das A, et al. Endoscopic treatment of anastomotic biliary strictures after deceased donor liver transplantation: outcomes after maximal stent therapy. Gastrointest Endosc 2007;66(1):44–51.
68. Haapamäki C, Udd M, Halttunen J, et al. Endoscopic treatment of anastomotic biliary complications after liver transplantation using removable, covered, self-expandable metallic stents. Scand J Gastroenterol 2012;47(1):116–21.
69. Hu B, Gao DJ, Yu FH, et al. Endoscopic stenting for post-transplant biliary stricture: usefulness of a novel removable covered metal stent. J Hepatobiliary Pancreat Sci 2011;18(5):640–5.
70. Sung MJ, Jo JH, Lee HS, et al. Optimal drainage of anastomosis stricture after living donor liver transplantation. Surg Endosc 2021;35(11):6307–17 [published correction appears in Surg Endosc 2021].
71. Rerknimitr R, Sherman S, Fogel EL, et al. Biliary tract complications after orthotopic liver transplantation with choledochocholedochostomy anastomosis: endoscopic findings and results of therapy. Gastrointest Endosc 2002;55(2): 224–31.
72. Moench C, Moench K, Lohse AW, et al. Prevention of ischemic-type biliary lesions by arterial back-table pressure perfusion. Liver Transpl 2003;9(3):285–9.
73. Rizk RS, McVicar JP, Emond MJ, et al. Endoscopic management of biliary strictures in liver transplant recipients: effect on patient and graft survival. Gastrointest Endosc 1998;47(2):128–35.
74. Verdonk RC, Buis CI, van der Jagt EJ, et al. Nonanastomotic biliary strictures after liver transplantation, part 2: Management, outcome, and risk factors for disease progression. Liver Transpl 2007;13(5):725–32.
75. Vijungco JD, Prinz RA. Management of biliary and duodenal complications of chronic pancreatitis. World J Surg 2003;27(11):1258–70.
76. Lygidakis NJ. Biliary stricture as a complication of chronic relapsing pancreatitis. Am J Surg 1983;145(6):804–6.
77. Dumonceau JM, Delhaye M, Tringali A, et al. Endoscopic treatment of chronic pancreatitis: European Society of Gastrointestinal Endoscopy (ESGE) Guideline - Updated August 2018. Endoscopy 2019;51(2):179–93.
78. Regimbeau JM, Fuks D, Bartoli E, et al. A comparative study of surgery and endoscopy for the treatment of bile duct stricture in patients with chronic pancreatitis. Surg Endosc 2012;26(10):2902–8.
79. Siriwardana HP, Siriwardena AK. Systematic appraisal of the role of metallic endobiliary stents in the treatment of benign bile duct stricture. Ann Surg 2005; 242(1):10–9.
80. Cote GA, Xu H, Slivka A, et al. 1057 fully covered metallic stents achieve comparable efficacy in a shorter time to plastic stents for the first-line endoscopic

treatment of benign biliary strictures: interim results of a multicenter, randomized, controlled trial. Gastrointest Endosc 2015. https://doi.org/10.1016/j.gie.2015.03.1950.

81. Ramchandani M, Lakhtakia S, Costamagna G, et al. Fully covered self-expanding metal stent vs multiple plastic stents to treat benign biliary strictures secondary to chronic pancreatitis: a multicenter randomized trial. Gastroenterology 2021;161(1):185–95.

82. Behm B, Brock A, Clarke BW, et al. Partially covered self-expandable metallic stents for benign biliary strictures due to chronic pancreatitis. Endoscopy 2009;41(6):547–51.

83. Dyson JK, Beuers U, Jones DEJ, et al. Primary sclerosing cholangitis. Lancet 2018;391(10139):2547–59.

84. Hilscher MB, Tabibian JH, Carey EJ, et al. Dominant strictures in primary sclerosing cholangitis: A multicenter survey of clinical definitions and practices. Hepatol Commun 2018;2(7):836–44, 4.

85. Prokopič M, Beuers U. Management of primary sclerosing cholangitis and its complications: an algorithmic approach. Hepatol Int 2021;15(1):6–20.

86. Aabakken L, Karlsen TH, Albert J, et al. Role of endoscopy in primary sclerosing cholangitis: European Society of Gastrointestinal Endoscopy (ESGE) and European Association for the Study of the Liver (EASL) Clinical Guideline. Endoscopy 2017;49(6):588–608.

87. Kaya M, Petersen BT, Angulo P, et al. Balloon dilation compared to stenting of dominant strictures in primary sclerosing cholangitis. Am J Gastroenterol 2001;96(4):1059–66.

88. Gotthardt DN, Rudolph G, Klöters-Plachky P, et al. Endoscopic dilation of dominant stenoses in primary sclerosing cholangitis: outcome after long-term treatment. Gastrointest Endosc 2010;71(3):527–34.

89. Ponsioen CY, Lam K, van Milligen de Wit AW, et al. Four years experience with short term stenting in primary sclerosing cholangitis. Am J Gastroenterol 1999;94(9):2403–7.

90. van Milligen de Wit AW, van Bracht J, Rauws EA, et al. Endoscopic stent therapy for dominant extrahepatic bile duct strictures in primary sclerosing cholangitis. Gastrointest Endosc 1996;44(3):293–9.

91. Allison MC, Sandoe JA, Tighe R, et al. Antibiotic prophylaxis in gastrointestinal endoscopy. Gut 2009;58(6):869–80.

92. Kamisawa T, Nakazawa T, Tazuma S, et al. Clinical practice guidelines for IgG4-related sclerosing cholangitis. J Hepatobiliary Pancreat Sci 2019;26(1):9–42.

93. Kamisawa T, Zen Y, Nakazawa T, et al. Advances in IgG4-related pancreatobiliary diseases. Lancet Gastroenterol Hepatol 2018;3(8):575–85.

94. Hart PA, Kamisawa T, Brugge WR, et al. Long-term outcomes of autoimmune pancreatitis: a multicentre, international analysis. Gut 2013;62(12):1771–6.

95. Okazaki K, Chari ST, Frulloni L, et al. International consensus for the treatment of autoimmune pancreatitis. Pancreatology 2017;17(1):1–6.

96. Bill JG, Mullady DK. Stenting for benign and malignant biliary strictures. Gastrointest Endosc Clin N Am 2019;29(2):215–35.

97. Nakai Y, Isayama H, Wang HP, et al. International consensus statements for endoscopic management of distal biliary stricture. J Gastroenterol Hepatol 2020;35(6):967–79.

98. Tarantino I, Amata M, Cicchese N, et al. Sequential multistenting protocol in biliary stenosis after liver transplantation: a prospective analysis. Endoscopy 2019;51(12):1130–5.

99. Bartel MJ, Higa JT, Tokar JL. The Status of SEMS versus plastic stents for benign biliary strictures. Curr Gastroenterol Rep 2019;21(7):29.

100. Pausawasadi N, Soontornmanokul T, Rerknimitr R. Role of fully covered self-expandable metal stent for treatment of benign biliary strictures and bile leaks. Korean J Radiol 2012;13(Suppl 1):S67–73.

101. Li Y, Sun H, Yan X, et al. Magnetic compression anastomosis for the treatment of benign biliary strictures: a clinical study from China. Surg Endosc 2020;34(6): 2541–50.

Endoscopic Management of Complex Biliary Stones

Simon Phillpotts, MBBS, MRCP[a], George Webster, MD, FRCP[a],*,
Marianna Arvanitakis, MD, PhD[b]

KEYWORDS

- ERCP • Papillary balloon dilatation • Cholangioscopy • Lithotripsy

KEY POINTS

- Complex biliary stones include a range of factors, including large size (≥15 mm), multiple stones, high stone:duct ratio, and stones proximal to strictures.
- Endoscopic techniques to extract large stones includes endoscopic papillary large balloon dilatation, mechanical lithotripsy, cholangioscopy-directed lithotripsy, and temporary biliary endoprosthesis.
- Endoscopic papillary large balloon dilatation after sphincterotomy is recommended when extracting large (≥15 mm) stones.
- Cholangioscopic visually directed lithotripsy allows a high stone clearance rate when conventional endoscopic retrograde cholangiopancreatography has failed or has low predicted success, including for large stones and those in difficult anatomic positions.

 Video content accompanies this article at http://www.giendo.theclinics.com.

INTRODUCTION

Gallstones are common, present in 20% of the adult population.[1] Stones migrating into the bile duct are a major cause of symptoms.[2] Biliary or common bile duct (CBD) stones are seen in 7% to 12% of patients with known cholelithiasis[3] and account for 10% to 20% of patients with symptomatic gallstones.[4,5] Complications from biliary stones occur in 1% to 3% of patients per year, including emergency scenarios: obstructive jaundice, cholangitis, and pancreatitis.[5] In patients who undergo cholecystectomy without clearing bile duct stones, unfavorable outcomes may be seen in 25% of patients,[6] including cholangitis, biliary pancreatitis, and cholangitis.[7]

[a] Department of Gastroenterology, University College London Hospitals, 250 Euston Road, London, England; [b] Department of Gastroenterology, Hepatopancreatology, and Digestive Oncology, CUB Hôpital Erasme, Université Libre de Bruxelles, Route de Lennik 808, Brussels 1070, Belgium
* Corresponding author.
E-mail address: george.webster1@nhs.net

Gastrointest Endoscopy Clin N Am 32 (2022) 477–492
https://doi.org/10.1016/j.giec.2022.02.002
1052-5157/22/© 2022 Elsevier Inc. All rights reserved.

Once biliary stones are confirmed stone extraction should be advised.[2,4] Endoscopic retrograde cholangiopancreatography (ERCP) with biliary endoscopic sphincterotomy (EST) enables stone removal with extraction balloons or baskets. This procedure was first described in 1974[8] and was subsequently demonstrated to be an effective technique in large observational studies.[9,10] Bile duct clearance is achieved in 85% to 90%, with little reported change over the past 4 decades.[9,11,12]

Failure to extract stones can be due to a range of factors, including large stone size, multiple stones, the location of the stones, the presence of strictures distal to stones, angulation of the distal bile duct, composition of stones and altered upper gastrointestinal anatomy (**Box 1**). Complex biliary stones is a generic term that refers to stones that are likely to be challenging to remove endoscopically; this article addresses the factors linked to difficulty and steps to overcome them.

FACTORS RELATED TO COMPLEX BILIARY STONES
Stone Size, Number, and Type

CBD stones 10 mm or less in size can generally be extracted after EST.[14] However, as the size of the largest stone increases, the success of removal decreases. Lauri and colleagues[19] found that there was a significant difference between success and stone size (successful, median size 10 mm; unsuccessful, median size, 18 mm; $P < .001$), with only 12% of stones greater than 15 mm being successfully removed with standard EST + balloon/basket alone. This finding was supported by Kim and colleagues,[3] who showed that CBD stone 15 mm or larger contributed to difficulty of clearance ($P = .002$), and Riemann and colleagues[20] described the need for mechanical lithotripsy (ML) for particularly large stones (median size, 22.8 mm). In general, a size of 15 mm or larger is most predictive of a complex biliary stone.

The presence of multiple CBD stones also limits the success at duct clearance,[2,13–16] although there does not seem to be a consensus on the number of stones that significantly predicts this correlation. Stone shape also affects success, with barrel[2,16] (**Fig. 1**) or irregularly[15] shaped stones being more challenging (**Fig. 2**).

Box 1
Factors associated with complex biliary stones

- Stone characteristics
  - Size: Large,[13,14] greater than 10 mm,[15] greater than 15 mm[2,3,16,17]
  - Multiple stones[2,13–16]
  - Stone shape: Barrell shaped,[2,16] irregular[15]
  - Stone composition[18]

- Stone location
  - Cystic duct insertion or intrahepatic[2,13–16]
  - Above strictures[2,3,14–16]

- Anatomic considerations
  - Narrow distal duct/high stone:duct ratio[2,15,16]
  - Angulated distal duct[2,3,15]
  - Short distal CBD[2,3,15]
  - Duodenal diverticulum[13,14]
  - Sigmoid distal CBD[2,13]

- Patient-related factors
  - Increasing age[3,14]
  - Performance status (eg, American Society of Anesthesiologists grade)[13,14]
  - Bleeding risk[14]
  - Altered surgical anatomy[3,13–16]

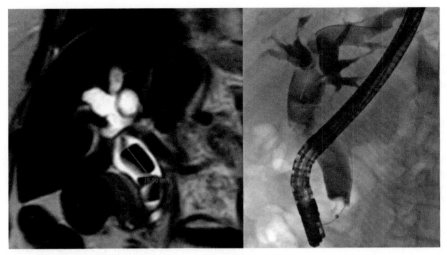

Fig. 1. MRCP and ERCP cholangiogram of large CBD stones.

The type of stone may also affect the ease of extraction. Cholesterol stones found more commonly in Western countries are generally much harder and more difficult to fragment than calcium stones found in Asian patients.[18]

Stone Location

Stones located within the cystic duct, including those leading to bile duct obstruction (ie, Mirizzi syndrome), present challenges in conventional extraction owing to difficulties passing a guidewire alongside the stone or an extraction balloon above it and/or difficulty capturing stones within a basket or lithotripter (Video 1). Intrahepatic stones may also prove difficult owing to similar problems, in addition to the presence

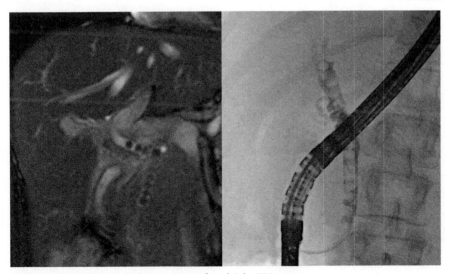

Fig. 2. MRCP and ERCP cholangiogram of multiple CBD stones.

of strictures distal to the calculi, angulation of intrahepatic ducts, and selective access to intrahepatic ducts. The presence of strictures distal to stones in all parts of the biliary tree may make stone extraction complex, as stone extraction is rarely possible without significant stone fragmentation or stricture remodeling. This situation can be particularly challenging in patients with coexisting cholangiopathy. Not only are these stones difficult to remove, they can also cause significant problems with recurrent cholangitis, and atrophy of the affected lobe[21] (**Fig. 3**).

Anatomic Considerations

There are a variety of different anatomic differences that may result in complex stone extraction.[2,3,13–16] The most important relationship may be the stone:duct ratio. A large stone relative to a narrow distal duct (stone:duct ratio of >1.0)[2,15,16] can result in significant challenges with extraction, similar to those presented by distal strictures (**Fig. 4**).

Kim and colleagues[3] showed significant correlations between technical difficulty of extraction and previous gastrojejunostomy (*P* = .004), short (≤36 mm) distal CBD arm downstream the stone (*P* < .001), and the presence of an acute (≤135°) distal CBD angle (*P* < .001). Through multivariate analysis, it has been shown CBD angle (*P* < .001) and short CBD length (*P* = .006) are important factors.[3] Duodenal diverticulum did not seem to correlate with difficulty; however, this entity is still described by others as a factor in stone complexity.[13,14]

Patient-related Factors

CBD stones are common in the elderly, affecting up to 30% of patients.[22] Age greater than 65 years is a significant factor in the difficulty of CBD stone removal (*P* = .004),[3] likely owing to larger and stacked stones being more common[13] as well as the presence of other patient-related factors, such as poor performance status, comorbidities, and the presence of duodenal diverticula. Elderly patients also have risk factors for

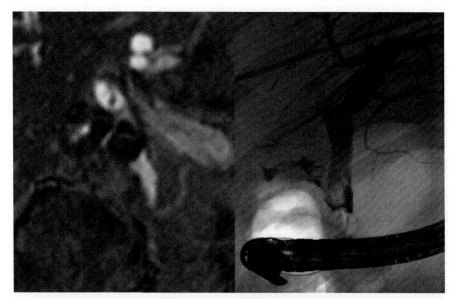

Fig. 3. MRCP and ERCP cholangiogram of a large stone at the junction of the cystic and CBDs, resulting in bile duct obstruction (Mirizzi syndrome).

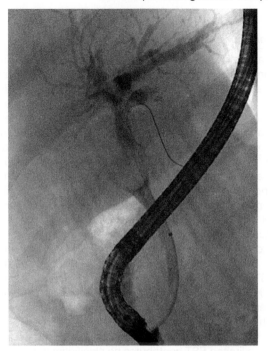

Fig. 4. ERCP cholangiogram of a large stone above a narrow distal duct, representing high stone: duct ratio.

stone recurrence despite EST (CBD dilatation, periampullary diverticulum, prior biliary surgery, and CBD angulation).[22] Another important consideration is the ability to reach the ampulla with an endoscope. This process may be very challenging in patients with surgically altered anatomy,[3,13–16] such as Billroth II partial gastrectomy and Roux-en-Y gastric bypass.

ENDOSCOPIC MANAGEMENT
Long-Term Biliary Stenting

When presented with a patient with complex stones that cannot be removed by standard techniques, biliary stents may be considered to provide drainage and prevent cholangitis. In patients with comorbidities that increase endoscopic or surgical risk, long-term stenting might be seen as a preferable solution. The effect of long-term biliary stenting in such patients has been investigated. Two studies from the 1990s compared the outcomes for patients undergoing plastic biliary stenting as a definitive treatment compared with either temporary stenting[23] or bile duct clearance[24] in elderly and high-risk patients. Both studies showed a less favorable outcome in patients who had stents placed as a long-term treatment. When compared with temporary stenting, Bergman and colleagues[23] showed a higher rate of complications ($\leq 40\%$), and mortality (23% vs 0%) in the long-term stented group. Equally, when randomized to long-term stenting or bile duct clearance, Chopra and colleagues[24] showed that there was significantly lower proportions of biliary complications in the bile duct clearance group (65% vs 86%; $P = .03$). The complications observed were mainly cholangitis and due to the significantly higher incidence of this in the long-term stented group, the study was terminated prematurely. Both authors concluded that long-term stenting should only be considered in high-risk elderly patients with a short life expectancy. Even in this clinical setting, regular stent exchange to avoid cholangitis should be considered.

Endoscopic Papillary Large Balloon Dilatation

Endoscopic papillary balloon dilation (EPBD) was first described as alternative to EST in 1982.[25] When compared with EST, EPBD has been shown to have a significantly increased risk of acute pancreatitis and mortality,[26] and as such is avoided as the default method of sphincter ablation therapy. However, in some settings EPBD may be preferred (eg, coagulopathy or altered anatomy) over EST; in these situations, it is recommended as an alternative for extracting CBD stones less than 8 mm in diameter.[27]

Endoscopic papillary large balloon dilatation (EPLBD) refers to sphincter dilatation of 12 mm or more.[28] First described by Ersoz and colleagues[29] in 2003, this is an effective (89% stone clearance after EPLBD) and safe way to extract difficult stones (large stones >15 mm and presence of a tapered distal duct) when performed after EST. This technique is recommended by both the European Society of Gastrointestinal Endoscopy (ESGE) and American Society of Gastrointestinal Endoscopy (ASGE) as an important approach to managing difficult or large CBD stones.[2,21]

The approach to EPLBD is debated, in particular the requirement for EST before balloon dilatation. Some authors describe equal effectiveness of stone clearance of EPBLD without EST (88.0%–97.2%) compared with the usual standard of EPLBD after EST (92.0%–96.5%), with no difference in complications.[28,30,31] However, we would caution against performing a balloon dilatation without EST in light of the proven association between EPBD and pancreatitis.[26] A large EST before EPLBD has been associated with a significant increased risk of bleeding compared with limited or no EST.[30,32] However, a limited EST contributes no significant increased risk of bleeding compared with EPLBD alone.[30,32]

EPLBD with EST compared with EST alone reduces the need for ML,[21,33–36] particularly for large stones (>15 mm),[34] although overall duct clearance rates do not seem to differ.[17,34,36] There is also a higher reported complication rate, in particular cholangitis, when EST alone is followed by ML compared with EST combined with EPLBD.[33] Other benefits include significantly shorter procedure and fluoroscopy time[36] and lower costs.[34]

Aside from the risk of bleeding associated with larger EST, there is also a recognized risk of perforation. A retrospective study by Park and colleagues[32] identified a link between perforation and continued balloon inflation despite persistence of balloon waisting on fluoroscopy. To avoid this risk, we do not recommend EPLBD as a treatment when there is a presence of a distal stricture or dilating the balloon wider than the diameter of the distal CBD.[27,28]

One final consideration is the duration of balloon inflation from the resolution of the balloon waisting. Liao and colleagues[37] suggest that longer dilatations of 5 minutes were more favorable than 1 minute, but this only related to 10-mm balloons. In contrast, Meng and colleagues[38] showed a significantly higher rate of post-ERCP pancreatitis in those having dilatations for 300 seconds or 0 second compared with 30 seconds after balloon waisting had disappeared, resulting in the conclusion that 30 seconds is the optimal dilatation time for removing CBD stones. When dilating to larger diameters (≤20 mm) shorter inflation duration (30 seconds) was as effective as a longer duration (60 seconds).[39] The ESGE[2] recommends that EPLBD dilatation should last for at least 30 seconds.

Cholangioscopy-assisted Lithotripsy

Cholangioscopy provides an opportunity for direct visualization and targeted intraductal therapy. In the setting of difficult stones, this modality is used to deliver visually directed lithotripsy to fragment the stones. This technique has been shown to have an overall stone clearance rate of 88% to 99% when conventional ERCP has failed.[40,41]

Per oral cholangioscopy was developed in the 1970s with the initial mother and baby scopes requiring 2 operators. The first generation of these devices had no facility for cholangioscope tip angulation, and only a small channel for irrigation.[42] As the technology developed the scopes became wider, which enabled a working channel (≤1.2 mm) to be included and also the ability to angulate the tip.[43] A significant leap forward was made with the development of a single operator cholangioscope (SpyGlass; Boston Scientific, Marlborough, MA), which was launched in 2007 and overcame some of the challenges faced by the traditional dual operator system. However, as with the dual operator scopes, the first generation of these scopes relied on fiber optic technology which had suboptimal image quality.[44] In 2015 a digital version of cholangioscope was released (Spyglass DS), which provided significant improvement in visualisation.[44] This was superseded by the SpyGlass DS II system in 2018, which has further improved resolution and field of view.

After stone visualization, a lithotripsy probe can be passed through the 1.2-mm working channel of the single operator cholangioscope to allow fragmentation. There are 2 types of lithotripsy, laser lithotripsy and electrohydraulic lithotripsy (EHL). Both technologies work by generating a shock wave that fragments the stone. In the case of EHL, the probe must be within an aqueous medium of normal saline. A charge generator discharges a spark at the end of the probe, which produces a high-pressure hydraulic wave within the saline which is directed at the stone. The probe should be positioned between 1 and 2 mm of the stone for optimum effect.[41] Laser lithotripsy works by generating plasma within the fluid adjacent to the stone. This rapid expansion of this plasma creates a shock wave that fragments it.[41] The immediate advantage of EHL over laser is that the equipment is compact and requires no special protective gear or electrical equipment.[45] However, there is some evidence that laser lithotripsy may be more success in stone clearance when compared with EHL (95.1%. vs 88.4%) and also stone fragmentation rate (92.5% vs 75.5%),[45] while also having a significantly shorter procedure duration (49.9 minutes vs 73.9 minutes; $P < .001$)[41] and a lower complication rate (9.6% vs 13.8%).[45] These studies were both retrospective and hence there is a need for prospective randomized studies to definitively conclude the benefits and risks of each modality.

When comparing intraductal laser lithotripsy with conventional therapies (balloon extraction, EPBD, and ML) to clear the duct of large (>1 cm) stones, laser lithotripsy performed significantly better (93% vs 67%; $P = .009$); however, these procedures were also significantly longer (120.7 minutes vs 81.2 minutes; $P = .0008$).[46] These differences were also seen when laser lithotripsy was compared directly to ML, with a significantly higher stone clearance rate in the first session (100% vs 63%; $P < .01$) and significantly lower radiation exposure ($P = .04$). Furthermore, laser lithotripsy rescued 60% of patients with failed ML by achieving complete stone clearance within the same session.[47]

Cholangioscopy-guided lithotripsy may be of particular benefit in aiding the extraction of stones in difficult anatomic locations, such as with Mirizzi syndrome (Video 2) or intrahepatic calculi. In Mirizzi syndrome, success rates with cholangioscopy guided therapy range from 60% to 91%,[48,49] which is considerably higher than the success rate with conventional ERCP (40%).[48] Equally, intrahepatic stones can be difficult to treat with conventional ERCP and stones in these locations are particularly complex because they often coexist with biliary strictures and cholangiopathy. Cholangioscopy-guided lithotripsy provides a useful opportunity to both assess the stricture and target treatment by enabling stone extraction.

With regard to health care resources, Deprez and colleagues[50] studied the impact of cholangioscopy-guided lithotripsy in treating difficult stones. They showed a decrease in the total number of procedures (27% relative reduction) and overall costs (11% relative reduction) compared with conventional therapy.

Cholangioscopy-directed lithotripsy carries an estimated adverse event rate of 7%, most frequently cholangitis (4%), as well as pancreatitis (2%), perforation (1%), and others (3%).[40] Owing to the risk of cholangitis, the ESGE recommend routine antibiotic prophylaxis for cholangitis in all patients undergoing cholangioscopy.[51]

Cholangioscopy-directed lithotripsy is an extremely useful method to successfully clear complex stones and its use is recommended depending on local availability, a recommendation also supported by the ESGE.[2] However, we acknowledge that the ASGE recommend either intraductal (cholangioscopy) or conventional therapy for difficult stones, the choice of therapy depending on local expertise and cost, as well as patient and physician preference.[21]

Mechanical Lithotripsy

ML was first described in 1982 as a technique for fragmenting and removing large (17–30 mm) CBD stones.[20] In the absence of any other method of stone fragmentation this was a popular technique, and likely remains so in areas without ready access to cholangioscopy and intraductal lithotripsy. The mechanical lithotripter device has a metal wire basket that can be advanced out of a plastic catheter, over which a metal sheath lies. The catheter is directed freehand into the bile duct before the basket is opened to capture the stone. The calculus can then be extracted with the basket alone, or fragmented by advancing the metal sheath so the wires of the basket progressively crush the calculus. Success with this technique varies from 76% to 90%,[18,52,53] although patients may often need repeat procedures.

The most important factor that may affect the success of ML is stone size, with a 90% success with stones less than 10 mm and only 68% of those greater than 28 mm ($P < .02$),[53] and a significant likelihood of failure if a stone is greater than 30 mm.[52] Other predictive factors of failure are a high stone:duct diameter ratio (>1.0)[52] and stone impaction ($P < .001$), as well multiple large stones, extremely hard stones, and patient intolerance during the procedure.[18]

The incidence of adverse events range from 1.4% to 3.3% for a single procedure, but increase to 19.6% for repeat procedures.[54] In 1 study, there was a reported 4-fold risk of stone recurrence and further hepaticobiliary complications when ML is used, possibly owing to small stone fragments remaining, which then generate new stone formation.[55] Fortunately, it seems that the risk of lithotripter malfunction with basket entrapment, broken handle, or wire fracture, is rare, occurring in only 3.6% of procedures.[56] If these complications occur then they can usually be rectified by using a salvage lithotripter, extending the sphincterotomy or intraductal lithotripsy with EHL.[56]

Salvage lithotripsy may be required when a mechanical lithotripter becomes trapped on a calculus within the duct (Video 3). Once the ML catheter has been removed from the endoscope the metal sheath of the salvage lithotripsy is advanced over it. Gradual traction is then applied via the salvage lithotripter to the ML wires, pulling the ML basket into the salvage lithotripsy sheath, crushing any impacted calculi and allowing removal of the lithotripter from the duct.

Extracorporeal Shockwave Lithotripsy

First described as a modality to treat bile duct stones in 1985,[57] extracorporeal shockwave lithotripsy provides an option to treat particularly challenging stones that have failed extraction with the techniques already described. Shock waves are delivered through the body either by electrohydraulic or electromagnetic energy to fragment the stones. A retrospective analysis of 392 extracorporeal shockwave lithotripsy procedures found CBD stone clearance rates of 89%,[58] and after failed endoscopic clearance extracorporeal shockwave lithotripsy achieved complete clearance in 83% of patients.[59]

Biliary Endoprosthesis

Long-term biliary stenting should only be considered a treatment option for patients with a short life expectancy. However, short-term stenting can be used a bridge to further therapy and as a treatment for large stones.

If a temporary plastic stenting approach is to be adopted, then stents need to be changed regularly, rather than doing so only when a patient develops symptoms. Di Giorgio and colleagues[60] showed that changing stents every 3 months significantly decreased the rate of cholangitis (3% vs 14%; $P = .03$) when compared with an on-demand approach. In the setting of complex stones, it may be that stents not only ensure drainage, but also act to progressively decrease stone load, making subsequent extraction easier. Horiuchi and associates[61] showed that plastic stenting (7F double pigtail) for large ($\geq$20 mm), or multiple ($\geq$3) stones, for 2 months resulted in a significant reduction in the number and size of stones at subsequent ERCP ($P < .0001$).

There is also some evidence that fully covered self-expandable metal stents (fcSEMS) can help in managing difficult stones. In 2 retrospective series, the use of fcSEMS for patients with difficult stones that had failed extraction with conventional techniques was assessed.[62,63] Stents were placed for an average of 45 and 56 days, and at repeat ERCP the ducts were cleared in 83% and 82%, respectively. The most common adverse event was stent migration, all of which were noted at repeat ERCP.

These options are worth trialing in the setting of complex stones, and are recommended by the ASGE to facilitate stone removal.[21] However, it is crucial that these are only used as temporary treatment options and, should they prove unsuccessful, it is important to consider other modalities.

SPECIFIC SITUATIONS
Stones above Strictures

This scenario presents difficulties in using the previously described techniques. As highlighted, the presence of a distal CBD stricture increases the risk of perforation when performing EPLBD.[32] If a tight stricture is encountered, we recommend placement of biliary endoprosthesis to widen or remodel the stricture to allow subsequent extraction, with or without fragmentation. The ESGE recommends either multiple temporary plastic stents (maximum number possible, replaced every 3–4 months) or a removable 8 to 10 mm diameter fcSEMS (for $\leq$6 months).[64]

There is a theoretic risk that, when using a fcSEMS, a mobile stone could come to sit immediately on top of the proximal end of the stent, causing obstruction. To avoid this eventuality, a double pigtail plastic stent can be placed through the SEMS, preventing stone impaction in the proximal flange.

If a stenting approach is used, there needs to be a robust process for following up these patients to avoid them being left with stents in situ for extended periods and the risks this caries of either stent obstruction or failure of stent removal owing to tissue ingrowth despite the fully covered design. The ESGE recommends keeping a registry of stented patients to avoid this adverse outcome.[64]

Surgically Altered Anatomy

This complexity will be covered in more detail in a different article. The difficulty lies in the ability to reach the ampulla or ducts above a choledochoenteric anastomosis with a conventional endoscope. **Table 1** highlights the common upper gastrointestinal surgery procedures and the approaches to biliary access.

PLANNING AND PREPARATION

Decision-making before treating complex stones can be as challenging as the procedural aspects. As highlighted, there are several factors that make stones complex and the different factors that influence treatment options. We recommend a careful consideration of each case depending on these different factors and the impact these have on what is to be attempted.

Before the Procedure

Multidisciplinary meetings have a key role in shared decision making about complex decisions in healthcare and are well established as part of cancer pathways and complex disease management. In the case of pancreatobiliary disease, and specifically complex stones, a collaborative meeting with gastroenterologists/endoscopists, pancreatobiliary radiologists and hepatopancreaticobiliary surgeons is invaluable. Advantages of these type of multidisciplinary meetings include timely review of urgent cases, imaging review before patient contact, sharing of alternative procedural approaches (eg, surgical, endoscopic, radiological), decreased administration costs, as well as teaching and training opportunities.[65] A full review of complex stone cases in such meetings is recommended to enable a detailed assessment of all the factors that have contributed to the stone's complexity and allow subsequent procedure planning.

Table 1
Methods of biliary access after upper gastrointestinal surgery

Previous Surgery	Primary Approaches for Biliary Access
Gastric band	Conventional ERCP
Sleeve gastrectomy	Conventional ERCP
Roux-en-Y gastric bypass	LAP-ERCP EDGE DAE-ERCP PTD ± cholangioscopy
Billroth I partial gastrectomy	Conventional ERCP
Billroth II partial gastrectomy	Conventional ERCP (via afferent limb) DAE-ERCP PTD ± cholangioscopy
Total—gastrectomy with Roux-en-Y anastomosis	DAE-ERCP PTD ± cholangioscopy
Pancreaticoduodenectomy (Whipple)	DAE-ERCP PTD ± cholangioscopy

DAE-ERCP, device assisted enteroscopy-assisted endoscopic retrograde cholangiopancreatography; EDGE, endoscopic ultrasound-directed transgastric endoscopic retrograde cholangiopancreatography; LAP-ERCP, laparoscopic-assisted ERCP; PTD, percutaneous transhepatic drainage.
Adapted from Martin H, El Menabawey T, Webster O, et al. Endoscopic biliary therapy in the era of bariatric surgery. *Frontline Gastroenterology* Published Online First: 24 February 2021. https://doi.org/10.1136/flgastro-2020-101755.

Once a conclusion is reached about how to proceed it is important the patient understands the complexity of the situation to make an informed decision and consent to the procedure being planned. Part of this consent process should include the chances of success and failure, as well as the alternative treatments available. These alternatives may include different types of stone therapy available, locally or elsewhere, as well as nonendoscopic options (medications or surgery), as well as abstaining from treatment and the risks this choice carries.

Procedural Considerations

Depending on the treatment modality to be undertaken, there are important considerations about how the procedure should be performed. As highlighted, ERCP with cholangioscopy-guided lithotripsy can be of long duration; therefore, appropriate sedation or anesthesia is required. If performed with general anesthesia and endotracheal intubation, it may be preferable for the airway management for the patient to be supine. However, it is often easier to obtain biliary cannulation with the patients in the prone position compared with supine ($P = .0047$), with a higher failure rate in the supine group ($P = .052$).[66] The supine position can result in fluid pooling in D2, and often over-the-scope tip and papilla, obscuring the endoscopic view, and this may particularly by the case with cholangioscopy, involving the infusion of significant volumes of normal saline.

After the Procedure

After stone extraction, patients should be referred for cholecystectomy if the gallbladder is still in place, owing to the significantly higher recurrence of biliary symptoms in patients not undergoing surgery.[67] However, ERCP can make laparoscopic cholecystectomy more complex and longer.[68] Adverse events at surgery are lower if

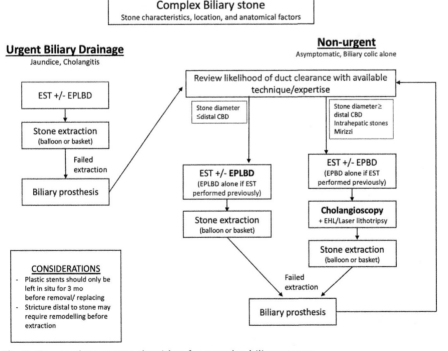

Fig. 5. Proposed treatment algorithm for complex biliary stones.

surgery is performed early, rather than delayed, and the ESGE recommend cholecystectomy within 2 weeks of patients presenting with choledocholithiasis.[2]

Some patients are at risk of recurrent stones despite clearance and hence pose an ongoing challenge, even when stones are cleared. Significant independent risk factors for stone recurrence include a dilated CBD of 13 mm or larger ($P = .017$); an angulated distal duct $\leq 145°$ ($P = .0002$); and the presence of a previous cholecystectomy ($P = .0117$). In such patients, close monitoring for further symptomatic stone disease may be recommended.

For patients with persistent stones and high procedural risk from comorbidities or age, there is some evidence that medical therapy alongside biliary stenting can reduce stone size and success of stone removal at subsequent ERCP. Han and colleagues[69] showed that ursodeoxycholic acid with stenting resulted in a significant decrease in stone size ($P < .01$), but this was not a comparative study. Other authors showed no significant difference in stone clearance[70,71] and fragmentation[70] between stenting with ursodeoxycholic acid and stenting alone.

SUMMARY

Complex stones provide a challenge in deciding on appropriate management, depending on patient characteristics and the availability of resources. Endoscopic therapy is long established as the preferable way to remove stones; however, the different techniques are not available universally. It is important to understand the chances of duct clearance at each planned procedure to facilitate decision-making for the patient, as well as determining health care resources (**Fig. 5**).

CLINICS CARE POINTS

- High-quality cross-sectional imaging is vital to correctly and safely plan endoscopic stone management.

- Complex biliary stones require careful decision-making. These cases warrant discussion in multidisciplinary team meetings to decide on the most appropriate therapy to enable informed discussions with the patient.

- Biliary endoprosthesis should be used as a short-term treatment as a bridge to further therapy, but the aim should to achieve definitive bile duct stone clearance.

- In the setting of failed stone extraction with conventional ERCP, early referral for advanced techniques should be considered, to avoid repeated incomplete procedures.

DISCLOSURE STATEMENT

S. Phillpotts reports no conflicts. G. Webster is an advisory board member and invited speaker for Boston Scientific, Cook Medical, Olympus, and Pentax Medical. M. Arvanitakis reports lecture fees from Olympus and Fujifilm, and consultant fees from Ambu.

SUPPLEMENTARY DATA

Supplementary data related to this article can be found online at https://doi.org/10.1016/j.giec.2022.02.002.

REFERENCES

1. Lammert F, Gurusamy K, Ko CW, et al. Gallstones. Nat Rev Dis Prim 2016;2: 16024.

2. Manes G, Paspatis G, Aabakken L, et al. Endoscopic management of common bile duct stones: European Society of Gastrointestinal Endoscopy (ESGE) guideline. Endoscopy 2019;51:472–91.

3. Kim HJ, Choi HS, Park JH, et al. Factors influencing the technical difficulty of endoscopic clearance of bile duct stones. Gastrointest Endosc 2007;66: 1154–60.

4. Williams E, Beckingham I, El Sayed G, et al. Updated guideline on the management of common bile duct stones (CBDS). Gut 2017;66:765–82.

5. Friedman GD. Natural history of asymptomatic and symptomatic gallstones. Am J Surg 1993;165:399–404.

6. Möller M, Gustafsson U, Rasmussen F, et al. Natural course vs interventions to clear common bile duct stones: data from the Swedish Registry for Gallstone Surgery and Endoscopic Retrograde Cholangiopancreatography (GallRiks). JAMA Surg 2014;149:1008–13.

7. Cox MR, Budge JPO, Eslick GD. Timing and nature of presentation of unsuspected retained common bile duct stones after laparoscopic cholecystectomy: a retrospective study. Surg Endosc 2015;29:2033–8.

8. Kawai K, Akasaka Y, Murakami K, et al. Endoscopic sphincterotomy of the ampulla of Vater. Gastrointest Endosc 1974;20:148–51.

9. Vaira D, D'Anna L, Ainley C, et al. Endoscopic sphincterotomy in 1000 consecutive patients. Lancet 1989;2:431–4.

10. Siegel JH. Endoscopic papillotomy in the treatment of biliary tract disease: 258 procedures and results. Dig Dis Sci 1981;26:1057–64.

11. Trikudanathan G, Navaneethan U, Parsi MA. Endoscopic management of difficult common bile duct stones. World J Gastroenterol 2013;19:165–73.

12. Sivak MVJ. Endoscopic management of bile duct stones. Am J Surg 1989;158: 228–40.

13. Hoshi K, Irisawa A, Tominaga K, et al. Association of long-term endoscopic biliary stent placement with choledocholithiasis: a literature review. Clin J Gastroenterol 2021;14:1303–7.

14. Yasuda I, Itoi T. Recent advances in endoscopic management of difficult bile duct stones. Dig Endosc 2013;25:376–85.

15. Kedia P, Tarnasky PR. Endoscopic management of complex biliary stone disease. Gastrointest Endosc Clin N Am 2019;29:257–75.

16. Galetti F, Moura DTH, Ribeiro IB, et al. Cholangioscopy-guided lithotripsy vs. conventional therapy for complex bile duct stones: a systematic review and meta-analysis. Arq Bras Cir Dig 2020;33:e1491.

17. Kim HG, Cheon YK, Cho YD, et al. Small sphincterotomy combined with endoscopic papillary large balloon dilation versus sphincterotomy. World J Gastroenterol 2009;15:4298–304.

18. Garg PK, Tandon RK, Ahuja V, et al. Predictors of unsuccessful mechanical lithotripsy and endoscopic clearance of large bile duct stones. Gastrointest Endosc 2004;59:601–5.

19. Lauri A, Horton RC, Davidson BR, et al. Endoscopic extraction of bile duct stones: management related to stone size. Gut 1993;34:1718–21.

20. Riemann JF, Seuberth K, Demling L. Clinical application of a new mechanical lithotripter for smashing common bile duct stones. Endoscopy 1982;14:226–30.

21. Buxbaum JL, Abbas Fehmi SM, Sultan S, et al. ASGE guideline on the role of endoscopy in the evaluation and management of choledocholithiasis. Gastrointest Endosc 2019;89:1075–105.e15.

22. Keizman D, Ish Shalom M, Konikoff FM. Recurrent symptomatic common bile duct stones after endoscopic stone extraction in elderly patients. Gastrointest Endosc 2006;64:60–5.
23. Bergman JJ, Rauws EA, Tijssen JG, et al. Biliary endoprostheses in elderly patients with endoscopically irretrievable common bile duct stones: report on 117 patients. Gastrointest Endosc 1995;42:195–201.
24. Chopra KB, Peters RA, O'Toole PA, et al. Randomised study of endoscopic biliary endoprosthesis versus duct clearance for bile duct stones in high-risk patients. Lancet (London, England) 1996;348:791–3.
25. Staritz M, Ewe K, Meyer zum Büschenfelde KH. Endoscopic papillary dilatation, a possible alternative to endoscopic papillotomy. Lancet (London, England) 1982; 1:1306–7.
26. Disario JA, Freeman ML, Bjorkman DJ, et al. Endoscopic balloon dilation compared with sphincterotomy for extraction of bile duct stones. Gastroenterology 2004;127:1291–9.
27. Testoni PA, Mariani A, Abakken L, et al. Papillary cannulation and sphincterotomy techniques at ERCP: European Society of Gastrointestinal Endoscopy (ESGE) Clinical Guideline. Endoscopy 2016;48:657–83.
28. Kim TH, Kim JH, Seo DW, et al. International consensus guidelines for endoscopic papillary large-balloon dilation. Gastrointest Endosc 2016;83:37–47.
29. Ersoz G, Tekesin O, Ozutemiz AO, et al. Biliary sphincterotomy plus dilation with a large balloon for bile duct stones that are difficult to extract. Gastrointest Endosc 2003;57:156–9.
30. Kim JH, Yang MJ, Hwang JC, et al. Endoscopic papillary large balloon dilation for the removal of bile duct stones. World J Gastroenterol 2013;19:8580–94.
31. Park J-S, Jeong S, Lee DK, et al. Comparison of endoscopic papillary large balloon dilation with or without endoscopic sphincterotomy for the treatment of large bile duct stones. Endoscopy 2019;51:125–32.
32. Park SJ, Kim JH, Hwang JC, et al. Factors predictive of adverse events following endoscopic papillary large balloon dilation: results from a multicenter series. Dig Dis Sci 2013;58:1100–9.
33. Stefanidis G, Viazis N, Pleskow D, et al. Large balloon dilation vs. mechanical lithotripsy for the management of large bile duct stones: a prospective randomized study. Am J Gastroenterol 2011;106:278–85.
34. Teoh AYB, Cheung FKY, Hu B, et al. Randomized trial of endoscopic sphincterotomy with balloon dilation versus endoscopic sphincterotomy alone for removal of bile duct stones. Gastroenterology 2013;144:341–5.e1.
35. Madhoun MF, Wani S, Hong S, et al. Endoscopic papillary large balloon dilation reduces the need for mechanical lithotripsy in patients with large bile duct stones: a systematic review and meta-analysis. Diagn Ther Endosc 2014;2014:309618.
36. Itoi T, Itokawa F, Sofuni A, et al. Endoscopic sphincterotomy combined with large balloon dilation can reduce the procedure time and fluoroscopy time for removal of large bile duct stones. Am J Gastroenterol 2009;104:560–5.
37. Liao W-C, Lee C-T, Chang C-Y, et al. Randomized trial of 1-minute versus 5-minute endoscopic balloon dilation for extraction of bile duct stones. Gastrointest Endosc 2010;72:1154–62.
38. Meng W, Leung JW, Zhang K, et al. Optimal dilation time for combined small endoscopic sphincterotomy and balloon dilation for common bile duct stones: a multicentre, single-blinded, randomised controlled trial. Lancet Gastroenterol Hepatol 2019;4:425–34.

39. Paspatis GA, Konstantinidis K, Tribonias G, et al. Sixty- versus thirty-seconds papillary balloon dilation after sphincterotomy for the treatment of large bile duct stones: a randomized controlled trial. Dig Liver Dis 2013;45:301–4.

40. Korrapati P, Ciolino J, Wani S, et al. The efficacy of peroral cholangioscopy for difficult bile duct stones and indeterminate strictures: a systematic review and meta-analysis. Endosc Int Open 2016;4:E263–75.

41. Brewer Gutierrez OI, Bekkali NLH, Rajiman I, et al. Efficacy and safety of digital single-operator cholangioscopy for difficult biliary stones. Clin Gastroenterol Hepatol 2018;16:918–26.e1.

42. Nakajima M, Akasaka Y, Fukumoto K, et al. Peroral cholangiopancreatosocopy (PCPS) under duodenoscopic guidance. Am J Gastroenterol 1976;66:241–7.

43. Komanduri S, Thosani N, Abu Dayyeh BK, et al. Cholangiopancreatoscopy. Gastrointest Endosc 2016;84:209–21.

44. Navaneethan U, Hasan MK, Kommaraju K, et al. Digital, single-operator cholangiopancreatoscopy in the diagnosis and management of pancreatobiliary disorders: a multicenter clinical experience (with video). Gastrointest Endosc 2016;84: 649–55.

45. Veld JV, ven Huijgevoort NCM, Boermeester MA, et al. A systematic review of advanced endoscopy-assisted lithotripsy for retained biliary tract stones: laser, electrohydraulic or extracorporeal shock wave. Endoscopy 2018;50:896–909.

46. Buxbaum J, Sahakian A, Ko C, et al. Randomized trial of cholangioscopy-guided laser lithotripsy versus conventional therapy for large bile duct stones (with videos). Gastrointest Endosc 2018;87:1050–60.

47. Angsuwatcharakon P, Kulpatcharapong S, Ridtitid W, et al. Digital cholangioscopy-guided laser versus mechanical lithotripsy for large bile duct stone removal after failed papillary large-balloon dilation: a randomized study. Endoscopy 2019;51:1066–73.

48. Bhandari S, Bathini R, Sharma A, et al. Usefulness of single-operator cholangioscopy-guided laser lithotripsy in patients with Mirizzi syndrome and cystic duct stones: experience at a tertiary care center. Gastrointest Endosc 2016;84:56–61.

49. Tsuyuguchi T, Sakai Y, Sugiyama H, et al. Long-term follow-up after peroral cholangioscopy-directed lithotripsy in patients with difficult bile duct stones, including Mirizzi syndrome: an analysis of risk factors predicting stone recurrence. Surg Endosc 2011;25:2179–85.

50. Deprez PH, Garces Duran R, Moreels T, et al. The economic impact of using single-operator cholangioscopy for the treatment of difficult bile duct stones and diagnosis of indeterminate bile duct strictures. Endoscopy 2018;50:109–18.

51. Dumonceau J-M, Kapral C, Aabakken L, et al. ERCP-related adverse events: European Society of Gastrointestinal Endoscopy (ESGE) Guideline. Endoscopy 2020;52:127–49.

52. Lee SH, Park JK, Yoon WJ, et al. How to predict the outcome of endoscopic mechanical lithotripsy in patients with difficult bile duct stones? Scand J Gastroenterol 2007;42:1006–10.

53. Cipolletta L, Costamagna G, Bianco MA, et al. Endoscopic mechanical lithotripsy of difficult common bile duct stones. Br J Surg 1997;84:1407–9.

54. Chang W-H, Chu C-H, Wang T-E, et al. Outcome of simple use of mechanical lithotripsy of difficult common bile duct stones. World J Gastroenterol 2005;11: 593–6.

55. Kuo Y-T, Wang H-P, Chang C-Y, et al. Comparable long-term outcomes of 1-minute vs 5-minute endoscopic papillary balloon dilation for bile duct stones. Clin Gastroenterol Hepatol 2017;15:1768–75.

56. Thomas M, Howell DA, Carr-Locke D, et al. Mechanical lithotripsy of pancreatic and biliary stones: complications and available treatment options collected from expert centers. Am J Gastroenterol 2007;102:1896–902.
57. Sauerbruch T, Holl J, Sackmann M, et al. Fragmentation of bile duct stones by extracorporeal shock-wave lithotripsy: a five-year experience. Hepatology 1992;15:208–14.
58. Cecinato P, Fuccio L, Azzaroli F, et al. Extracorporeal shock wave lithotripsy for difficult common bile duct stones: a comparison between 2 different lithotripters in a large cohort of patients. Gastrointest Endosc 2015;81:402–9.
59. Ellis RD, Jenkins AP, Thompson RP, et al. Clearance of refractory bile duct stones with extracorporeal shockwave lithotripsy. Gut 2000;47:728–31.
60. Di Giorgio P, Manes G, Grimaldi E, et al. Endoscopic plastic stenting for bile duct stones: stent changing on demand or every 3 months. A prospective comparison study. Endoscopy 2013;45:1014–7.
61. Horiuchi A, Nakayama Y, Kajiyama M, et al. Biliary stenting in the management of large or multiple common bile duct stones. Gastrointest Endosc 2010;71: 1200–3.e2.
62. Cerefice M, Sauer B, Javaid M, et al. Complex biliary stones: treatment with removable self-expandable metal stents: a new approach (with videos). Gastrointest Endosc 2011;74:520–6.
63. Hartery K, Lee CS, Doherty GA, et al. Covered self-expanding metal stents for the management of common bile duct stones. Gastrointest Endosc 2017;85:181–6.
64. Dumonceau J-M, Tringali A, Papanikolaou IS, et al. Endoscopic biliary stenting: indications, choice of stents, and results: European Society of Gastrointestinal Endoscopy (ESGE) Clinical Guideline - Updated October 2017. Endoscopy 2018;50:910–30.
65. Bekkali NLH, Murray S, Winter L, et al. The role of multidisciplinary meetings for benign pancreatobiliary diseases: a tertiary centre experience. Frontline Gastroenterol 2017;8:210–3.
66. Terruzzi V, Radaelli F, Meucci G, et al. Is the supine position as safe and effective as the prone position for endoscopic retrograde cholangiopancreatography? A prospective randomized study. Endoscopy 2005;37:1211–4.
67. Boerma D, et al. Wait-and-see policy or laparoscopic cholecystectomy after endoscopic sphincterotomy for bile-duct stones: a randomised trial. Lancet (London, England) 2002;360:761–5.
68. Reinders JSK, Gouma DJ, Heisterkamp J, et al. Laparoscopic cholecystectomy is more difficult after a previous endoscopic retrograde cholangiography. HPB (Oxford) 2013;15:230–4.
69. Han J, Moon JH, Koo HC, et al. Effect of biliary stenting combined with ursodeoxycholic acid and terpene treatment on retained common bile duct stones in elderly patients: a multicenter study. Am J Gastroenterol 2009;104:2418–21.
70. Katsinelos P, Kountouras J, Paroutoglou G, et al. Combination of endoprostheses and oral ursodeoxycholic acid or placebo in the treatment of difficult to extract common bile duct stones. Dig Liver Dis 2008;40:453–9.
71. Lee TH, Han J-H, Kim HJ, et al. Is the addition of choleretic agents in multiple double-pigtail biliary stents effective for difficult common bile duct stones in elderly patients? A prospective, multicenter study. Gastrointest Endosc 2011; 74:96–102.

Percutaneous Biliary Interventions

Clinical Indications, Comparative Effectiveness, Technical Considerations, Complications, and Outcomes

Nima Hafezi-Nejad, MD, Robert P. Liddell, MD*

KEYWORDS

- Percutaneous biliary interventions • Percutaneous transhepatic cholangiogram
- External biliary drain • Percutaneous biliary endoscopy

KEY POINTS

- Percutaneous biliary interventions are commonly performed by interventional radiologists for diagnostic evaluation and treatment of various hepatobiliary disorders.
- Indications, effectiveness, technical considerations, complications, and outcomes of percutaneous biliary interventions are discussed.
- Percutaneous brush and forceps biopsies often aid when imaging findings and endoscopic means of tissue diagnosis are equivocal.
- Percutaneously placed external biliary drains and stents can be used for both benign and malignant biliary strictures.
- Percutaneous biliary endoscopy is increasingly being used by interventional radiologists to help diagnose and treat biliary pathology.

INTRODUCTION

Percutaneous biliary interventions (PBIs) are commonly performed by interventional radiologists for diagnostic evaluation and treatment of various hepatobiliary disorders.[1,2] PBIs can be categorized into 2 main groups: (1) percutaneous transhepatic cholangiography (PTC) and percutaneous biliary drainage (PBD), (2) percutaneous cholecystostomy (PC) and biliary endoscopy.

Division of Vascular and Interventional Radiology, Department of Radiology and Radiological Sciences, Johns Hopkins School of Medicine, 1800 Orleans Street, Sheik Zayed Tower, Suite 7203, Baltimore, MD 21287, USA
* Corresponding author.
E-mail address: rliddel1@jhmi.edu

Gastrointest Endoscopy Clin N Am 32 (2022) 493–505
https://doi.org/10.1016/j.giec.2022.02.005
1052-5157/22/© 2022 Elsevier Inc. All rights reserved.

In this narrative review, we overview common clinical indications, technical considerations, complications, and outcomes related to PBIs. We highlight the role of PBIs in relation to endoscopic and surgical techniques and provide a detailed evaluation of outcomes in transplant patients.

CLINICAL INDICATIONS

PTC/PBD is commonly performed for benign and malignant biliary obstruction of intrahepatic and extrahepatic bile ducts.[3–5] Management of biliary leaks, cholangitis, and biopsy of the biliary tree are other common indications.[6] Malignant causes of biliary obstruction are commonly due to metastases, hepatocellular carcinoma, and cholangiocarcinoma (CC).[7] In patients with metastatic disease, PTC/PBD can be of therapeutic and prognostic value. Liver is the second most common site for solid organ metastasis. In several malignancies, including colorectal and neuroendocrine malignancies, liver disease can be a cause of death. Thus, optimal biliary drainage and preservation of liver function can improve long-term outcomes.[8] Moreover, adequate biliary drainage may be necessary before systemic and locoregional treatment in oncologic patients. The most common non-neoplastic and benign disorders requiring PTC/PBD include biliary stones, infectious (ie, cholangitis), and inflammatory disorders of the biliary tree.[6]

PERCUTANEOUS TRANSHEPATIC CHOLANGIOGRAPHY/PERCUTANEOUS BILIARY DRAINAGE VERSUS MAGNETIC RESONANCE CHOLANGIOPANCREATOGRAPHY AND ENDOSCOPIC RETROGRADE CHOLANGIOPANCREATOGRAPHY

Owing to advances in MRI techniques, resulting in shorter acquisition times with greater contrast and spatial resolution, PTC/PBD is usually reserved for patients requiring therapeutic intervention in addition to diagnostic evaluation. Magnetic resonance cholangiopancreatography (MRCP) protocols with heavily T2-weighted sequences have obviated the need for intravenous gadolinium contrast administration and provide a noninvasive alternative to PTC/PBD with superior diagnostic accuracy.[9,10] PTC/PBD can be of diagnostic value when results from MRCP and endoscopic retrograde cholangiopancreatography (ERCP) are indeterminate. For therapeutic purposes, ERCP provides a less invasive approach to biliary drainage through the natural orifice with lower periprocedural complication rates. However, the efficacy of ERCP may be limited for intrahepatic biliary drainage and when cannulation of the sphincter of Oddi is not possible. Overall, 10% to 20% of patients may have difficult biliary cannulation in ERCP requiring multiple attempts using several advanced endoscopic techniques.[11] Moreover, patients with altered anatomy like gastrojejunostomy or hepaticojejunostomy (HJ) may not be candidates for ERCP. Depending on availability and institutional preference, a wide range of alternatives may be pursued including laparoscopy-assisted ERCP, balloon-assisted enteroscopy, endoscopic ultrasound (EUS)-directed transgastric ERCP, laparoscopic common bile duct exploration, or EUS-guided intrahepatic puncture. Finally, when less invasive methods fail, PTC/PBD and rendezvous guidewire-associated ERCP are pursued as the last resort before surgical intervention.[12,13]

PERCUTANEOUS TRANSHEPATIC CHOLANGIOGRAPHY/PERCUTANEOUS BILIARY DRAINAGE VERSUS ENDOSCOPIC ULTRASOUND–GUIDED DRAINAGE

Several prior studies have compared the technical and clinical success as well as adverse events and reintervention rates between EUS-guided drainage and

PTC/PBD.[14,15] EUS-guided drainage and PTC/PBD are alternative methods of biliary drainage when ERCP fails.[16] In patients with distal biliary obstruction and comparable baseline demographics and similar etiology of biliary obstruction, both EUS-guided drainage and PTC/PBD are highly successful in relieving the obstruction (100% vs 97%). Nevertheless, EUS-guided drainage is associated with higher clinical success (85% vs 62%) and lower rates of postprocedural adverse events (14% vs 29%). EUS-guided drainage is associated with remarkably lower rates of reintervention (11% vs 78%), most importantly in patients with a life expectancy of more than 50 days. Overall, although both EUS-guided drainage and PTC/PBD are effective methods, EUS-guided drainage has a superior safety profile when it comes to procedural and overall adverse events.[15] Given the lack of prospective high-quality randomized clinical trials, further research is needed to provide a more granular comparative evaluation of EUS-guided drainage versus PTC/PBD.[16]

MANAGEMENT OF POSTOPERATIVE COMPLICATIONS AFTER HEPATOBILIARY SURGERY

Biliary obstruction and leaks are 2 of the most common postsurgical complications after hepatobiliary resections[17] and liver transplantation.[12] PTC/PBD can relieve the obstruction, bypass the area of stricture, and divert bile leaks. Clinical course and prognosis often depend on the underlying diagnosis, primary surgical procedure, and existing comorbidities.[6] When the etiology of obstruction or leak is procedure-related, usually in the setting of Whipple's procedure[18] or liver transplantation,[19] nonsurgical management with PTC/PBD for 3 to 6 months is the standard of care in our institution.

A multicenter analysis from the Society of Pediatric Liver Transplantation (SPLIT) registry found clinically significant biliary strictures in 4% to 12% of cases.[19] Left untreated, biliary strictures can lead to graft failure. However, stricture resolution was achieved in 96% of cases with isolated biliary stricture and graft survival was patent in 92% of cases in 3-year follow-up.[19] Compared with PTC/PBD, ERCP was more likely to result in optimal biliary outcome (75% vs 59%) and longer time intervals between procedures.[19] In a large single-center cohort study, 26% of pediatric liver transplantations had complications that were managed by interventional radiologists.[20] Most common complications included biliary strictures in 17.3% and bile leaks in 6.3%. Less common complications included biliary stones, iatrogenic obstruction, and vanishing syndrome. Although biliary complications are more common in the early posttransplantation period, some complications may arise several years after the original transplantation. Technical success with relatively low postprocedural complications was achieved in all cases. Similar figures were reported by other investigators and in adult populations. In a case series of 443 patients undergoing pancreaticoduodenectomy, 10% had clinical HJ stenosis associated with intrahepatic biliary dilatation.[18] A hepatic duct diameter of less than 8 mm was associated with a higher likelihood of HJ stricture. Most cases were successfully treated with endoscopic drainage (31 of 40). PTC/PBD and reanastomosis were pursued in the remaining cases.[18]

More recently, endoscopic balloon dilatation for benign HJ strictures has gained traction, with a technical success of more than 90% and 3- to 5-year patency of around 50%.[21–23] Similarly, benign HJ strictures treated with a 3-session protocol (3 consecutive balloon dilatation sessions following a fixed time interval) had a high rate of clinical success, long-term patency, as well as a clinical, biochemical, and radiological response.[24] In another series of 52 patients, benign HJ strictures treated with percutaneous biliary balloon dilatation had 87% and 70% patency in 1- and 5-year follow-ups.[25] Postsurgical complications after liver transplantation requiring reintervention under general anesthesia or advanced life support were the main predictors of HJ stricture recurrence.[25]

Although HJ is a more common method of biliary–bowel anastomosis, duct to duct anastomosis is an alternative method used in living donor liver transplantation.[26] In a series of 112 patients, multiple strictures requiring multiple drainage catheters were commonly needed after duct-to-duct anastomosis (in about 70% of patients). In the absence of hepatic artery stenosis, biliary drainage catheters were successfully removed in the majority of patients (95%) during an 8-month follow-up period. Although more than 85% of patients remained drain-free at the 1-year interval, about 32% of patients had recurrent biliary stricture, commonly in the setting of untreated isolated sectoral duct or concurrent bile leak.[26] For refractory biliary leaks persisting after long-lasting PBD, endoscopic or percutaneous injection of sclerosing agents and/or coiling can be useful. Novel investigative techniques incorporate microcatheter-mediated percutaneous or endoscopic argon plasma coagulation.[27]

PERCUTANEOUS TRANSHEPATIC CHOLANGIOGRAPHY/PERCUTANEOUS BILIARY DRAINAGE, BIOPSY, AND TISSUE DIAGNOSIS

Tissue sampling is often an essential component of the management of indeterminant biliary obstructions.[28] Brush cytology and intraductal biopsy are the 2 most common procedures that are performed during ERCP or PTC/PBD (**Fig. 1**). In peripheral and hilar strictures, the diagnostic yield of tissue sampling during ERCP can be markedly limited, and percutaneous sampling may be the only viable option. A meta-analysis

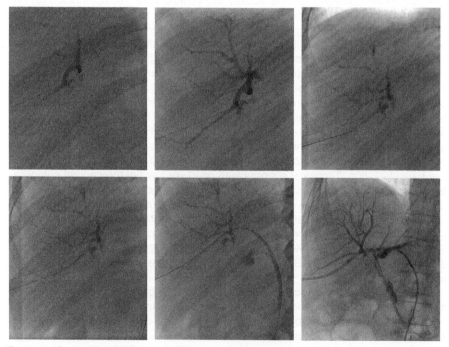

Fig. 1. Brush cytology device: cholangiogram showing filling defect at the hilum which was targeted for brush cytology sampling. Final cytology results were inconclusive.

of diagnostic accuracy studies conducted in 2015 revealed a sensitivity of 45% and 48% for percutaneous brush cytology and intraductal biopsy, respectively. When combined, the sensitivity may increase to up to 59%, whereas the specificity was typically greater than 99%.[28] Advances in interventional techniques and device development may have changed the paradigm in the past decade. A more recent meta-analysis of studies using forceps/clam-shell biopsy devices found sensitivity and specificity of 81% and 100%, respectively[29] (**Fig. 2**). The sensitivity was higher for intrinsic compressions (ie, CC, especially in the upper parts of the biliary tree[30]) and the minor and major complication rates were observed in 10% and 3% of cases, respectively. Biliary leak, hemobilia, and pneumoperitoneum were some of the most common complications after forceps biopsy.[30] Biopsy devices with larger diameters (6 mm vs 4.5 mm) were able to provide superior samples with fewer passes and a similar risk of complications.[31]

Biopsy using cholangioscopy with direct visualization has been a topic of new studies. Although cholangioscopy-guided biopsy has a similar sensitivity to fluoroscopy-guided biopsy, the combination of the 2 techniques can increase the sensitivity to up to 80%.[32]

Percutaneous Transhepatic Cholangiography/Percutaneous Biliary Drainage–Related Complications

With technical advances in imaging and periprocedural care of interventional radiology patients, PTC/PBD is considered a safe and effective treatment with a relatively low rate of postprocedural complications. Common complications include bleeding, cholangitis, tube dislocation, pancreatitis, perforation, intra-abdominal abscess, and biloma.[33] Severity of complications can be classified as major (Clavien-Dindo I and II) or minor (Clavien-Dindo III and IV). In a large series of 599 patients, minor and major complications occurred in 19% and 4% of patients, respectively. The most common major complication was early drain dislocation requiring reintervention in 3% of cases. Only 1 case of death (0.2%) was reported in their series.[33] PTC/PBD-related complications were more frequent in a large series of 822 pancreatoduodenectomies.[17] Overall, 35% of patients had a procedure-related complication with cholangitis

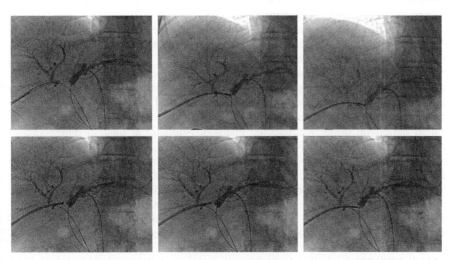

Fig. 2. Clamshell biopsy using a forceps device: cholangiogram showing filling defect at the hilum which was biopsied resulting in the diagnosis of cholangiocarcinoma.

(21%) and hemobilia (11%) being the most common complications. About 6% of patients required reintervention and 2 deaths (6%) were attributed to the procedure.[17]

Owing to the percutaneous nature of the PTC/PBD techniques, procedure-related complications are more common and more severe than ERCP and/or endoscopic techniques.[34] Bleeding is the most dreaded complication associated with PTC/PBD. Although prior studies were suggesting that right-sided drain placement (vs left side), more peripheral access site (vs central), and ultrasound (US) guidance may potentially decrease the risk of bleeding, a recent meta-analysis found no significant difference with either of these variables.[35] Similarly, drain placement in a nondilated system was shown to have a risk of bleeding similar to dilated systems.[36] Overall, the risk of injury to the hepatic artery branches and hemobilia requiring transcatheter embolization is higher with left-sided drain placement.[37] The risk of intraperitoneal bile leak and duodenal injury were similar between PTC/PBD and endoscopic techniques while pancreatitis was more common after endoscopic drainage.[4] Overall complication rates, 30-day mortality, and long-term patency are likely to be determined by the underlying diagnosis, comorbidity profile, and patient's performance status.[7] From a practical standpoint in a clinical setting, other factors such as the location of the obstruction, purpose of drainage, and level of experience may dictate the desirable approach.[4]

A STEP-BY-STEP DESCRIPTION OF THE PROCEDURE

In the absence of a localized pathology, right-sided biliary drainage is commonly preferred due to a lower risk of bleeding due to the anterior position of the branches of the left hepatic artery. A peripheral side branch is commonly selected as the access site to the biliary tree. Peripheral access sites have a lower risk of bleeding and allow for optimal drainage of other side branches. Access to the right posterior biliary duct or a ventral branch of the left biliary tree is usually desired. Variability of the right posterior duct's anatomy can be of clinical importance. Special attention should be paid to the origin of the right posterior duct with regard to the left biliary duct and the cystic duct at the time of cholangiography and before drain placement. Finally, having a smooth curve without sharp turns can be essential for optimal drainage and to avoid complications at the time of tube exchange.

Advances in US imaging have significantly changed the common approach to PTC/PBD. Left-sided drains are commonly accessed with the help of US. Although right-sided drain placement can benefit from US evaluation, access to the biliary tree is commonly established under fluoroscopic guidance. From a lateral approach, horizontal to the floor with the patient's right arm placed inferiorly by an arm board, a 22-gauge needle is advanced superiorly and centrally. The inner stylet of the needle is then removed, and contrast is gently injected while retracting the needle, from central to peripheral under fluoroscopic imaging. Attention is paid to differences in contrast opacification of the hepatic veins, portal veins, and the biliary tree. Once a biliary duct is identified, the remainder of the biliary tree is opacified by continued contrast injection. If the access site is central, a two-stick approach is pursued to get second access into a more peripheral side branch (**Fig. 3**). Multiple adjustments by moving back and forth to an oblique projection may be necessary to achieve an accurate ventral/dorsal needle positioning. An oblique view can provide positioning information on the third plane that cannot be appreciated on anteroposterior views alone.

Next, a 0.018-inch wire is advanced to the biliary tree, the needle is removed and a skin incision is made. Using a triaxial introducer system, the 0.018 system is converted

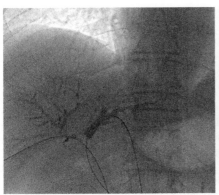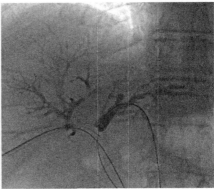

Fig. 3. Percutaneous biliary drain placement with "two-stick" method: the biliary tree is opacified on the first stick and accessed using a second needle.

to a 0.035 system. The inner portion of the triaxial introducer set is advanced to the peripheral biliary duct and then removed. The outer provides 0.035 access and can accommodate a Glide wire and 4-5F catheter. The catheter is advanced to the small bowel and the wire is exchanged for a stiff wire. The catheter and the triaxial introducer set are removed, and a biliary drain is advanced over a stiff wire. Previous studies have shown lower complication rates with drainage catheters that are 10F or smaller in size. The biliary drains may be destringed, preventing the locking mechanism of the tips from forming a knot when more than one biliary drain is placed.

PERCUTANEOUS BILIARY DRAINAGE

An external biliary drain (EBD), or anchor, is a drainage catheter that terminates within the biliary system above a tight biliary stricture or obstruction. The EBD is most often connected to an external drainage bag and most often placed in the setting of: (1) an obstruction which cannot be crossed on initial attempt, (2) a cholangitic patient in which significant catheter manipulation may further cause clinical deterioration, (3) a biliary stricture had been relieved, via surgical bypass or stent placement, and a drain may be left in place to initiate a clinical trial. An internal/external biliary drain (IEBD) is a catheter with multiple side holes above and below the level of obstruction to allow for both internal and external drainage, often with a locking distal loop positioned in the bowel. Side holes placed above and below the obstruction allow bile to drain into the bowel when the drain is capped externally. Serial upsizing of IEBD allows for better bile drainage and patency rates in benign strictures after the drain is removed. In benign disease states (postoperative anastomotic strictures), IEBDs are often left in place for 3 to 6 months with exchanges occurring every 6 to 8 weeks to prevent clogging and cholangitis.

PERCUTANEOUS BILIARY STENTS

Percutaneous biliary stents (PBS) are indicated in patients with malignant strictures with a limited life expectancy (<9 months), or in patients with no other option. The mean stent patency for malignant stricture is 8.5 months.[38] These stents may be bare-metal stents or covered. Closed-cell bare-metal stents (Wallstent, Boston Scientific, Marlborough, MA) have been shown to slow the ingrowth of tumors through the stent interstices, like covered stents (Viabil, Gore Medical, Flagstaff, AR; WallFlex Biliary RX Stent, Boston Scientific). Stents placed for benign strictures are most often covered metallic stents as they are more easily removed compared with bare-metal stents (**Fig. 4**).

PERCUTANEOUS CHOLECYSTOSTOMY AND BILIARY ENDOSCOPY

PC is a minimally invasive procedure that is commonly used in patients with cholecystitis who are not candidates for surgical cholecystectomy.[39] Percutaneous biliary endoscopy, including cholecystoscopy, choledochoscopy, and cholangioscopy, can be used for direct visualization of the biliary tree and provide percutaneous access for biliary interventions (**Fig. 5**). Interventions like tissue biopsy, lithotripsy, stone removal, as well as stent placement and removal, are usually performed under moderate sedation and are deemed to be safer than surgical alternatives in patients with multiple comorbidities.[39,40] The Tokyo guidelines for acute cholangitis and cholecystitis provide validity-tested diagnostic criteria and severity grading system that has been adopted globally in the past two decades.[41,42] The timing of the procedure depends on the severity of the presentation and patients' clinical condition.

First, percutaneous access to the biliary system (usually the gallbladder) is established via standard technique. This is followed by drain upsize in a 3- to 6-week period, allowing the passage of endoscopic instruments. Lithotripsy and stone removal is

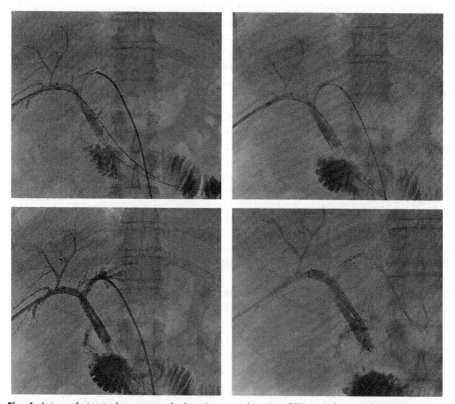

Fig. 4. Internal stent placement: cholangiogram showing filling defect at the hilum. Given limited life expectancy, patient preference, and potential for improved quality of life, the decision was made to place bilateral bare-metal stents centered over the area of obstruction. Measurements of length were performed using a marker catheter and stents were deployed consecutively.

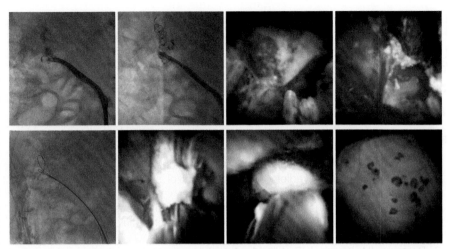

Fig. 5. Percutaneous cholecystostomy and biliary endoscopy: contrast injection through percutaneous cholecystostomy catheter showing several stones in the gallbladder preventing the pigtail tip of the catheter to form. Catheter is exchanged with a sheath and contrast injection shows the stones to a better advantage. The cystic duct was only partially visualized. Cholangioscopy was performed showing gallstones and inflammatory changes of the mucosa followed by stone retrieval using a basket device.

effective in reducing the risk of systemic infection and improving patients' quality of life.[43,44] The technical process has improved and has become more accessible by the use of single-use endoscopes in the past few years.[45] In addition to diagnosis and treatment of cholelithiasis, percutaneous biliary endoscopy can be useful in the identification and biopsy of biliary neoplasms and providing symptomatic relief in stone-mimicking pathologies.[43] Percutaneous biliary endoscopy is a viable alternative when conventional ERCP and/or PTC/PBD procedures fail.[46] Given its potential, percutaneous biliary endoscopy can add a new dimension to fluoroscopic guided procedures performed by interventional radiologists and is underutilized in clinical practice to date.[44]

SUMMARY

PBIs consist of PTC/PBD, PC, and biliary endoscopy and can be accompanied by a variety of procedures that can aid in clinical problem-solving in patients with biliary infections, strictures, leaks, and postoperative complications. PBIs have high technical and clinical success rates and are relatively safe when compared with more invasive surgical techniques.

CLINICS CARE POINTS

- When MRCP and ERCP are indeterminate for diagnosis of biliary stricture, percutaneous transhepatic cholangiography may offer both diagnostic and therapeutic benefits.
- When an ERCP placed stent is not technically feasible, a percutaneously placed biliary stent placement may offer relief of malignant biliary obstruction in patients whose life expectancy is less than 9 months.

> • When a patient with cholelithiasis is not a surgical candidate, one should consider percutaneous biliary endoscopy and lithotripsy after a cholecystostomy drain has been placed.

DISCLOSURE

The authors have nothing to disclose.

REFERENCES

1. Expert Panel on Interventional R, Fairchild AH, Hohenwalter EJ, et al. ACR appropriateness criteria((r)) radiologic management of biliary obstruction. J Am Coll Radiol 2019;16:S196–213.
2. Hatzidakis A, Venetucci P, Krokidis M, et al. Percutaneous biliary interventions through the gallbladder and the cystic duct: what radiologists need to know. Clin Radiol 2014;69:1304–11.
3. Peregrin JH, Kovac J, Prchlik M, et al. Interventional radiological treatment of paediatric liver transplantation complications. Cardiovasc Intervent Radiol 2020;43(5):765–74.
4. Duan F, Cui L, Bai Y, et al. Comparison of efficacy and complications of endoscopic and percutaneous biliary drainage in malignant obstructive jaundice: a systematic review and meta-analysis. Cancer Imaging 2017;17:27.
5. O'Shea SJ, Martin DF. Percutaneous removal of retained calculi from the abdomen. Cardiovasc Intervent Radiol 2003;26:81–4.
6. Hafezi-Nejad N, Bailey CR, Areda MA, et al. Characteristics and outcomes of percutaneous biliary interventions in the United States. J Am Coll Radiol 2021; 18:1059–68.
7. Liu JG, Wu J, Wang J, et al. Endoscopic biliary drainage versus percutaneous transhepatic biliary drainage in patients with resectable hilar cholangiocarcinoma: a systematic review and meta-analysis. J Laparoendosc Adv Surg Tech A 2018;28:1053–60.
8. Mahnken AH, Pereira PL, de Baere T. Interventional oncologic approaches to liver metastases. Radiology 2013;266:407–30.
9. Garg B, Rastogi R, Gupta S, et al. Evaluation of biliary complications on magnetic resonance cholangiopancreatography and comparison with direct cholangiography after living-donor liver transplantation. Clin Radiol 2017;72:518.e9–15.
10. Shanmugam V, Beattie GC, Yule SR, et al. Is magnetic resonance cholangiopancreatography the new gold standard in biliary imaging? Br J Radiol 2005;78: 888–93.
11. Dalal A, Gandhi C, Patil G, et al. Safety and efficacy of different techniques in difficult biliary cannulation at endoscopic retrograde cholangiopancreatography. Hosp Pract 1995;2022:1–7.
12. Karatoprak S, Kutlu R, Karatoprak NB, et al. Percutaneous radiological biliary interventions after failed endoscopic treatment in living liver donors: experience of a high-volume transplantation center. Transpl Int 2021;34:2846–55.
13. Connell M, Sun WYL, Mocanu V, et al. Management of choledocholithiasis after Roux-en-Y gastric bypass: a systematic review and pooled proportion meta-analysis. Surg Endosc 2022;PMID:35041054. https://doi.org/10.1007/s00464-022-09018-y.
14. Sawas T, Bailey NJ, Yeung K, et al. Comparison of EUS-guided choledochoduodenostomy and percutaneous drainage for distal biliary obstruction: a multicenter

cohort study. Endosc Ultrasound 2022;35102902. https://doi.org/10.4103/EUS-D-21-00031.

15. Hayat U, Bakker C, Dirweesh A, et al. EUS-guided versus percutaneous transhepatic cholangiography biliary drainage for obstructed distal malignant biliary strictures in patients who have failed endoscopic retrograde cholangiopancreatography: a systematic review and meta-analysis. Endosc Ultrasound 2022; 11(1):4–16.

16. Wang Y, Lyu Y, Li T, et al. Comparing outcomes following endoscopic ultrasound-guided biliary drainage versus percutaneous transhepatic biliary drainage for malignant biliary obstruction: a systematic review and meta-analysis. J Laparoendosc Adv Surg Tech A 2021;PMID:34677099. https://doi.org/10.1089/lap.2021.0587.

17. Henry AC, Smits FJ, van Lienden K, et al. Biliopancreatic and biliary leak after pancreatoduodenectomy treated by percutaneous transhepatic biliary drainage. Oxford: HPB; 2021.

18. Yamaki S, Satoi S, Yamamoto T, et al. Risk factors and treatment strategy for clinical hepatico-jejunostomy stenosis defined with intrahepatic bile duct dilatation after pancreaticoduodenectomy: a retrospective study. J Hepatobiliary Pancreat Sci 2021;PMID:34882986. https://doi.org/10.1002/jhbp.1095.

19. Valentino PL, Wang T, Shabanova V, et al. North American biliary stricture management strategies in children after liver transplantation: a multicenter analysis from the society of pediatric liver transplantation (SPLIT) registry. Liver Transpl 2021;PMID:34837468. https://doi.org/10.1002/lt.26379.

20. Dulcetta L, Marra P, Carbone FS, et al. Biliary complications in pediatric liver transplantation: findings of percutaneous transhepatic cholangiography in a large single-center cohort. Pediatr Radiol 2022;PMID:35107594. https://doi.org/10.1007/s00247-021-05278-3.

21. Sato T, Kogure H, Nakai Y, et al. Double-balloon endoscopy-assisted treatment of hepaticojejunostomy anastomotic strictures and predictive factors for treatment success. Surg Endosc 2020;34:1612–20.

22. Mizukawa S, Tsutsumi K, Kato H, et al. Endoscopic balloon dilatation for benign hepaticojejunostomy anastomotic stricture using short double-balloon enteroscopy in patients with a prior Whipple's procedure: a retrospective study. BMC Gastroenterol 2018;18:14.

23. Tomoda T, Kato H, Miyamoto K, et al. Comparison between endoscopic biliary stenting combined with balloon dilation and balloon dilation alone for the treatment of benign hepaticojejunostomy anastomotic stricture. J Gastrointest Surg 2020;24:1352–8.

24. Czerwonko ME, Huespe P, Mazza O, et al. Percutaneous biliary balloon dilation: impact of an institutional three-session protocol on patients with benign anastomotic strictures of hepatojejunostomy. Dig Surg 2018;35:397–405.

25. Oggero AS, Bruballa RC, Huespe PE, et al. percutaneous balloon dilatation for hepaticojejunostomy stricture following paediatric liver transplantation: long-term results of an institutional "Three-Session" protocol. Cardiovasc Intervent Radiol 2021;45(3):330–6.

26. Lee IJ, Lee JH, Kim SH, et al. Percutaneous transhepatic treatment for biliary stricture after duct-to-duct biliary anastomosis in living donor liver transplantation: a 9-year single-center experience. Eur Radiol 2022;32(4):2414–25.

27. Perez Lafuente M, Camacho Oviedo JA, Diez Miranda I, et al. Percutaneous or endoscopic treatment of peripheral bile duct leaks: initial experience with an

innovative approach of microcatheter-delivered argon plasma coagulation. Cardiovasc Intervent Radiol 2022;45(3):365–70.

28. Navaneethan U, Njei B, Lourdusamy V, et al. Comparative effectiveness of biliary brush cytology and intraductal biopsy for detection of malignant biliary strictures: a systematic review and meta-analysis. Gastrointest Endosc 2015;81:168–76.

29. Jeon TY, Choi MH, Yoon SB, et al. Systematic review and meta-analysis of percutaneous transluminal forceps biopsy for diagnosing malignant biliary strictures. Eur Radiol 2022;32:1747–56.

30. Fohlen A, Bazille C, Menahem B, et al. Transhepatic forceps biopsy combined with biliary drainage in obstructive jaundice: safety and accuracy. Eur Radiol 2019;29:2426–35.

31. Wu ZY, Jiao DC, Guo FF, et al. Treatment of biliary stenosis using percutaneous transhepatic cholangiobiopsy with biopsy forceps of varying diameter. Quant Imaging Med Surg 2022;12:207–14.

32. Sekine K, Yasuda I, Doi S, et al. Peroral cholangioscopy-guided targeted biopsy versus conventional endoscopic transpapillary forceps biopsy for biliary stricture with suspected bile duct cancer. J Clin Med 2022;11(2):289.

33. Kokas B, Szijarto A, Farkas N, et al. Percutaneous transhepatic drainage is safe and effective in biliary obstruction-a single-center experience of 599 patients. PLoS One 2021;16:e0260223.

34. Zhao XQ, Dong JH, Jiang K, et al. Comparison of percutaneous transhepatic biliary drainage and endoscopic biliary drainage in the management of malignant biliary tract obstruction: a meta-analysis. Dig Endosc 2015;27:137–45.

35. Lee YT, Yen KC, Liang PC, et al. Procedure-related risk factors for bleeding after percutaneous transhepatic biliary drainage: a systematic review and meta-analysis. J Formos Med Assoc 2021;PMID:34903432. https://doi.org/10.1016/j.jfma.2021.11.013.

36. Pedersoli F, Schroder A, Zimmermann M, et al. Percutaneous transhepatic biliary drainage (PTBD) in patients with dilated vs. nondilated bile ducts: technical considerations and complications. Eur Radiol 2021;31:3035–41.

37. Rivera-Sanfeliz GM, Assar OS, LaBerge JM, et al. Incidence of important hemobilia following transhepatic biliary drainage: left-sided versus right-sided approaches. Cardiovasc Intervent Radiol 2004;27:137–9.

38. Thornton RH, Frank BS, Covey AM, et al. Catheter-free survival after primary percutaneous stenting of malignant bile duct obstruction. AJR Am J Roentgenol 2011;197:W514–8.

39. Ahmed S, Schlachter TR, Hong K. Percutaneous transhepatic cholangioscopy. Tech Vasc Interv Radiol 2015;18:201–9.

40. Venbrux AC, McCormick CD. Percutaneous endoscopy for biliary radiologic interventions. Tech Vasc Interv Radiol 2001;4:186–92.

41. Nagino M, Takada T, Kawarada Y, et al. Methods and timing of biliary drainage for acute cholangitis: Tokyo guidelines. J Hepatobiliary Pancreat Surg 2007;14:68–77.

42. Yokoe M, Hata J, Takada T, et al. Tokyo Guidelines 2018: diagnostic criteria and severity grading of acute cholecystitis (with videos). J Hepatobiliary Pancreat Sci 2018;25:41–54.

43. Herr A, Collins D, White M, et al. Percutaneous biliary endoscopy for stones. Tech Vasc Interv Radiol 2019;22:127–34.

44. Srinivasa RN, Chick JFB, Cooper K, et al. Interventional radiology-operated endoscopy as an adjunct to image-guided interventions. Curr Probl Diagn Radiol 2019;48:184–8.

45. Pang S, England RW, Solomon A, et al. Single-use versus reusable endoscopes for percutaneous biliary endoscopy with lithotripsy: technical metrics, clinical outcomes, and cost comparison. J Vasc Interv Radiol 2021;PMID:34958859. https://doi.org/10.1016/j.jvir.2021.12.028.

46. Tejaswi S, Pillai RM, Grandhe S, et al. Disposable digital percutaneous cholangioscope-aided retrieval of a plastic biliary stent after failed retrieval at ERCP. VideoGIE 2021;6:413–5.

Endoscopic Ultrasound–Guided Biliary Interventions

Vinay Dhir, MD, FASGE*, Rahul Shah, MRCP, Priyanka Udawat, MD

KEYWORDS

- EUS • ERCP • Biliary drainage • Obstructive jaundice

KEY POINTS

- EUS-guided biliary drainage is an acceptable alternative at expert centers for patients with failed ERCP or altered surgical anatomy.
- EUS-BD allows biliary drainage into the stomach or duodenum depending on the procedure used
- Randomized studies have shown EUS-BD to have equivalent safety and efficacy to ERCP in patients with distal malignant biliary obstruction.
- A variety of EUS-BD procedures are described depending on the access and exit points of the stents.
- There is a learning curve, and these procedures should be attempted at expert pancreaticobiliary endoscopy centers.

INTRODUCTION

Endoscopic retrograde cholangiopancreatography (ERCP) is considered the gold standard for the management of biliary obstruction caused by bile duct stones or benign and malignant biliary strictures.[1-3] The success rate for ERCP has been quoted as more than 90%; however, this varies with expertise.[4] Should the ERCP fail, a repeat ERCP by a more experienced endoscopist at a high-volume center at an interval is suggested, provided there is no clinical emergency for biliary drainage, that is, cholangitis.[5] However, ERCP can be challenging even in expert hands because of the pathology encountered (gastric outlet obstruction, periampullary diverticulum, etc) or surgically altered anatomy (ie, Whipple, Roux en-Y gastric bypass, Billroth II surgery) and techniques such as double wire technique or precut sphincterotomy have been used in patients with difficult access.[6-8]

Alternative options for biliary drainage after the failure of ERCP include percutaneous transhepatic biliary drainage (PTBD), endoscopic ultrasound (EUS)-guided biliary drainage (EUS-BD), and surgical drainage[9-12] (**Table 1**). PTBD is widely available; however, complication rates have been estimated as high as 23%, including

Division of Endosonography, Institute of Digestive and Liver Care, SL Raheja Hospital-A Fortis Associate, Mumbai 400016, India
* Corresponding author.
E-mail address: vinaydhir@gmail.com

Gastrointest Endoscopy Clin N Am 32 (2022) 507–525
https://doi.org/10.1016/j.giec.2022.02.003
1052-5157/22/© 2022 Elsevier Inc. All rights reserved.

Table 1			
Various procedures for biliary drainage			
	PTBD	**ERCP**	**EUS-BD**
Access	Blind	Semiblind	Under vision
Difficult access	Rare	Relatively common	Rare
Access points	Liver	Papilla	Liver, duodenum
Stent placement	External/antegrade	Retrograde	Antegrade/Retrograde
Postsurgical anatomy Duodenal stenosis	Easy access	Difficult access	Easy access
Gall bladder	Easy access	Difficult access	Easy access

cholangitis, dislocation, or blocked catheters. PTBD is associated with higher morbidity, repeated procedures, and poor patient compliance.[13–15]

Wiersema and colleagues[16] described the first EUS-guided cholangiopancreatography in 1996 on patients who had failed ERCP. The world's first EUS-guided biliary drainage was published by Giovannini and colleagues[17] in 2001. Since then, several studies have been published proving its safety and efficacy.[18–21] EUS-BD is accepted as a safe and effective alternative for biliary drainage. The procedure is attractive as it can be performed via multiple routes, and access to papilla is not necessary. A variety of procedures are clubbed under EUS-BD, each with its own advantages.

INDICATIONS

EUS biliary interventions have been used for both benign and malignant indications, although most publications deal with malignant obstruction. The indications may broadly be classified depending on access to papilla.

Accessible Papilla

Failed ERCP (at an expert center), periampullary diverticulum, or neoplastic infiltration of the ampulla.

Inaccessible Papilla

Normal anatomy
Peptic duodenal strictures, malignant outlet obstructions, duodenal strictures from chronic pancreatitis.

Altered anatomy
Bariatric Roux-en Y gastric bypass surgery, Billroth II gastroenterostomy, Whipples surgery.

CONTRAINDICATIONS

Absolute contraindications would be tumor infiltration along the luminal surface and relative contraindications include massive ascites, coagulopathy, and lack of ductal dilatation.

TECHNIQUES

Currently, EUS-BD is used as a salvage technique for failed conventional ERCP, which could be due to anatomic constraints or the underlying pathology. The choice of EUS-BD depends on the indication for biliary drainage and operator preference.[22] There are 4 well-described techniques for performing EUS-BD: EUS-rendezvous (EUS-RV; **Fig. 1**), EUS-choledochoduodenostomy (EUS-CDS; **Fig. 2**), EUS-hepaticogastrostomy (EUS-HGS; **Fig. 3**), and EUS-antegrade (EUS-AG; **Fig. 4**). EUS-hepaticoduodenostomy (EUS-HDS) is not yet fully established. All the procedures essentially follow the same principles as described in the following sections other than the rendezvous procedure. With the advent of "Hot stent," EUS-BD may be performed as a single-step procedure.

Biliary Access

A therapeutic linear echoendoscope is used. The first step in biliary access is scope position, which is paramount to the success of the procedure. The scope position for CDS should be in the long/semilong loop in the duodenum looking toward the liver hilum, so as to ensure that the needle punctures in the axis of the bile duct. For HGS, the transgastric puncture is made after ascertaining the needle direction toward

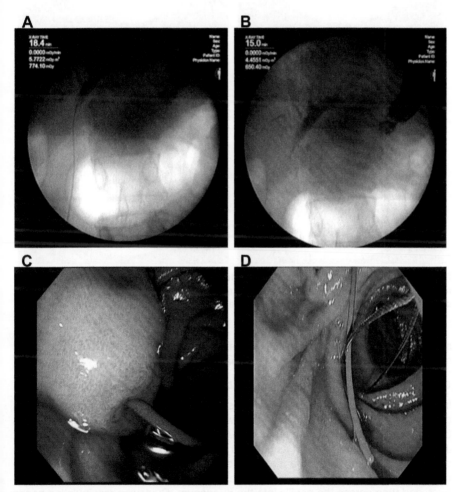

Fig. 1. EUS-Rendezvous procedure. (*A*) Transhepatic puncture with 19-gauge needle into the left duct. (*B*) Manipulation of the hydrophilic guidewire into the duodenum. (*C*) Guidewire seen extruding from the papilla with a side-viewing scope. (*D*) Guidewire retrieval with a snare.

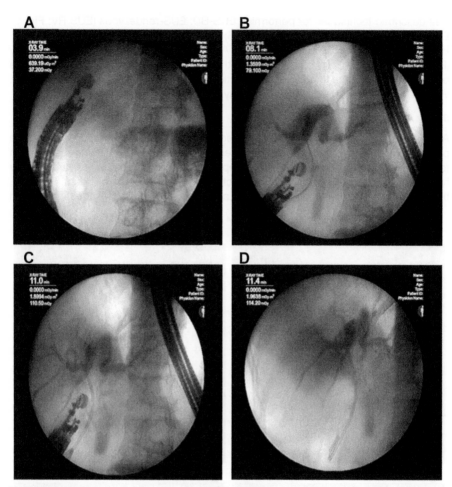

Fig. 2. EUS-Choledochoduodenostomy procedure. (*A*) Scope position for choledochoduode-nostomy. (*B*) Needle puncture and guidewire manipulation in the bile duct. (*C*) Plastic stent placement with the aid of fluoroscopy. (*D*) Final choledochoduodenostomy stent placement.

segment B2/B3 biliary radicles. A 19-gauge needle is used in most cases, although 22 gauge may be used in patients with minimally dilated ducts.

Guidewire Manipulation into the Desired Duct

In cases of HGS and antegrade procedures, dilated left hepatic ducts are targeted as close to the hilum as possible to aid guidewire manipulation usually in segment B3. A 0.032″J tip Terumo (Radiofocus, Inc, USA) or 0.025″Visiglide 2 (Olympus, Tokyo, Japan) is preferred because of its flexible hydrophilic tip, which can negotiate bends and tight strictures. Guidewire manipulation could be challenging in the antegrade procedure as the wire has to be negotiated across the hilum down into the bile duct, and then across the papilla into the duodenum. Guidewire manipulation needs experience and patience, but can be successfully performed in most patients. Trans-luminal procedures like CDS and HGS do not require complex guidewire manipula-tions. Wire shearing may occur if the manipulation is done too fast.

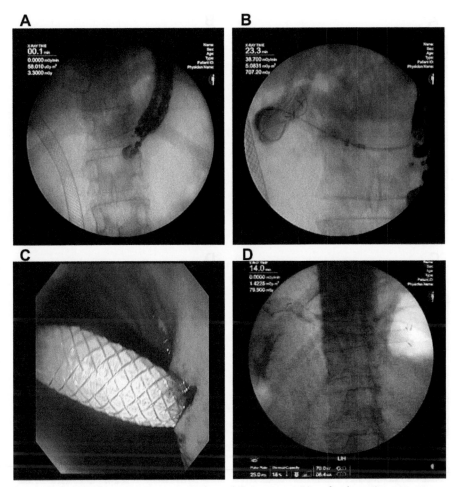

Fig. 3. EUS-Hepaticogastrostomy procedure. (A) Scope position for hepaticogastrostomy. (Note previously placed right-sided metal stent.) (B) Guidewire and cystotome manipulation within the left intrahepatic ducts. (C) EUS-Hepatico gastrostomy with Giobor stent placement in the stomach. (Note the long length in the stomach-covered portion.) (D) Hepaticogastrostomy Giobor stent placement as seen on fluoroscopy.

Tract Dilatation

After access has been secured with the guidewire in place, a 6-mm CRE biliary balloon or a 6-French cystotome is used to dilate the desired tract. Precut papillotomy or knife has been used, but has been shown to increase adverse events, as the cautery is not coaxial.

Stent Placement

Once the tract is dilated, a plastic or metal stent is inserted under endoscopy and fluoroscopy guidance. Our choice of stents is indicated in the chart (**Table 2**). There should be good coordination between the endoscopist and the gastrointestinal assistant, as the guidewire will need to be held tightly when the stent is traversing a tight stricture or an angulated duct.

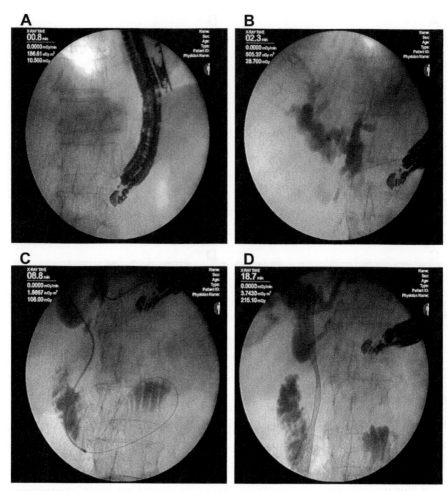

Fig. 4. EUS-Antegrade stenting procedure. (*A*) Scope position for antegrade puncture of intrahepatic ducts. (*B*) Antegrade puncture of the left ducts with contrast injection. (*C*) Antegrade wire manipulation into the duodenum and cystotome dilatation. (Note the contrast in the duodenal and jejunal loops to confirm the wire placement.) (*D*) Antegrade metal stent placement.

The hot stents have an inbuilt cautery device and the procedure of puncturing, dilatation, and stent placement is performed in a single step. This is usually easy when the bile duct is significantly dilated, but may be challenging in the minimally dilated bile duct, and a guidewire placement is advised in such situation to prevent injury to the opposite bile duct wall.

The rendezvous procedure can be attempted via the transgastric or transduodenal route. The position of the echoendoscope and direction of needle puncture are crucial to the success of the procedure. After needle puncture (transhepatic or transduodenal), a soft tip 0.032″ wire (Terumo or Visiglide 2) is passed and manipulated across the papilla into the duodenum (see **Fig. 1**). The echoendoscope is then withdrawn, leaving the guidewire in place under fluoroscopy control. A duodenoscope is inserted by the side of the guidewire, and cannulation is attempted either by the side of the wire

Table 2
Suggested stent choice for EUS-guided procedures

		Stent Type			
Procedure	Plastic	Uncovered Metal	Covered Metal	LAMS	Tubular
Rendezvous	✔	✔	✔	×	×
Transluminal CDS (CBD<15 mm)	?	×	✔	?	×
Transluminal CDS(CBD>15 mm)	?	×	✔	✔	×
Transluminal HGS	✔	×	?	×	✔
Antegrade	×	✔	×	×	×

coming out of the papilla (see **Fig. 1**) or if this does not succeed, the wire is pulled through the biopsy channel with the aid of a cannula through the duodenoscope, with the help of a snare (see **Fig. 1**) or a rat tooth forceps. ERCP is then completed in the usual way.

TECHNICAL TIPS AND TRICKS

Scope position is the key to various EUS-guided procedures (see **Figs. 1A, 2A, 3A,** and **4A**). A sharp needle with flexible and echo visible tip is preferred to target the duct. Although soft guide wires are a great boon to negotiate tight strictures, they can shear within the 19-gauge needle due to repeated to and fro movements within the biliary tract. This must be avoided as this will lead to a sheared wire within the duct and difficult subsequent fluoroscopic visualization. After the initial intended cannulation, it is imperative to change the wire to a kink-resistant stiff wire as this will aid tract dilatation and most importantly stent placement. Optimal saline flush of accessories is required as the wires are hydrophilic.

Coaxial instruments should only be used to safely dilate the tract. Cystotome seems to outscore balloon dilatation and precut knife in safety and gives a clean cut. Needle knives/papillotomy should be avoided because of lack of control and bleeding. The choice of stent and its placement must be deployed under utmost care with radiological and endoscopic guidance to prevent malpositioning of stents and subsequent complications. Care must be taken to visualize the proximal, middle, and distal markers before final deployment, and often the stent can be partially deployed within the scope to prevent inward migration. Lumen apposing stents offer good anchorage, low migration rates. With antegrade procedures, it is important to identify the papilla on fluoroscopy with contrast injection as the stent placement is purely fluoroscopy guided. The key in the rendezvous procedure is to get the wire past the papilla hence. If the duct is dilated beyond 15 mm, then wire manipulation can become tricky and care must be taken to puncture the bile duct near the ampulla with the needle facing in the downward fashion.

APPROACH AND CHOICE OF STENTS

Several algorithms are available regarding the choice of EUS-BD procedure. There is no significant difference in the success rate and adverse event rate of the various EUS-BD procedures in expert hands. In general, transpapillary approaches (rendezvous or antegrade stenting) are used first probably due to the comfort level of deploying a stent through the papilla and familiarity with the accessories in using conventional ERCP specific stents. Transluminal approaches are used if transpapillary procedures fail; however, as accessories evolve and experience of EUS-BD increases, this may change with time. A learning curve effect was also suggested by the cumulative experience of 101 salvage EUS procedures carried out at a single center after failed ERCP.[23] In another study by Vila and colleagues,[24] endoscopists with more than 500 EUS procedures had higher success rates than endoscopists who had performed fewer than 500 EUS procedures.

In a recent study, patients were divided based on cross-sectional imaging. If intrahepatic biliary radicals were dilated on imaging, an antegrade procedure was the first choice. If intrahepatic biliary radicals were not dilated, rendezvous procedure was the first choice. Transluminal procedures were used in the event of failure of transpapillary procedures (hepaticogastrostomy for dilated radicals, and choledochoduodenostomy for nondilated radicals).[25]

EUS-SPECIFIC STENTS

Traditional ERCP stents do not serve the purpose of EUS-guided transluminal stenting in all cases due to the length of the stent, no anchoring mechanism, and the chance of migration.

As the experience with interventional EUS increased, the specific requirements from stents became clear. The most important distinction was the need for a covered stent, full or partial, as EUS-guided stents need to traverse across organs like stomach, liver, jejunum, duodenum, bile duct, or gallbladder. In the absence of a covered stent, the probability of leaks between organs is high. The extent of covered portion was different in different organs. For example, hepaticogastrostomy needs long tubular stents with a distal uncovered portion in the intrahepatic ducts to prevent side branch obstruction, and fully covered portion between the liver capsule and stomach to prevent bile leak.[26,27]

The second issue was the stent length. Stents used in ERCP are usually 4 cm or longer. Such a long stent is not needed for many indications with EUS like choledochoduodenostomy, gastroenterostomy, or pancreatic fluid collection drainage. A short stent length like 1 to 2 cm is usually sufficient to bring the 2 walls close together.[26] A longer stent has a propensity to migration, as well as separation of the 2 anastomosed walls leading to bleeding and complications. The third issue was migration. As these stents do not traverse through any stricture or tumor, they can migrate easily. Thus antimigration mechanisms in the form of wide flanges or other anchoring mechanisms were needed. In a study by Umeda and colleagues,[28] newly designed plastic stent has been used for EUS-guided hepaticogastrostomy.

Several stents have been designed specific to EUS therapies, which have been summarized in **Tables 3** and **4**.

ADVERSE EVENT AND MANAGEMENT

alOutcomes and complications in EUS-BD have been well documented in sever large studies as summarized in **Table 5**.[21,23–25,29–40] EUS-BD has a similar profile of adverse events to ERCP. In a meta-analysis, an overall pooled rate of adverse events was 17.9%, the commonest being biliary leak and infection.[41] The pooled rate of biliary leaks was 4%, and the pooled rate of infection and stent migration was 3.8%.[42]

Bleeding

This is the most common adverse event, 10% to 15% of cases[43–45] largely prevented by checking the coagulation parameters before the procedure and puncturing with Doppler control. Bleeding is more with needle knives rather than coaxial instruments

Table 3
Comparative data of LAMS stents

Stent Type	Flange Diameter (mm)	Length (mm)	Catheter Diameter (French)	Lumen Apposing Force (Newton)	Studied Applications
AXIOS	6–20	8,10	10.8	2.29	GJ, CDS, PFC, GG, GBD
SPAXUS	8–16	20	10	1.76	PFC, GBD, GJ
NAGI	10–16	10,20,30	9,10	1.08	PFC, GBD
AIXSTENT	10–15	30	10	NA	PFC
PLUMBER	12–16	10,20,30	10.2	NA	PFC

like cystotome or balloon dilators. Bleeding is managed with usual endoscopic methods such as metallic clips, injection of epinephrine solution (1:10,000), and use of coagulation devices, balloon compression, and hemostatic spray powder. SEMS or LAMS can stop bleeding in the great majority of cases by sheer mechanical compression.

Perforation, Peritonitis

If identified, early intervention is necessary either with clip closure or placement of a new LAMS in the same place, provided the trajectory and site is identified. Even if closure is not possible generally conservative treatment with intravenous (IV) antibiotics, IV fluids, and NBM status heals most perforations.[29,46] Rarely in the presence of peritonitis, surgical intervention may be required.

Malpositioned Stent

Usually, rat tooth forceps are good enough to remove or reposition the stents. Malpositioned stents into the peritoneum usually need surgical intervention.

Cholangitis

Cholangitis reportedly occurs in 1.9% to 31.0% of patients undergoing EUS-guided drainage[45,47] and usually indicates partial drainage. An imaging study should be done to look for residual biliary system dilation. IV antibiotics should be administered. In some patients, particularly those with hilar obstruction, additional drainage may be needed.

Table 4
Comparative data of hybrid stents

Stent Type	Stent Diameter (mm)	Stent Covered Length (mm)	Stent Length (cm)	Catheter Diameter (French)	Studied Applications	Stent Type
Giobor	8,10	40,50	8,10	8.5	HGS	Giobor
Hanaro	10	30	8,10	8.5	HGS	Hanaro
Deus delivery premounted stent	6	35–85	5,10	7	HGS, CDS	Deus delivery premounted stent

Table 5
Outcome of EUS-BD in studies with greater than 50 patients

Study	No. Patients	Technical Success	Complications
Dhir et al[21]	104	97 (93.3%)	9 (8.6%)
Poincloux et al[23]	101	99 (98.0%)	12 (11.9%)
Vila et al[24]	106	73 (68.9%)	29 (27.3%)
Tyberg et al[25]	52	50 (96.2%)	5 (9.6%)
Park et al[29]	57	55 (96.5%)	22 (38.6%)
Khashab et al[30]	121	112 (92.6%)	20 (17.8%)
Dhir et al[31]	58	57 (98.3%)	2 (3.4%)
Kawakubo et al[32]	64	61 (95.3%)	12 (18.7%)
Gupta et al[33]	240	207 (86.2%)	81 (33.7%)
Cho et al[34]	54	54 (100%)	9 (16.7%)
Shah et al[35]	66	50 (75.7%)	6 (9.1%)
Kunda et al[36]	57	56 (98.2%)	4 (7.0%)
Khashab et al[37]	96	92 (95.8%)	10 (10.4%)
Minaga et al[38]	54	46 (85.1%)	10 (5.4%)
Will et al[39]	94	80 (85.1%)	15 (15.9%)
Paik et al[40]	64	60 (93.8%)	4 (6.3%)
Total	1520	1432 (87.2%)	266 (16.7%)

Bile Leak

Incidence of bile leaks in various studies have been shown in **Table-6**,[21,23–25,32–35,37–39,48] which often tend to cause self-limiting abdominal pain and provided there are no signs of peritonitis or sepsis can be managed conservatively with analgesics, IV antibiotics, and fluids. Choosing the right stent size and type is

Table 6
Incidence of bile leak in EUS-BD procedures

Author	Number of Patients	Bile Leak
Dhir et al[21]	104	3
Poincloux et al[23]	101	5
Vila et al[24]	125	6
Tyberg et al[25]	52	0
Kawakubo et al[32]	64	5
Gupta et al[33]	234	27
Shah et al[35]	88	1
Khashab et al[37]	96	3
Minaga et al[38]	54	1
Will et al[39]	94	0
Dhir et al[48]	68	4
Total	1115	55 (4.9%)

important to prevent bile leaks (see **Table 2**). Patients with significant bile leaks may need surgical intervention.

STENT OBSTRUCTION

The mean stent patency of EUS-BD is equivalent to that of ERCP, and has been summarized in **Table 7**.[34,37,49,50] Stents found blocked during follow-up may need additional therapy in the form of a plastic stent through the blocked stent or a fresh metal stent.

OUTCOMES

Comparative studies between EUS-BD and other techniques are primarily available for distal malignant obstruction.

In a recent systemic review and meta-analysis of EUS-BD versus ERCP, 9 studies involving 634 patients were included. There were no significant differences between the technical and clinical success of EUS-BD and ERCP-BD. EUS-BD was associated with significantly less reintervention versus ERCP-BD and regarding adverse events, the rates were similar for EUS-BD and ERCP-BD. There were no significant differences in the types of adverse events (stent occlusion, stent migration, stent dysfunction, and duration of stent patency) between the 2 techniques. EUS-BD was associated with lower reintervention rates compared with ERCP-BD, with comparable safety and efficacy outcomes[51]

EUS-BD versus PTBD

There is level 1 evidence for EUS-BD in the distal biliary malignant block. A recent systematic review and meta-analysis by Sharaiha and colleagues[41] included 9 studies comparing the efficacy and safety of EUS-BD and PTBD: 3 randomized controlled trials (RCTs) and 6 retrospective studies. EUS-BD and PTBD showed equivalent technical success. However, EUS-BD was associated with better clinical success, fewer postprocedure adverse events, and lower reintervention rates as shown in **Table 8**.[12,50,52–54] No significant differences were observed for the duration of hospital stay between EUS-BD and PTBD, but EUS-BD was more cost-effective. In another systemic review and meta-analysis, 20 independent cohort studies and 3 RCTs with a total of 1437 patients were included, which showed a calculated pooled rate of reintervention was 6.5%.[42] In another RCT, EUS-BD had similar outcomes and adverse events to ERCP for primary biliary decompression.[55]

EUS-BD versus ERCP

In a recent systemic review and meta-analysis, 9 studies (3 RCTs and 6 retrospective analyses) involving 634 patients were included. There were no significant differences

Table 7 Average stent patency of EUS-specific stents	
Author	**Stent Patency in Days**
Cho et al[34]	166 - HGS 329 - CDS
Khashab et al[37]	>365
Nakai et al[49]	255
Lee et al[50]	228

Table 8
Studies comparing EUS-BD versus PTBD

Author	Study Type	Study	Success	P Value	AE	P Value
Giovannini et al[12]	RCT	EUS[20]	19 (95%)	NS	11	
		PTBD[21]	17 (80.9%)		18	
Lee et al[50]	RCT	EUS (32)	32 (100%)	NS	3 (8.8%)	.022
		PTBD (34)	31 (91.1%)		10 (31.2%)	
Ginestet et al[52]	Retrospective	EUS[50]	49 (98.2%)	<.0001	(2.12%)	0.003
		PTBD[45]	41 (89.3%)		(22.7%)	
Huang et al[53]	Prospective	EUS[36]	29 (94.4%)	>0.05	(5.5%)	
		PTBD[30]	26 (86.6%)		(23.3%)	
Artifon et al[54]	RCT	EUS 13	13 (100%)	NS	2	
		PTBD 12	12 (100%)		3	

between EUS-BD and ERCP-BD in the technical and clinical success. There were no significant differences in the types of adverse events (stent occlusion, stent migration, stent dysfunction, and duration of stent patency) between the 2 techniques. EUS-BD was associated with lower reintervention rates compared with ERCP-BD, with comparable safety and efficacy outcomes.[51] Adverse events rates were similar for EUS-BD and ERCP-BD in various studies shown in **Table 9**.[21,32,40,55,56]

EUS-HGS and CDS

In a systemic review and meta-analysis published recently, 13 studies were included. This showed that EUS-CDS and EUS-HGS have comparable technical and clinical success rates, adverse events, and overall survival. However, EUS-CDS has less reintervention and stent obstruction.[57] In another systemic review, a total of 10 studies with 434 patients were included with similar outcomes. This showed that the technical success for CDS and HGS was 94.1% and 93.7%, respectively, and clinical success was 88.5% in CDS and 84.5% in HGS. There was no difference for adverse events[47]

In an international multicenter trial, both EUS-CDS and EUS-HG were effective and safe techniques for the treatment of distal biliary obstruction after failed ERCP. CDS was associated with shorter hospital stay, improved stent patency, and fewer procedure and stent-related complications.[30]

Table 9
Studies comparing EUS-BD versus ERCP

Author	Study Type	Study	Success	P Value	AE	P Value
Dhir et al[21]	Retrospective	EUS (104)	93.3%	NS	8.6	NS
		ERCP (104)	94.2%		8.6	
Kawakubo et al[32]	Retrospective	EUS[26]	96.2%	NS	26.9	NS
		ERCP[56]	98.2%		35.7	
Paik et al[40]	RCT	EUS[64]	93.8%	NS	6.3	P = 0.03
		ERCP[61]	90.2%		19.7	
Bang et al[55]	RCT	EUS[33]	90.9%	NS	21.2	NS
		ERP[34]	94.1%		14.7	
Park et al[56]	RCT	EUS[15]	93%	NS	-	NA
		ERCP[15]	100%		-	

EUS-Rendezvous

This procedure can be cumbersome but in cases where ERCP fails with an accessible ampulla in a potentially benign condition then it is an invaluable technique. There have been studies evaluating the technique itself,[58] rendezvous with short hydrophilic guidewire,[59] extrahepatic versus transhepatic route[60] and comparing it with precut papillotomy[31] suggestive of good outcomes. In a recent meta-analysis, 12 studies reporting a total of 342 patients were included. The pooled rates of technical success, clinical success, and overall adverse events were 86.1%, 80.8%, and 14%, respectively.[61]

EUS-BD with LAMS

LAMS stents have been a major advance in EUS-guided procedures. The main advantage is that their deployment is a single-step process that significantly shortens procedural time with lower adverse events. A recent meta-analysis examined 7 studies including 284 patients who underwent EUS-BD using LAMS after a failed ERCP. The pooled rates of technical success, clinical success, and postprocedure adverse events were 95.7%, 95.9%, and 5.2%, respectively.[62]

EUS-BD in Malignant Hilar Block

Malignant hilar block (MHO) is a challenging problem needing drainage of various segments of the liver to achieve clinical success. ERCP has been the standard of care with percutaneous biliary drainage as the rescue option. Recently, EUS-BD has been shown to be an alternative for MHO.

In one of the largest series of 30 patients by Minaga and colleagues, 40% had type IV block, 43.3% had type III block, and 16.6% had type II block.[63] Technical success was 96.6% and clinical success in those with technical success was 75.9%. In this series, 28 patients underwent EUS-HGS and 2 patients underwent EUS-HDS. Bismuth type IV block was the only factor associated with the clinical ineffectiveness of EUS-BD on multivariate analysis. Systemic review and meta-analysis is lacking. **Table 10** summarizes recent studies.[63–68]

EUS-Guided Stone Extraction

EUS-guided AG stone extraction is an alternative to enteroscopy-assisted ERCP in patients with altered anatomy. In EUS-AG stone extraction, biliary access is achieved

Table 10
EUS-guided biliary drainage in patients with malignant hilar block

Author	Patient Number	Technical Success	Clinical Success	Adverse Events	Reintervention Days
Minaga et al[63]	30	29/30 (96.6%)	22/29 (75.95)	3 - Early (10%) 7 - Late (23.3%)	NA
Bories et al[64]	11	10/11(90.9%)	10/11(90.9%)	3 (27.2%)	NA
Ogura et al[65]	11	11/11 (100%)	11/11 (100%)	0	NA
Ogura et al[66]	10	10/10 (100%)	9/10 (90%)	0	NA
Moryoussef et al[67]	18	17/18 (94.4%)	14/18 (72.2%)	3 (16.7%)	NA
Kongkam et al[68]	36	CERES 16/19 (84%)	CERES 15/18 (78.9%)	5/19 (26.3%)	92 d

Abbreviation: CERES, combined EUS and ERCP.

through the puncture of the left intrahepatic bile duct, followed by guidewire advancement through the ampulla into the duodenum. Then, balloon dilatation of the ampulla is performed, and stones are extracted with a balloon catheter. A plastic stent is placed in antegrade fashion through the ampulla. Intrahepatic duct dilatation is minimal in these cases and duct puncture, guidewire manipulation can be challenging. Large stones may not be amenable to extraction through the papilla, in which case a mechanical lithotripter, electrohydrolithotripsy, or spy cholangioscope may be needed in staged sessions. In these cases, a fistula is formed with either an HGS or CDS metal stent. In a recent study, the overall technical success of the creation of the hepatoenteric tract by EUS was 91.9% with modest adverse events were observed in 8.1%.[69] In a prospective study of 103 patients, the technical success was 96%, clinical success 100%, reintervention rates were 18%, and adverse events of 25%.[70]

Training in EUS-Guided Interventions

There are several studies involving training in EUS-guided biopsy but interventional EUS training is lacking because of the inadequate training facilities, low volumes even in tertiary centers, and no formal training program. However, with the training models like the "Mumbai EUS," "hybrid model (Mumbai Endoscopic Ultrasound II)" and the "EUS Magic Box" trainees can achieve competence in various interventional EUS procedures.[71–73] During the COVID-19 epidemic, virtual training courses have been trialed with good success.[74]

SUMMARY

EUS-BD has evolved as a safe viable technique for patients with failed ERCP and seems to have lower adverse events and similar technical and clinical success compared to PTBD. However, techniques and accessories need to be refined to tailor specifically to EUS-guided interventions.

CLINICS CARE POINTS

- Establishing a good echoendoscope position and maintaining it throughout the procedure is critical to the success of procedure
- Learning guidewire manipulation helps in procedures especially antegrade and rendezvous procedures
- A balloon dilator or a coaxial cautery dilator is preferred for track dilation
- It is advisable to deploy the final part of the stent within the echoendoscope for better control of the final stent position
- Early recognition of postprocedure adverse events and a backup interventional radiology or surgical team is essential for better outcomes

DISCLOSURE

The authors have nothing to disclose.

REFERENCES

1. Fogel EL, Sherman S, Devereaux B, et al. Therapeutic biliary endoscopy. Endoscopy 2003;35:156–63.
2. Carr-Locke DL. Overview of the role of ERCP in the management of diseases of the biliary tract and the pancreas. Gastrointest Endosc 2002;56:S157–60.

3. Schöfl R. Diagnostic endoscopic retrograde cholangiopancreatography. Endoscopy 2001;33:147–57.
4. Wani S, Han S, Simon V, et al. Setting minimum standards for training in EUS and ERCP: Results from a prospective multicenter study evaluating learning curves and competence among advanced endoscopy trainees. Gastrointest Endosc 2019;89:1160–8, e9.
5. Kumar S, Sherman S, Hawes RH, et al. Success and yield of second attempt ERCP. Gastrointest Endosc 1995;41:445–7.
6. Baron TH, Petersen BT, Mergener K, et al. Quality indicators for endoscopic retrograde cholangiopancreatography. Am J Gastroenterol 2006;101:892–7.
7. Enochsson L, Swahn F, Arnelo F, et al. Nationwide, population-based data from 11,074 ERCP procedures from the Swedish Registry for Gallstone Surgery and ERCP. Gastrointest Endosc 2010;72:1175–84.
8. Coté GA, Singh S, Bucksot LG, et al. Association between volume of endoscopic retrograde cholangiopancreatography at an academic medical center and use of pancreatobiliary therapy. Clin Gastroenterol Hepatol 2012;10:920–4.
9. Voegeli DR, Crummy AB, Weese JL. Percutaneous transhepatic cholangiography drainage, and biopsy in patients with malignant biliary obstruction: an alternative to surgery. Am J Surg 1985;150:243–7.
10. Sharaiha RZ, Kumta NA, Desai AP, et al. Endoscopic ultrasound-guided biliary drainage versus percutaneous transhepatic biliary drainage: predictors of successful outcome in patients who fail endoscopic retrograde cholangiopancreatography. Surg Endosc 2016;30:5500–5.
11. Holt BA, Hawes R, Hasan M, et al. Biliary drainage: role of EUS guidance. Gastrointest Endosc 2016;83:160–5.
12. Minaga K, Kitano M. Recent advances in endoscopic ultrasound-guided biliary drainage. Dig Endosc 2018;30:38–47.
13. Giovannini M, Napoleon B, Barthet M, et al. Multicenter randomized phase ii study: percutaneous biliary drainage vs eus guided biliary drainage. results of the intermediate analysis. Gastrointest Endosc 2015;81:AB174.
14. Oh HC, Lee SK, Lee TY, et al. Analysis of percutaneous transhepatic cholangioscopy-related complications and the risk factors for those complications. Endoscopy 2007;39:731–6.
15. Nennstiel S, Weber A, Frick G, et al. Drainage-related complications in percutaneous transhepatic biliary drainage: an analysis over 10 years. J Clin Gastroenterol 2015;49:764–70.
16. Wiersema MJ, Sandusky D, Carr R, et al. Endosonography-guided cholangiopancreatography. Gastrointest Endosc 1996;43:102–6.
17. Giovannini M, Moutardier V, Pesenti C, et al. Endoscopic ultrasound-guided bilioduodenal anastomosis: a new technique for biliary drainage. Endoscopy 2001;33:898–900.
18. Dhir V, Isayama H, Itoi T, et al. Endoscopic ultrasonography-guided biliary and pancreatic duct interventions. Dig Endosc 2017;29:472–85.
19. Itoi T, Dhir V, Moon JH. EUS-guided biliary drainage: moving into a new era of biliary drainage. Gastrointest Endosc 2017;85:915–7.
20. Dhir V, Khashab MA. EUS-guided biliary drainage: moving beyond the cliché of prime time. Endosc Ultrasound 2019;8(Suppl 1):S1–2.
21. Dhir V, Itoi T, Khashab MA, et al. Multicenter comparative evaluation of endoscopic placement of expandable metal stents for malignant distal common bile duct obstruction by ERCP or EUS-guided approach. Gastrointest Endosc 2015;81:913–23.

22. Boulay BR, Lo SK. Endoscopic ultrasound-guided biliary drainage. Gastrointest Endosc Clin N Am 2018;28:171–85.
23. Poincloux L, Rouquette O, Buc E, et al. Endoscopic ultrasound guided biliary drainage after failed ERCP: Cumulative experience of 101 procedures at a single center. Endoscopy 2015;47:794–801.
24. Vila JJ, Pérez-Miranda M, Vazquez-Sequeiros E, et al. Initial experience with EUS-guided cholangiopancreatography for biliary and pancreatic duct drainage: a spanish national survey. Gastrointest Endosc 2012;76:1133–41.
25. Tyberg A, Desai AP, Kumta NA, et al. EUS-guided biliary drainage after failed ERCP: a novel algorithm individualized based on patient anatomy. Gastrointest Endosc 2016;84:941–6.
26. Weilert F, Binmoeller KF. Specially designed stents for transluminal drainage. Gastrointest Interv 2015;4:40–5.
27. Mangiavillano B, Pagano N, Baron TH, et al. Biliary and pancreatic stenting: devices and insertion techniques in therapeutic endoscopic retrograde cholangio-pancreatography and endoscopic ultrasonography. World J Gastrointest Endosc 2016;8:143–56.
28. Umeda J, Itoi T, Tsuchiya T, et al. A newly designed plastic stent for EUS-guided hepaticogastrostomy: a prospective preliminary feasibility study (with videos). Gastrointest Endosc 2015;82:390–6.e2.
29. Park DH, Jang JW, Lee SS, et al. EUS-guided biliary drainage with transluminal stenting after failed ERCP: predictors of adverse events and long-term results. Gastrointest Endosc 2011;74:1276–84.
30. Khashab M, Messallam A, Penas I, et al. International multicenter comparative trial of transluminal EUS-guided biliary drainage via hepatogastrostomy vs. choledochoduodenostomy approaches. Endosc Int Open 2016;4:E175–81.
31. Dhir V, Bhandari S, Bapat M, et al. Comparison of EUS-guided rendezvous and precut papillotomy techniques for biliary access (with videos). Gastrointest Endosc 2012;75:354–9.
32. Kawakubo K, Isayama H, Kato H, et al. Multicenter retrospective study of endoscopic ultrasound-guided biliary drainage for malignant biliary obstruction in Japan. J Hepatobiliary Pancreat Sci 2014;21:328–34.
33. Gupta K, Perez-Miranda M, Kahaleh M, et al. Endoscopic ultrasound-assisted bile duct access and drainage: multicenter, long-term analysis of approach, outcomes, and complications of a technique in evolution. J Clin Gastroenterol 2014; 48:80–7.
34. Cho DH, Lee SS, Oh D, et al. Long term outcomes of a newly developed hybrid metal stent for EUS-guided biliary drainage (with videos). Gastrointest Endosc 2016. https://doi.org/10.1016/j.gie.2016.09.010. Published Online: 17 Sep.
35. Shah JN, Marson F, Weilert F, et al. Single-operator, single- session EUS-guided anterograde cholangiopancreatography in failed ERCP or inaccessible papilla. Gastrointest Endosc 2012;75:56–64.
36. Kunda R, Perez-Miranda M, Will U, et al. EUS-guided choledochoduodenostomy for malignant distal biliary obstruction using a lumen apposing fully covered metal stent after failed ERCP. Surg Endosc 2016;30:5002–8.
37. Khashab MA, Van der Merwe S, Kunda R, et al. Prospective international multicenter study on endoscopic ultrasound- guided biliary drainage for patients with malignant distal biliary obstruction after failed endoscopic retrograde cholangiopancreatography. Endosc Int Open 2016;4:E487–96.
38. Minaga K, Ogura T, Shiomi H, et al. Comparison of the efficacy and safety of endoscopic ultrasound-guided choledochoduodenostomy and

hepaticogastrostomy for malignant distal biliary obstruction: Multicenter, randomized, clinical trial. Dig Endosc 2019;31:575–82.

39. Will U, Fueldner F, Kern C, et al. EUS-guided bile duct drainage (EUBD) in 95 patients. Ultraschall Med 2015;36:276–83.

40. Paik WH, Lee TH, Park DH, et al. EUS-guided biliary drainage versus ercp for the primary palliation of malignant biliary obstruction: a multicenter randomized clinical trial. Am J Gastroenterol 2018;113:987–97.

41. Sharaiha RZ, Khan MA, Kamal F, et al. Efficacy and safety of EUS-guided biliary drainage in comparison with percutaneous biliary drainage when ERCP fails: a systematic review and meta-analysis. Gastrointest Endosc 2017;85:904–14.

42. Dhindsa BS, Mashiana HS, Dhaliwal A, et al. EUS-guided biliary drainage: a systematic review and meta-analysis. Endosc Ultrasound 2020;9:101–9.

43. Siddiqui UD, Levy MJ. EUS-guided transluminal interventions. Gastroenterology 2018;154:1911–24.

44. Hedjoudje A, Sportes A, Grabar S, et al. Outcomes of endoscopic ultrasound-guided biliary drainage: A systematic review and meta-analysis. United European Gastroenterol J 2019;7:60–8.

45. De Rezende DT, Brunaldi VO, Bernardo WM, et al. Use of hemostatic powder in treatment of upper gastrointestinal bleeding: a systematic review and meta-analysis. Endosc Int Open 2019;7:E1704–13.

46. Artifon LE, Ferreira FC, Otoch JP, et al. EUS-guided biliary drainage: a review article. JOP 2012;13:7–17.

47. Uemura RS, Khan MA, Otoch JP, et al. EUS-guided choledochoduodenostomy versus hepaticogastrostomy: a systematic review and meta-analysis. J Clin Gastroenterol 2018;52:123–30.

48. Dhir V, Artifon EL, Gupta K, et al. Multicenter study on endoscopic ultrasound-guided expandable biliary metal stent placement: choice of access route, direction of stent insertion, and drainage route. Dig Endosc 2014;26:430–5.

49. Nakai Y, Isayama H, Yamamoto N, et al. Safety and effective- ness of a long partially covered metal stent for endoscopic ultrasound-guided hepaticogastrostomy in patients with malignant biliary obstruction. Endoscopy 2016;48:1125–8.

50. Lee TH, Choi JH, Park DH, et al. Similar efficacies of endoscopic ultrasound-guided transmural and percutaneous drainage for malignant distal biliary obstruction. Clin Gastroenterol Hepatol 2016;14:1011–9.

51. Lyu Y, Li T, Cheng Y, et al. Endoscopic ultrasound-guided vs ERCP-guided biliary drainage for malignant biliary obstruction: a up-to-date meta-analysis and systematic review. Dig Liver Dis 2021;53:1247–53.

52. Ginestet C, Sanglier F, Hummel V, et al. EUS-guided biliary drainage with electrocautery-enhanced lumen-apposing metal stent placement should replace PTBD after ERCP failure in patients with distal tumoral biliary obstruction: a large real-life study. Surg Endosc 2021. https://doi.org/10.1007/s00464-021-08653-1.

53. Huang P, Zhang H, Zhang XF, et al. Comparison of endoscopic ultrasonography guided biliary drainage and percutaneous transhepatic biliary drainage in the management of malignant obstructive jaundice after failed ERCP. Surg Laparosc Endosc Percutan Tech 2017;27:e127–31.

54. Artifon EL, Aparicio D, Paione JB, et al. Biliary drainage in patients with unresectable, malignant obstruction where ERCP fails: endoscopic ultrasonography-guided choledochoduodenostomy versus percutaneous drainage. J Clin Gastroenterol 2012;46:768–74.

55. Bang JY, Navaneethan U, Hasan M, et al. Stent placement by EUS or ERCP for primary biliary decompression in pancreatic cancer: a randomized trial. Gastrointest Endosc 2018;88:9–17.

56. Park JK, Woo YS, Noh DH, et al. Efficacy of EUS-guided and ERCP-guided biliary drainage for malignant biliary obstruction: prospective randomized controlled study. Gastrointest Endosc 2018;88:277–82.

57. Mao K, Hu B, Sun F, et al. Choledochoduodenostomy versus hepaticogastrostomy in endoscopic ultrasound-guided drainage for malignant biliary obstruction: a meta-analysis and systematic review. Surg Laparosc Endosc Percutan Tech 2021. https://doi.org/10.1097/SLE.0000000000000992.

58. Itoi T, Dhir V. EUS-guided biliary rendezvous: slow, hesitant, baby steps forward. Gastrointest Endosc 2016;83:401–3.

59. Dhir V, Kwek BEA, Bhandari S, et al. EUS-guided biliary rendezvous using a short hydrophilic guidewire. J Interv Gastroenterol 2011;1:153–9.

60. Dhir V, Bhandari S, Bapat M, et al. Comparison of transhepatic and extrahepatic routes for EUS-guided rendezvous procedure for distal CBD obstruction. United European Gastroenterol J 2013;1:103–8.

61. Klair JS, Zafar Y, Ashat M, et al. Effectiveness and safety of EUS rendezvous after failed biliary cannulation with ERCP: a systematic review and proportion meta-analysis. J Clin Gastroenterol 2021. https://doi.org/10.1097/MCG.0000000000001543.

62. Krishnamoorthi R, Dasari CS, Chandrasekar VT, et al. Effectiveness and safety of EUS-guided choledochoduodenostomy using lumen-apposing metal stents (LAMS): a systematic review and meta-analysis. Surg Endosc 2020;34:2866–77.

63. Minaga K, Takenaka M, Kitano M, et al. Rescue EUS-guided intrahepatic biliary drainage for malignant hilar biliary stricture after failed transpapillary re-intervention. Surg Endosc 2017;31:4764–72.

64. Bories E, Pesenti C, Caillol F, et al. Transgastric endoscopic ultrasonography-guided biliary drainage: Results of a pilot study. Endoscopy 2007;39:287–91.

65. Ogura T, Sano T, Onda S, et al. Endoscopic ultrasound-guided biliary drainage for right hepatic bile duct obstruction: Novel technical tips. Endoscopy 2015;47:72–5.

66. Ogura T, Onda S, Takagi W, et al. Clinical utility of endoscopic ultrasound-guided biliary drainage as a rescue of re-intervention procedure for high-grade hilar stricture. J Gastroenterol Hepatol 2017;32:163–8.

67. Moryoussef F, Sportes A, Leblanc S, et al. Is EUS-guided drainage a suitable alternative technique in case of proxi- mal biliary obstruction? Therap Adv Gastroenterol 2017;10:537–44.

68. Kongkam P, Orprayoon T, Boonmee C, et al. ERCP plus endoscopic ultrasound-guided biliary drainage versus percutaneous transhepatic biliary drainage for malignant hilar biliary obstruction: A multicenter observational open-label study. Endoscopy 2021;53:55–62.

69. Mukai S, Takao Itoi T, Sofuni A, et al. EUS-guided antegrade intervention for benign biliary diseases in patients with surgically altered anatomy. Gastrointest Endosc 2019;89:399–407.

70. Füldner F, Meyer F, Will U. EUS-guided biliary interventions for benign diseases and unsuccessful ERCP - a prospective unicenter feasibility study on a large consecutive patient cohort. Z Gastroenterol 2021;59:933–43.

71. Dhir V, Itoi T, Fockens P, et al. Novel ex vivo model for hands-on teaching of and training in EUS-guided biliary drainage: creation of "Mumbai EUS" stereolithography/3D printing bile duct prototype. Gastrointest Endosc 2015;81:440–6.

72. Dhir V, Maydeo A, Itoi T, et al. Evaluation of a novel, easily reproducible, hybrid model (Mumbai Endoscopic Ultrasound II) for teaching and training endoscopic ultrasound-guided biliary drainage and rendezvous procedure. Endosc Int Open 2017;5:E1087–95.
73. Dhir V, Udawat P. Shah R et al.Evaluation of all in one hybrid model (EUS Magic Box) for stepwise teaching and training in multiple interventional EUS procedures. Endosc Int Open, in press.
74. Dhir V, Udawat P, Shah R, et al. Prospective evaluation of feasibility of structured EUS training with a virtual EUS course with live cases. Endosc Int Open 2021; 09:E1–6.

Endoscopic Management of Acute Cholecystitis

Xiaobei Luo, MD[a], Reem Sharaiha, MD[b], Anthony Yuen Bun Teoh, FRCSEd[c],*

KEYWORDS

- Acute cholecystitis • EUS-guided gallbladder drainage
- Endoscopic transpapillary gallbladder drainage
- Percutaneous transhepatic gallbladder drainage

KEY POINTS

- Endoscopic management of acute cholecystitis in high surgical risk patients is recommended in tertiary hospitals whereby expertise, resources, and technical support are available.
- In patients who are not fit for surgery, percutaneous transhepatic gallbladder drainage (PTGBD), endoscopic transpapillary-gallbladder drainage (ET-GBD), and endoscopic ultrasound-guided gallbladder drainage (EUS-GBD) are effective and safe alternative procedures to cholecystectomy (CCY).
- EUS-GBD is preferred over PTGBD due to similar rates of technical success and reduced rates of reintervention and unplanned readmissions.
- Lumen-apposing metal stents (LAMS) are associated with reduced risks of AEs such as bile peritonitis and perforation as compared with plastic stents and these stents should be used for EUS-GBD.
- EUS-GBD is associated with a steeper learning curve and should be performed in high-volume endoscopy centers whereby expertise is available.

INTRODUCTION

Early laparoscopic cholecystectomy (CCY) is considered the standard treatment of patients with acute cholecystitis.[1,2] Nevertheless, for patients with high surgical risks, such as elderly patients and patients with multiple comorbidities, hemodynamic instability or intraabdominal malignancies, gallbladder drainage (GBD) with concomitant antibiotic treatment is recommended.[3] The GBD approaches for these nonsurgical candidates include percutaneous transhepatic gallbladder drainage (PTGBD) and endoscopic gallbladder drainage (EGBD). PTGBD is often recommended as the first

[a] Department of Gastroenterology, Nanfang Hospital, Southern Medical University, Guangzhou, China; [b] Division of Gastroenterology and Hepatology, New York Presbyterian Hospital/Weill Cornell Medical Centre, New York, NY, USA; [c] Department of Surgery, Prince of Wales Hospital, The Chinese University of Hong Kong, Shatin, Hong Kong
* Corresponding author. Department of Surgery, Prince of Wales Hospital, The Chinese University of Hong Kong.
E-mail address: anthonyteoh@surgery.cuhk.edu.hk

Gastrointest Endoscopy Clin N Am 32 (2022) 527–543
https://doi.org/10.1016/j.giec.2022.02.004
1052-5157/22/© 2022 Elsevier Inc. All rights reserved.

alternative to surgical intervention in these patients.[4] PTGBD is technically less challenging and can be performed in most medical institutions with access to interventional radiology. Contraindications to PTGBD include severe ascites, untreated coagulopathy, or an anatomically inaccessible position. Adverse events (AEs) which include bile peritonitis, recurrent cholecystitis, bleeding, pneumothorax, catheter dislodgement, and inadvertent removal have been reported in up to 14% of patients undergoing PTGBD.[5] Additionally, PTGBD can cause physical discomfort to patients and adversely affect their quality of life. With the advancements in endoscopic techniques and accessories, endoscopic approaches for GBD including endoscopic transpapillary gallbladder drainage (ET-GBD) and endoscopic ultrasound (EUS)-guided gallbladder drainage (EUS-GBD) have gained popularity.[6] The Tokyo Guideline 2018 considers ET-GBD and EUS-GBD as effective alternative procedures to CCY in high-volume endoscopy centers whereby expertise is available.[4] The recently published European Society of Gastrointestinal Endoscopy (ESGE) therapeutic EUS guideline has also highlighted that when technically available, EUS-GBD should be preferred over PTGBD in view of lower rates of AEs and reinterventtion in EUS-GBD.[7] The aim of the present article is to review the current status of endoscopic approaches for GBD in patients with acute cholecystitis and to compare the efficacy, safety, and outcomes of these endoscopic approaches with PTGBD.

Endoscopic Transpapillary Gallbladder Drainage

The transpapillary approach for GBD via cystic duct cannulation during endoscopic retrograde cholangiopancreatography (ERCP) has been used for the treatment of acute cholecystitis for more than 20 years.[8] There are 2 methods of ET-GBD: endoscopic transpapillary naso-cholecystic drainage (endoscopic nasobiliary gallbladder drainage, ENGBD) and endoscopic transpapillary gallbladder stenting (ETGBS). The details of the procedures have been described previously.[3] In brief, a guidewire is advanced into the cystic duct and gallbladder after successful CBD cannulation. A 5-F or 8.5-F naso-cholecystic drainage tube (ENGBD) or a 6-Fr to 10-Fr double pigtail stent (ETGBS) is placed into the gallbladder to enable drainage and irrigation. However, cannulation of the gallbladder may be technically challenging due to the tortuosity of the cystic duct, obstruction by stones, or severe inflammation. Cholangioscopy can be used to facilitate cystic duct cannulation when necessary.[9]

Outcomes

As shown in **Table 1**, the ET-GBD is associated with acceptable rates of technical success (70.6%–96.0%), clinical success (82.8%–100%), and AEs (0%–18%).[10–19] It is a technically challenging procedure and requires proficiency in the cannulation of the cystic duct. Cannulation of the gallbladder may not always be feasible especially if the cystic duct cannot be well-visualized on cholangiography or when there is tortuosity or stenosis of the cystic duct. A retrospective study investigated factors affecting the technical success of ET-GBD and revealed that cystic duct stones, CBD dilation, and unfavorable cystic duct direction can be considered predictors for increased rates of technical failure.[20] Ridtitid and colleagues reported a 22% increment in ET-GBD technical success rates with the use of cholangioscopy combined with fluoroscopy for difficult cystic duct cannulation.[9] Other studies have shown an improved technique success rate in high-volume endoscopy centers.[10,21] Kjaer and colleagues reported an enhanced success rate from 50% in the first 4 years of the study to 89% in the subsequent 5 years, demonstrating a relatively long learning curve for the procedure.[10]

Exploiting the natural biliary tree, ET-GBD reduced complications related to externalized drainage. A recent meta-analysis of ET-GBD reported a pooled overall AE

Table 1
Outcomes of endoscopic transpapillary gallbladder drainage

Author, Year	Research Type	Treatment Options	No. of Patients	Technical Success	Clinical Success	No. of Adverse Events	No. of Recurrence
Kjaer et al,[10] 2007	Retrospective	ENGBD/ETGBS	34	70.6%	87.5%	4	-
Mutignani et al.[11], 2009	Retrospective	ENGBD/ETGBS	35	82.9%	82.8%	6	2
Lee et al.[12], 2011	Prospective	ETGBS	29	79.3%	100.0%	Early 4 + Late 4	-
Yang et al.[13], 2015	Prospective	ENGBD	17	82.4%	85.7%	3	-
	Prospective	ETGBS	18	88.9%	93.8%	2	-
Widmer et al.[14], 2015	Prospective	ETGBS	128	91.0%	100.0%	7	-
Itoi et al.[15], 2015	Prospective	ENGBD	37	91.9%	94.1%	2	-
	Prospective	ETGBS	36	86.1%	90.3%	1	-
McCarthy et al.[16], 2015	Retrospective	ETGBS	29	75.9%	90.0%	2	-
Inoue et al.[17], 2016	Retrospective	ETGBS	35	82.9%	94.3%	3	0
Kim et al.[18], 2020	Retrospective	ENGBD/ETGBS	171	90.6%	90.1%	21	1
Storm et al.[19], 2021	Retrospective	ENGBD/ETGBS	51	96.0%	100.0%	3	3

rate of 8.83% (95% confidence interval (CI): 7.42–10.34).[22] The most common AEs were post-ERCP pancreatitis (1.98%), recurrent cholecystitis or biliary colic (1.48%), bleeding (1.03%), perforation (0.78%) of the cystic duct or gallbladder, and peritonitis/bile leakage (0.45%). The pooled rates of stent occlusion and migration were 0.39% and 0.13%, respectively.

Similar to PTGBD, ENGBD usually serves as a temporary measure for controlling acute cholecystitis until the patient is eligible for subsequent surgery or internal stent placement. Although it allows repeated gallbladder irrigation, performance of a cholecystogram, and bile sampling via the drainage tube, ENGBD is less favored by the patient and inadvertent drain dislodgement can occur. In contrast, ETGBS is better tolerated by patients and can be used for long-term drainage in high-risk patients or patients with limited life expectancy. However, in ETGBS, the stent cannot be irrigated and carries risks of occlusion or migration.[23,24] A randomized trial that compared ENGBD versus ETGBS in the management of acute cholecystitis demonstrated comparable safety and efficacy of these 2 methods.[15] As the stent can be removed when required, the major advantage of long-term placement of ETGBS over other alternatives is that it avoids permanent anatomic distortion. A few studies evaluated the long-term outcome of ETGBS. Hatanaka and colleagues reported a recurrence cholecystitis rate of 15.7% with a median follow-up time of 229 days, and the cumulative recurrent cholecystitis rates were 10.5% at 1 year and 18.7% at 2 years.[25] A multicenter prospective study by Lee and colleagues investigated the long-term clinical outcomes for patients after ET-GBD and revealed a median stent patency of 760 days.[12] Maekawa and colleagues reported long-term recurrent cholecystitis rate was approximately 3.3%, and 93.5% of the patients remained asymptomatic until death or the end of the study period (1 month to 5 years) without stent exchanges.[26] A recent multicenter retrospective cohort study by Maruta and colleagues showed a similar recurrent cholecystitis rate of 5.0% with a median follow-up time of 375 days.[27] These data demonstrated the long-term effectiveness of ETGBS in surgically unfit patients with acute cholecystitis. However, the optimal duration of stenting and whether routine stent replacement is required for improved long-term outcomes are still undefined.[28] Some studies have suggested that capillary action alongside the stent enables adequate drainage of the gallbladder even when the stent is occluded, eliminating the need for frequent stent exchange. Nevertheless, further prospective trials with a larger number of patients are warranted to determine the optimal time for stent removal or exchange.[17]

Endoscopic ultrasound-guided gallbladder drainage

EUS-GBD has opened new avenues in the treatment of acute cholecystitis. Baron and Topazian and colleagues initially reported EUS-GBD using a plastic stent in 2007 as a palliative treatment of acute cholecystitis in a patient with cholangiocarcinoma after failed ET-GBD.[29] With parallel development in novel endoscopic devices such as fully covered self-expandable metal stents (FCSEMS) and lumen-apposing metal stents (LAMS), substantial technical progress has been made to enable subsequent interventional procedures such as magnifying endoscopy, gallstone removal and polypectomy.[30]

Previous reports have described the procedures in detail (**Fig. 1**).[3] EUS-GBD can be achieved via a transgastric or transduodenal approach with the placement of transmural stents. Generally, the procedure is performed using a linear array echoendoscope. After clear visualization under EUS, the gallbladder is punctured from the duodenal bulb or gastric body with a 19-gauge needle. A guidewire is then placed into the gallbladder through the needle. Thereafter, a double pigtail plastic stent, FCSEMS, or a

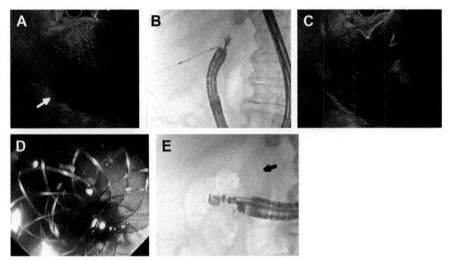

Fig. 1. (*A*) EUS noted a distended gallbladder as indicated by the white arrow. (*B*) Direct puncture with the cautery enhanced LAMS and insertion of a guidewire into the gallbladder. (*C*) Opening of the distal flange under EUS guidance. (*D*) Endoscopic view of the proximal flange. (*E*) X-ray image of a fully opened stent.

LAMS is inserted into the gallbladder for drainage and to allow subsequent interventional procedures if required.

Earlier EUS-GBD was performed with a double pigtail plastic stent with an acceptable technical success rate.[31] However, it was associated with a higher rate of advent events including pneumoperitoneum, bile peritonitis, stent occlusion, and migration. Subsequently, FCSEMS were used for EUS-GBD. These stents reduced the risk of bile leakage but were still not ideal for transmural drainage as the stents were too long, prone to migration. In light of these limitations, LAMSs were designed for transmural drainage of the gallbladder and pseudocysts.[32] With the anchoring function of the flanges and a shorter length, LAMS can generate adequate lumen-apposing force (LAF) to hold 2 organs in apposition and prevent stent migration.[33] The larger diameter of these LAMS also minimize the risk of stent obstruction and enable endoscopes to traverse the 2 organs for further interventional therapies including stone removal and polypectomy.

Recently, novel cautery-tipped stent delivery systems have been developed and enabled single-step EUS-guided gallbladder stenting.[34–36] Combining the functions of cystotomes, tract dilators, and stent delivery catheters, these devices decrease the need for a multistep procedure, instrument exchanges, and related AEs. Successful applications of these cautery-enhanced stents have been reported in the treatment of acute cholecystitis and peripancreatic fluid collection.[34]

Outcomes

As shown in **Table 2**, an increasing number of case series on EUS-GBD have been reported with high success rates and low AEs rates.[37–44] The technical success rate of EUS-GBD is 90% to 100%, the clinical success rate 86.4%–100%, and the procedure-related AE rate is 7.25%–12.80%. A retrospective international multicenter registry on EUS-GBD in 379 consecutive patients revealed technical and clinical success rates of 95.3% and 90.8% and 30-day AE and 30-day mortality rates of 15.3%

Table 2
Outcomes of endoscopic ultrasound-guided gallbladder drainage

Author, Year	Research Type	Number of Patients	Technical Success	Clinical Success	Number of Adverse Events	Number of Recurrence
Jang et al.[37], 2011	Prospective	15	100.0%	100.0%	2	0
Choi et al.[38], 2014	Retrospective	63	98.4%	98.4%	Early AE 3< Late AE 4	2
Walter et al.[39], 2015	Prospective	30	90.0%	86.7%	4	2
Dollhopf et al.[40], 2017	Retrospective	75	98.7%	95.9%	8	3
Ahmed et al.[41], 2018	Retrospective	13	100.0%	92.3%	1	1
Anderloni et al.[42], 2018	Retrospective	45	97.8%	86.4%	5	-
Oh et al.[43], 2019	Retrospective	83	99.3%	99.3%	6	2
Teoh et al.[44], 2019	Prospective (RCT)	39	97.4%	92.3%	30 d 5 1 year10	1

and 9.2%, respectively.[45] A recent meta-analysis reviewed a total of 558 patients from 17 EUS-GBD studies and the cumulative pooled technical success, clinical success and procedure-related AEs of 87.33% (95% CI: 84.42–89.77), 84.16% (95% CI: 80.30–87.38), and 11.00% (95% CI: 9.25–13.03), respectively.[46] Subgroup studies using only LAMS for EUS-GBD revealed superior outcomes; the technical success was 94.65% (95% CI: 91.54–96.67), clinical success was 92.06% (95% CI: 88.65–94.51), and AE rate was 11.71% (95% CI: 8.92–15.23). Data from these studies have shown definite benefits of EUS-GBD for the treatment of acute cholecystitis in surgically unfit patients.

Common AEs with EUS-GBD include pneumoperitoneum, bile leakage/peritonitis, bleeding, perforation, stent migration, and recurrent cholecystitis. A recent meta-analysis of EUS-GBD demonstrated pneumoperitoneum and bile leakage as the most common AEs in the procedure, which may potentially be caused by tract dilation and the placement of small diameter plastic stents. The use of self-expanding LAMS is, therefore, recommended to minimize tract dilation and reduce the risks of bile leakage and stent migration.[37,40] Another meta-analysis consisting of 8 studies with 393 patients evaluated AEs with LAMS in EUS-GBD.[47] The study reported an overall AE rate of 12.7% (95% CI: 8.4–18.7), an early AE risk of 6.5% (95% CI: 4.2–10), and a delayed AE risk of 8.3% (95% CI: 5.8–11.9). Common early AEs with LAMSs were bleeding (2.6%; 95% CI: 0.9-7.2), bile leakage (1.3%, 95% CI: 0.5-3.3), perforation (2.3%; 95% CI: 1.1-4.7) and stent migration (1.5%; 95% CI: 0.6-3.5), and common delayed AEs were stent occlusion (5.2%; 95% CI: 3-8.7), stent migration (3%; 95% 1.5-5.8), recurrent cholecystitis/cholangitis (4.6%; 95% CI: 2.6-9.5), and death (5%; 95% CI: 2.6-9.5), which were mainly attributed to patient comorbidities.

On the other hand, there is so far no consensus on when LAMS should be removed or replaced. Recent studies from Jang and colleagues and Saumoy and colleagues demonstrated that the presence of a LAMS did not interfere with subsequent CCY if required.[48,49] However, for patients with limited life expectancy and those that are too frail to undergo CCY or another endoscopic procedure for stent removal, LAMS may be left indefinitely after EUS-GBD. A multicenter, prospective, long-term study of EUS-GBD with LAMS reported the absence of stent-related AEs during a mean follow-up time of 364 days.[39] Similar results have also been observed in other studies using SEMS, LAMS, or cautery enhanced LAMS with long term stenting up to 3 years.[50] Although preliminary data suggested that LAMS might be considered for permanent placement in selected patients, more research should be carried out to improve stent patency and to avoid potential stent-induced AEs in the long term.

In addition, although high technical and clinical success were reported in the literature, most of these procedures have been performed in tertiary hospitals by endoscopists proficient in interventional EUS and ERCP. Some studies have suggested EUS-GBD is associated with a steep learning curve even when adopted by experienced endoscopists in high-volume centers.[45,51] Tyberg and colleagues and Teoh and colleagues concluded that the number of cases required to gain competency with EUS-GBD was 19 cases and 25 cases, respectively. Further effort is required to establish a standardized training program and accreditation system for more endoscopists to develop the required skills if EUS-GBD is to become the standard GBD procedure.

Interventions after endoscopic ultrasound-guided gallbladder drainage with lumen-apposing metal stents

EUS-GBD with LAMS has made subsequent advanced endoscopic assessment and interventions to the gallbladder and cystic duct possible. Exploiting the large diameter of the LAMS, endoscopes and different accessories can be directly advanced into the gallbladder for further treatment after EUS-GBD, such as stone removal, magnifying endoscopy, and polypectomy (**Fig. 2**).[30,52] Chan S et al. reported that stone clearance was achieved in 88% of patients after EUS-GBD.[30] Spontaneous passage of gallstones via the fistula was observed in 56% of these patients, and the remaining gallstones can be retrieved with water irrigation, basket, and laser lithotripsy.

In another report, a polypoid lesion in the gallbladder was assessed using magnified endoscopy. Irregular glands with a corkscrew microvascular pattern were observed, highly suggestive of a malignant lesion.[53] Biopsy confirmed adenocarcinoma of the gallbladder. Gallbladder polypectomy has also been described in a few studies using LAMS as a portal.[30,54] However, further studies with long-term follow-up are needed to investigate the clinical outcomes of these advanced interventional procedures.

COMPARATIVE STUDIES
Comparison of Endoscopic Transpapillary-Gallbladder Drainage and Endoscopic Ultrasound-Guided Gallbladder Drainage

The two endoscopic modalities for GBD have been compared in surgically unfit patients with acute cholecystitis in a few recent studies. A retrospective study consisting of 172 consecutive patients revealed significantly higher rates of technical (99.3% vs 86.6%, $P < 0.01$) and clinical success (99.3% vs 86%, $P < 0.01$) with EUS-GBD compared with ET-GBD (**Table 3**).[43] The AE rate (7.1% vs 19.3%, $P = 0.02$) and combined cholecystitis and cholangitis recurrence rate (3.2% vs 12.4% vs, $P = 0.04$) were also lower for EUS-GBD. A meta-analysis including 5 retrospective studies with 857 high-surgical risk patients noted a similar finding. Significantly higher rates of technical ($P < 0.01$) and clinical ($P < 0.01$) success were observed in the EUS-GBD group than in the ET-GBD group.[55] With similar rates of overall AEs, EUS-GBD is preferred over ET-GBD due to a lower rate of recurrent cholecystitis ($P < 0.01$). In view of the superior technical efficacy and clinical outcome of EUS-GBD, it may be favored over ET-GBD in nonsurgical patients with acute cholecystitis. The ESGE Guideline also recommends EUS-GBD over ET-GBD when both techniques are available.[7] However, most of the studies comparing EUS-GBD versus ET-GBD were conducted in a retrospective cohort, and well-designed prospective studies are needed to verify the current results.

Comparison of Endoscopic Transpapillary-Gallbladder Drainage and Percutaneous Transhepatic Gallbladder Drainage

Several studies compared the efficacy and outcomes of ET-GBD with PTGBD for the treatment of acute cholecystitis. An international multicenter comparative study involving 1764 patients suggested similar clinical success rates within 3 days

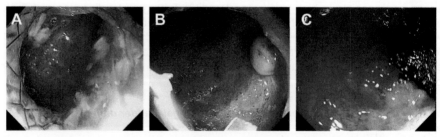

Fig. 2. (A) Endoscopic view of cholecystoscopy. (B) Inflammatory polyp noted in the gallbladder. (C) Gallstone noted in the cystic duct opening.

Table 3
Summary of results from comparative studies in gallbladder drainage

Study, Year	Research Type	Type of GBD	No. of Patients	Technical Success	Clinical Success	Adverse Effects	Notes
Teoh et al.[44], 2020	Randomized control trial	EUS-GBD	39	97.4%	92.3%	1 y: 25.6% 30 d: 12.8%	EUS-GBD significantly reduced 1-y AEs, 30 d AEs, re-interventions, unplanned readmissions, and recurrent cholecystitis
		PTGBD	40	100.0%	92.5%	1 y: 77.5% 30 d: 47.5%	
Jang et al.[48], 2012	Randomized control trial	EUS-GBD	30	97.0%	100.0%	7.0%	EUS-GBD significantly reduced postprocedure pain score
		PTGBD	29	97.0%	96.0%	3.0%	
Choi et al.[66], 2016	Retrospective	EUS-GBD	14	85.7%	100.0%	28.5%	EUS-GBD significantly reduced postprocedure cost and length of hospital stay
		PTGBD	19	91.7%	86.4%	21.1%	
Irani et al.[67], 2016	Retrospective	EUS-GBD	45	98.0%	96.0%	11.0%	EUS-GBD significantly reduced the length of hospital stay and postprocedure pain
		PTGBD	45	100.0%	91.0%	32.0%	
Tyberg et al.[60], 2018	Retrospective	EUS-GBD	42	95.0%	95.0%	11.0%	EUS-GBD was associated with a significantly decreased rate of re-interventions
		PTGBD	113	99.0%	86.0%	32.0%	
Iino et al.[58], 2018	Retrospective	ET-GBD	43	77.0%	–	9.3%	ET-GBD resulted in a significantly lower technique success rate but a shorter length of hospitalization
		PTGBD	32	100.0%	–	6.0%	
Itoi et al.[56], 2017	Retrospective	ET-GBD	333	–	7 d: 89.2%	8.2%	ET-GBD significantly increased the clinical success within 3 d
		PTGBD	333	–	7 d: 85.7%	5.6%	
Oh et al.[43], 2018	Retrospective	EUS-GBD	76	99.3%	99.3%	7.1%	EUS-GBD was associated with significantly higher rates of clinical success and technical success; and lower rates of AEs and recurrent cholecystitis or cholangitis
		ET-GBD	96	86.6%	86.0%	19.3%	

(continued on next page)

Table 3
(continued)

Study, Year	Research Type	Type of GBD	No. of Patients	Technical Success	Clinical Success	Adverse Effects	Notes
Higa et al.[68], 2019	Retrospective	EUS-GBD	40	97.5%	95.0%	17.9%	EUS-GBD resulted in significantly higher technical and clinical success, and less-frequent recurrent cholecystitis
		ET-GBD	38	84.2%	86.0%	9.4%	
Siddiqui et al.[62], 2019	Retrospective	EUS-GBD	102	94.0%	90.0%	2.0%	ET-GBD was associated with significantly lower technical and clinical success compared with PTGBD and EUS-GBD. EUS-GBD with LAMS had significantly lower AEs, length of hospital stays, and unplanned admissions compared with PTGBD.
		ET-GBD	124	88.0%	80.0%	5.0%	
		PTGBD	146	98.0%	97.0%	20.0%	

(62.5% and 69.8%, $P = 0.085$) and 7 days (87.6% and 89.2%, $P = 0.579$) and no significant difference in AE rates (4.8% and 8.2%, $P = 0.083$) between PTGBD and ET-GBD, respectively.[56] Contrast to the previous report, studies by Iino and colleagues and Kaura and colleagues demonstrated that ET-GBD was associated with a suboptimal technical success rate (77%–91% vs 100%; $P < 0.001$) compared with PTGBD.[57,58]

However, the long-term outcome was superior in the ET-GBD group versus PTGBD group; Inoue and colleagues revealed a significantly reduced rate of recurrent cholecystitis (0% vs 17.2%, $P = 0.043$) and reduced overall biliary event rates (9.1% vs 24.1%, albeit not statistically significant, $P = 0.207$) in the ET-GBD group.[17] Surgical outcomes post–ET-GBD versus PTGBD were also investigated and suggested comparable rates of conversion to open CCY and postoperative complications.[57,59] One recently published randomized controlled trial enrolled 22 high-surgical risk patients with acute cholecystitis who received CCY 2 to 3 months after ET-GBD or PTGBD drainage[59]; and showed significantly reduced abdominal pain ($P < 0.001$), less postoperative hemorrhage and abdominal drainage tube placement ($P = 0.03$), and better gallbladder pathologic grades ($P = 0.004$) in the ET-GBD group compared with PTGBD group.

Comparison of Endoscopic Ultrasound-Guided Gallbladder Drainage and Percutaneous Transhepatic Gallbladder Drainage

Several studies have compared EUS-GBD with PTGBD in nonsurgical candidates and have suggested that EUS-GBD may be associated with comparable technical success rates but improved clinical outcomes and fewer AEs than PTGBD.[6,48,60] An international randomized multicenter controlled superiority trial (DRAC 1) with 80 consecutive high-risk patients with acute calculous cholecystitis reported similar technical (97.4% vs 100%, $P = 0.494$) and clinical success rates (92.3% vs 92.5%, $P = 1.0$), 30-day mortality (7.7% vs 10%, $P = 0.68$) and hospital stays (8 vs 9 days; $P = 0.18$) in EUS-GBD and PTGBD.[44] The study also demonstrated that EUS-GBD was associated with significantly reduced 30-day AEs (12.8% vs 47.5%, $P = 0.010$) and 1-year AEs (25.6% vs 77.5%, $P = 0.001$), 30-day reinterventions (2.6% vs 30%, $P = 0.001$), unplanned readmissions (15.4% vs 50%, $P = 0.002$) and recurrent cholecystitis (2.6% vs 20%, $P = 0.029$). Similar results were reported in a recent meta-analysis including 5 comparative studies with a total of 495 patients with acute cholecystitis.[61] Comparable rates in technical and clinical success (odds ratio (OR): 0.43; $P = 0.21$) between the 2 modalities were demonstrated, while postprocedure AEs (OR: 0.43, $P = 0.05$), days of hospital stay (– 2.53; $P = 0.005$), reinterventions (OR: 0.16, $P < 0.001$) and readmissions (OR: 0.16, $P = 0.003$) were significantly lower for EUS-GBD than for PTGBD.

In addition, EUS-GBD might be considered an alternative modality to PTGBD as a bridging therapy to CCY, even though the technical challenges for closing the gastric/duodenal fistula in EUS-GBD have to be taken into consideration. A prospective randomized controlled trial reported that the conversion rate from laparoscopic to open CCY was comparable between patients post–EUS-GBD and PTGBD (9% vs 12%, $P = 0.99$).[48] A multicenter international retrospective study also reported similar open conversion rates and AEs between the 2 GBD modalities and demonstrated that interval CCY after EUD-GBD is safe and feasible.[49]

Overall, although larger comparative studies are warranted, EUS-GBD and PTGBD showed comparable technical and clinical success rates in the results of the above literature. In view of the lower rates of AEs and reduced readmission and reintervention rates, EUS-GBD should be favored over PTGBD when technically available.[7]

Comparison of Endoscopic Transpapillary-Gallbladder Drainage, Endoscopic Ultrasound-Guided Gallbladder Drainage, and Percutaneous Transhepatic Gallbladder Drainage

Three-way comparative studies were performed retrospectively to evaluate the clinical outcomes and efficacy of the 3 modalities.[62] An international multicenter study consisting of 372 high-risk surgical patients with acute cholecystitis compared EUS-GBD using LAMS, ET-GBD, and PTGBD. PTGBD and EUS-GBD had significantly higher technical (98% vs 94% vs 88%; $P = 0.004$) and clinical (97% vs 90% vs 80%; $P < 0.001$) success rates than ET-GBD. While significantly higher AEs (20% vs 2% vs 5%; $P = 0.01$) and additional surgical intervention (49% vs 4% vs 11%; $P < 0.0001$) were observed in the PTGBD group. The lowest overall AEs, hospital stay, and unplanned admissions were observed in the EUS-GBD group. Another network meta-analysis (10 studies, 1267 patients) comparing the 3 treatment options of GBD also reported similar outcomes.[63] In the network ranking estimate, PTGBD and EUS-GBD had higher rates of technical and clinical success compared with ET-GBD. While EUS-GBD had the lowest rate of recurrent cholecystitis and PTGBD had the highest reintervention and unplanned readmission.

Recently, a cost-effectiveness analysis in a hypothetical cohort of surgically unfit patients with acute cholecystitis illustrated that, compared with PTGBD, ET-GBD was associated with reduced cost and improved effectiveness and EUS-GBD was associated with higher expenses but improved effectiveness.[64] The study suggests that endoscopic approaches for GBD may be favored over PTGBD from an economical perspective.

Comparison of Endoscopic Ultrasound-Guided Gallbladder Drainage and Laparoscopic Cholecystectomy

One retrospective study compared the outcomes of EUS-GBD with laparoscopic CCY for acute cholecystitis in 60 patients.[65] A comparable technical (100% vs 100%) and clinical success (93.3% vs 100%, $P = 1$), mortality (6.7% vs 0%, $P = 0.492$), recurrent biliary events (10% vs 10%, $P = 0.784$), reintervention (13.3% vs 10%, $P = 1$) and 1-year unplanned readmission rate (10% vs 10%, $P = 0.784$) were reported. Although future prospective studies with a larger sample size is warranted, the results suggest that EUS-GBD may potentially be an alternative to laparoscopic CCY in a selected group of patients who may be suitable for definitive surgery.

SUMMARY

Endoscopic management of acute cholecystitis in high surgical risk patients is recommended in tertiary hospitals whereby expertise, resources, and technical support are available. The optimal treatment modality (PTGBD, ET-GBD, or EUS-GBD) should be individualized based on patient conditions and the techniques available in the facility. There are accumulating evidence that suggests that EUS-GBD should be favored over PTGBD or ET-GBD when the expertise is available due to the higher technical efficacy, lower rates of AEs, and reintervention in EUS-GBD. However, further prospective studies and long-term follow-up are necessary to clarify the optimal patient selection for each technique and to guide stent management after EUS-GBD/ET-GBD. Future research is also required to address the optimal stent, the duration of stenting, and the need for gallstone removal after stent placement for transmural GBD. Studies are also required to further elucidate the role of EUS-GBD as an alternative treatment to laparoscopic CCY for patients who might be fit for surgery. Finally, the endoscopic procedures for GBD need to be standardized and training programs are required to introduce the techniques effectively and safely to the wider endoscopic society.

CLINICS CARE POINTS

- In patients who are not fit for surgery, PTGBD, ET-GBD, and EUS-GBD are effective and safe alternative procedures to cholecystectomy (CCY).

- ET-GBD and EUS-GBD showed similar conversion rates from CCY to open surgery compared with PTGBD and can be considered as bridging therapies to CCY instead of PTGBD.

- EUS-GBD is preferred over PTGBD due to similar rates of technical success and reduced rates of reintervention and unplanned readmission.

- LAMS is associated with reduced risks of AEs such as bile peritonitis and perforation compared with plastic stents after EUS-GBD.

- EUS-GBD is associated with a steeper learning curve and should be performed in high-volume endoscopy centers whereby expertise is available.

DISCLOSURE

A.Y.B. Teoh is a consultant for Boston Scientific, Cook, Taewoong and Microtech Medical Corporations. R. Sharaiha is a consultant for Boston Scientific, Cook, Lumendi. Other co-authors do not have any conflicts of interest to disclose.

REFERENCES

1. Pisano M, Allievi N, Gurusamy K, et al. 2020 World society of emergency surgery updated guidelines for the diagnosis and treatment of acute calculus cholecystitis. World J Emerg Surg 2020;15(1):61.
2. Loozen CS, van Santvoort HC, van Duijvendijk P, et al. Laparoscopic cholecystectomy versus percutaneous catheter drainage for acute cholecystitis in high risk patients (CHOCOLATE): multicentre randomised clinical trial. BMJ 2018; 363:k3965.
3. Yeung B, Teoh AY. Endoscopic management of gallbladder stones: can we eliminate cholecystectomy? Curr Gastroenterol Rep 2016;18(8):42.
4. Mori Y, Itoi T, Baron TH, et al. Tokyo Guidelines 2018: management strategies for gallbladder drainage in patients with acute cholecystitis (with videos). J Hepatobiliary Pancreat Sci 2018;25(1):87–95.
5. Winbladh A, Gullstrand P, Svanvik J, et al. Systematic review of cholecystostomy as a treatment option in acute cholecystitis. HPB (Oxford) 2009;11(3):183–93.
6. Itoi T, Coelho-Prabhu N, Baron TH. Endoscopic gallbladder drainage for management of acute cholecystitis. Gastrointest Endosc 2010;71(6):1038–45.
7. van der Merwe SW, van Wanrooij RLJ, Bronswijk M, et al. Therapeutic endoscopic ultrasound: european society of gastrointestinal endoscopy (ESGE) guideline. Endoscopy 2022;54(2):185–205.
8. Feretis CB, Manouras AJ, Apostolidis NS, et al. Endoscopic transpapillary drainage of gallbladder empyema. Gastrointest Endosc 1990;36(5):523–5.
9. Ridtitid W, Piyachaturawat P, Teeratorn N, et al. Single-operator peroral cholangioscopy cystic duct cannulation for transpapillary gallbladder stent placement in patients with acute cholecystitis at moderate to high surgical risk (with videos). Gastrointest Endosc 2020;92(3):634–44.
10. Kjaer DW, Kruse A, Funch-Jensen P. Endoscopic gallbladder drainage of patients with acute cholecystitis. Endoscopy 2007;39(4):304–8.
11. Mutignani M, Iacopini F, Perri V, et al. Endoscopic gallbladder drainage for acute cholecystitis: technical and clinical results. Endoscopy 2009;41(6):539–46.

12. Lee TH, Park DH, Lee SS, et al. Outcomes of endoscopic transpapillary gall-bladder stenting for symptomatic gallbladder diseases: a multicenter prospective follow-up study. Endoscopy 2011;43(8):702–8.

13. Yang MJ, Yoo BM, Kim JH, et al. Endoscopic naso-gallbladder drainage versus gallbladder stenting before cholecystectomy in patients with acute cholecystitis and a high suspicion of choledocholithiasis: a prospective randomised preliminary study. Scand J Gastroenterol 2016;51(4):472–8.

14. Widmer J, Alvarez P, Sharaiha RZ, et al. Endoscopic gallbladder drainage for acute cholecystitis. Clin Endosc 2015;48(5):411–20.

15. Itoi T, Kawakami H, Katanuma A, et al. Endoscopic nasogallbladder tube or stent placement in acute cholecystitis: a preliminary prospective randomized trial in Japan (with videos). Gastrointest Endosc 2015;81(1):111–8.

16. McCarthy ST, Tujios S, Fontana RJ, et al. Endoscopic transpapillary gallbladder stent placement is safe and effective in high-risk patients without cirrhosis. Dig Dis Sci 2015;60(8):2516–22.

17. Inoue T, Okumura F, Kachi K, et al. Long-term outcomes of endoscopic gall-bladder stenting in high-risk surgical patients with calculous cholecystitis (with videos). Gastrointest Endosc 2016;83(5):905–13.

18. Kim TH, Park DE, Chon HK. Endoscopic transpapillary gallbladder drainage for the management of acute calculus cholecystitis patients unfit for urgent cholecystectomy. PLoS One 2020;15(10):e0240219.

19. Storm AC, Vargas EJ, Chin JY, et al. Transpapillary gallbladder stent placement for long-term therapy of acute cholecystitis. Gastrointest Endosc 2021;94(4):742–8.e1.

20. Maruta A, Iwata K, Iwashita T, et al. Factors affecting technical success of endoscopic transpapillary gallbladder drainage for acute cholecystitis. J Hepatobiliary Pancreat Sci 2020;27(7):429–36.

21. Khan MA, Atiq O, Kubiliun N, et al. Efficacy and safety of endoscopic gallbladder drainage in acute cholecystitis: Is it better than percutaneous gallbladder drainage? Gastrointest Endosc 2017;85(1):76–87, e3.

22. Jandura DM, Puli SR. Efficacy and safety of endoscopic transpapillary gall-bladder drainage in acute cholecystitis: An updated meta-analysis. World J Gastrointest Endosc 2021;13(8):345–55.

23. Lee DW, Chan AC, Lam YH, et al. Biliary decompression by nasobiliary catheter or biliary stent in acute suppurative cholangitis: a prospective randomized trial. Gastrointest Endosc 2002;56(3):361–5.

24. Sharma BC, Kumar R, Agarwal N, et al. Endoscopic biliary drainage by nasobiliary drain or by stent placement in patients with acute cholangitis. Endoscopy 2005;37(5):439–43.

25. Hatanaka T, Itoi T, Ijima M, et al. Efficacy and safety of endoscopic gallbladder stenting for acute cholecystitis in patients with concomitant unresectable cancer. Intern Med 2016;55(11):1411–7.

26. Maekawa S, Nomura R, Murase T, et al. Endoscopic gallbladder stenting for acute cholecystitis: a retrospective study of 46 elderly patients aged 65 years or older. BMC Gastroenterol 2013;13:65.

27. Maruta A, Iwashita T, Iwata K, et al. Permanent endoscopic gallbladder stenting versus removal of gallbladder drainage, long-term outcomes after management of acute cholecystitis in high-risk surgical patients for cholecystectomy: multi-center retrospective cohort study. J Hepatobiliary Pancreat Sci 2021;28(12):1138–46.

28. Elmunzer BJ, Novelli PM, Taylor JR, et al. Percutaneous cholecystostomy as a bridge to definitive endoscopic gallbladder stent placement. Clin Gastroenterol Hepatol 2011;9(1):18–20.

29. Baron TH, Topazian MD. Endoscopic transduodenal drainage of the gallbladder: implications for endoluminal treatment of gallbladder disease. Gastrointest Endosc 2007;65(4):735–7.

30. Chan SM, Teoh AYB, Yip HC, et al. Feasibility of per-oral cholecystoscopy and advanced gallbladder interventions after EUS-guided gallbladder stenting (with video). Gastrointest Endosc 2017;85(6):1225–32.

31. Song TJ, Park DH, Eum JB, et al. EUS-guided cholecystoenterostomy with single-step placement of a 7F double-pigtail plastic stent in patients who are unsuitable for cholecystectomy: a pilot study (with video). Gastrointest Endosc 2010;71(3): 634–40.

32. Binmoeller KF, Shah J. A novel lumen-apposing stent for transluminal drainage of nonadherent extraintestinal fluid collections. Endoscopy 2011;43(4):337–42.

33. Teoh AY, Ng EK, Chan SM, et al. Ex vivo comparison of the lumen-apposing properties of EUS-specific stents (with video). Gastrointest Endosc 2016;84(1):62–8.

34. Teoh AY, Binmoeller KF, Lau JY. Single-step EUS-guided puncture and delivery of a lumen-apposing stent for gallbladder drainage using a novel cautery-tipped stent delivery system. Gastrointest Endosc 2014;80(6):1171.

35. Park DH, Lee TH, Paik WH, et al. Feasibility and safety of a novel dedicated device for one-step EUS-guided biliary drainage: a randomized trial. J Gastroenterol Hepatol 2015;30(10):1461–6.

36. Ogura T, Ueno S, Okuda A, et al. One-step deployment for EUS-guided gallbladder drainage using a novel fully covered metal stent (with video). J Hepatobiliary Pancreat Sci 2021;28(2):e4–5.

37. Jang JW, Lee SS, Park DH, et al. Feasibility and safety of EUS-guided transgastric/transduodenal gallbladder drainage with single-step placement of a modified covered self-expandable metal stent in patients unsuitable for cholecystectomy. Gastrointest Endosc 2011;74(1):176–81.

38. Choi JH, Lee SS, Choi JH, et al. Long-term outcomes after endoscopic ultrasonography-guided gallbladder drainage for acute cholecystitis. Endoscopy 2014;46(8):656–61.

39. Walter D, Teoh AY, Itoi T, et al. EUS-guided gall bladder drainage with a lumen-apposing metal stent: a prospective long-term evaluation. Gut 2016;65(1):6–8.

40. Dollhopf M, Larghi A, Will U, et al. EUS-guided gallbladder drainage in patients with acute cholecystitis and high surgical risk using an electrocautery-enhanced lumen-apposing metal stent device. Gastrointest Endosc 2017;86(4): 636–43.

41. Ahmed O, Ogura T, Eldahrouty A, et al. Endoscopic ultrasound-guided gallbladder drainage: results of long-term follow-up. Saudi J Gastroenterol 2018; 24(3):183–8.

42. Anderloni A, Leo MD, Carrara S, et al. Endoscopic ultrasound-guided transmural drainage by cautery-tipped lumen-apposing metal stent: exploring the possible indications. Ann Gastroenterol 2018;31(6):735–41.

43. Oh D, Song TJ, Cho DH, et al. EUS-guided cholecystostomy versus endoscopic transpapillary cholecystostomy for acute cholecystitis in high-risk surgical patients. Gastrointest Endosc 2019;89(2):289–98.

44. Teoh AYB, Kitano M, Itoi T, et al. Endosonography-guided gallbladder drainage versus percutaneous cholecystostomy in very high-risk surgical patients with

acute cholecystitis: an international randomised multicentre controlled superiority trial (DRAC 1). Gut 2020;69(6):1085–91.

45. Teoh AY, Perez-Miranda M, Kunda R, et al. Outcomes of an international multi-center registry on EUS-guided gallbladder drainage in patients at high risk for cholecystectomy. Endosc Int Open 2019;7(8):E964–73.

46. McCarty TR, Hathorn KE, Bazarbashi AN, et al. Endoscopic gallbladder drainage for symptomatic gallbladder disease: a cumulative systematic review meta-analysis. Surg Endosc 2021;35(9):4964–85.

47. Mohan BP, Asokkumar R, Shakhatreh M, et al. Adverse events with lumen-apposing metal stents in endoscopic gallbladder drainage: A systematic review and meta-analysis. Endosc Ultrasound 2019;8(4):241–8.

48. Jang JW, Lee SS, Song TJ, et al. Endoscopic ultrasound-guided transmural and percutaneous transhepatic gallbladder drainage are comparable for acute cholecystitis. Gastroenterology 2012;142(4):805–11.

49. Saumoy M, Tyberg A, Brown E, et al. Successful cholecystectomy after endoscopic ultrasound gallbladder drainage compared with percutaneous cholecystostomy, can it be done? J Clin Gastroenterol 2019;53(3):231–5.

50. de la Serna-Higuera C, Pérez-Miranda M, Gil-Simón P, et al. EUS-guided transenteric gallbladder drainage with a new fistula-forming, lumen-apposing metal stent. Gastrointest Endosc 2013;77(2):303–8.

51. Tyberg A, Jha K, Shah S, et al. EUS-guided gallbladder drainage: a learning curve modified by technical progress. Endosc Int Open 2020;8(1):E92–6.

52. Ge N, Sun S, Sun S, et al. Endoscopic ultrasound-assisted transmural cholecystoduodenostomy or cholecystogastrostomy as a bridge for per-oral cholecystoscopy therapy using double-flanged fully covered metal stent. BMC Gastroenterol 2016;16:9.

53. Teoh AY, Chan AW, Chiu PW, et al. In vivo appearances of gallbladder carcinoma under magnifying endoscopy and probe-based confocal laser endomicroscopy after endosonographic gallbladder drainage. Endoscopy 2014;46(1):E13–4.

54. Tian L, Yang Y, Xiao D, et al. Resection of gallbladder polyps following endoscopic ultrasound-guided cholecystoduodenostomy using a lumen-apposing metal stent. Endoscopy 2018;50(10):E307–8.

55. Krishnamoorthi R, Jayaraj M, Thoguluva Chandrasekar V, et al. EUS-guided versus endoscopic transpapillary gallbladder drainage in high-risk surgical patients with acute cholecystitis: a systematic review and meta-analysis. Surg Endosc 2020;34(5):1904–13.

56. Itoi T, Takada T, Hwang TL, et al. Percutaneous and endoscopic gallbladder drainage for acute cholecystitis: international multicenter comparative study using propensity score-matched analysis. J Hepatobiliary Pancreat Sci 2017;24(6):362–8.

57. Kaura K, Bazerbachi F, Sawas T, et al. Surgical outcomes of ERCP-guided transpapillary gallbladder drainage versus percutaneous cholecystostomy as bridging therapies for acute cholecystitis followed by interval cholecystectomy. HPB (Oxford) 2020;22(7):996–1003.

58. Iino C, Shimoyama T, Igarashi T, et al. Comparable efficacy of endoscopic transpapillary gallbladder drainage and percutaneous transhepatic gallbladder drainage in acute cholecystitis. Endosc Int Open 2018;6(5):E594–601.

59. Mu P, Lin Y, Zhang X, et al. The evaluation of ENGBD versus PTGBD in high-risk acute cholecystitis: a single-center prospective randomized controlled trial. EClinicalMedicine 2021;31:100668.

60. Tyberg A, Saumoy M, Sequeiros EV, et al. EUS-guided versus percutaneous gall-bladder drainage: isn't it time to convert? J Clin Gastroenterol 2018;52(1):79–84.
61. Luk SW, Irani S, Krishnamoorthi R, et al. Endoscopic ultrasound-guided gall-bladder drainage versus percutaneous cholecystostomy for high risk surgical pa-tients with acute cholecystitis: a systematic review and meta-analysis. Endoscopy 2019;51(8):722–32.
62. Siddiqui A, Kunda R, Tyberg A, et al. Three-way comparative study of endoscopic ultrasound-guided transmural gallbladder drainage using lumen-apposing metal stents versus endoscopic transpapillary drainage versus percutaneous cholecys-tostomy for gallbladder drainage in high-risk surgical patients with acute cholecys-titis: clinical outcomes and success in an International, Multicenter Study. Surg Endosc 2019;33(4):1260–70.
63. Podboy A, Yuan J, Stave CD, et al. Comparison of EUS-guided endoscopic trans-papillary and percutaneous gallbladder drainage for acute cholecystitis: a sys-tematic review with network meta-analysis. Gastrointest Endosc 2021;93(4): 797–804.
64. Corral JE, Das A, Kröner PT, et al. Cost effectiveness of endoscopic gallbladder drainage to treat acute cholecystitis in poor surgical candidates. Surg Endosc 2019;33(11):3567–77.
65. Teoh AYB, Leung CH, Tam PTH, et al. EUS-guided gallbladder drainage versus laparoscopic cholecystectomy for acute cholecystitis: a propensity score anal-ysis with 1-year follow-up data. Gastrointest Endosc 2021;93(3):577–83.
66. Choi JH, Kim HW, Lee JC, et al. Percutaneous transhepatic versus EUS-guided gallbladder drainage for malignant cystic duct obstruction. Gastrointest Endosc 2017;85(2):357–64.
67. Irani S, Ngamruengphong S, Teoh A, et al. Similar efficacies of endoscopic ultra-sound gallbladder drainage with a lumen-apposing metal stent versus percuta-neous transhepatic gallbladder drainage for acute cholecystitis. Clin Gastroenterol Hepatol 2017;15(5):738–45.
68. Higa JT, Sahar N, Kozarek RA, et al. EUS-guided gallbladder drainage with a lumen-apposing metal stent versus endoscopic transpapillary gallbladder drainage for the treatment of acute cholecystitis (with videos). Gastrointest En-dosc 2019;90(3):483–92.

Endoscopic Papillectomy

Sara Teles de Campos, MD[a], Marco J. Bruno, MD, PhD[b],*

KEYWORDS

- Ampullary lesions • Endoscopic ultrasound
- Endoscopic retrograde cholangiopancreatography • Endoscopic papillectomy
- Radiofrequency ablation

KEY POINTS

- Endoscopic papillectomy is the first-line treatment for histology-proven ampullary lesions of the major papilla up to 20 to 30 mm in diameter, with benign endoscopic characteristics and with up to 20 mm intraductal extension.
- Initial diagnostic evaluation comprises side-viewing endoscopy with biopsies, EUS, and/ or MRCP.
- Endoscopic papillectomy is a complex procedure that requires ample endoscopic expertise and skills, proper equipment, and qualified support staff.
- Complications can occur but are most often mild to moderate and usually treated conservatively.
- There is a risk of recurrence and long-term follow-up after EP with a minimum of 5 years is recommended.

 Video content accompanies this article at http://www.giendo.theclinics.com

INTRODUCTION

Ampullary lesions (ALs) arise from the ampulla of Vater. Although considered to be rare with an incidence of less than 1 per 100,000 persons per year, representing only 0.6% to 0.8% of the digestive cancers[1,2] and 6% to 10% of lesions arising in the periampullary region,[3] they account for 20% of all tumor-related obstructions of the common bile duct (CBD).[4] The incidence of AL has remained stable in old age groups, but is increasing among young adults (<45 years).[5]

Most ALs are sporadic, involve the major papilla, and are premalignant (eg, adenomas).[6] Adenomatous precursor lesions arise from intestinal-type mucosa or pancreatic duct–type ampullary mucosa.[7] The intestinal-type AL follows the well-known

[a] Department of Gastroenterology, Digestive Unit, Champalimaud Foundation, Avenida de Brasília, Lisbon 1400-038, Portugal; [b] Department of Gastroenterology & Hepatology, Erasmus University Medical Center, Dr. Molewaterplein 40, Rotterdam 3015 GD, the Netherlands
* Corresponding author.
E-mail address: m.bruno@erasmusmc.nl

Gastrointest Endoscopy Clin N Am 32 (2022) 545–562
https://doi.org/10.1016/j.giec.2022.01.005
1052-5157/22/© 2022 Elsevier Inc. All rights reserved.

adenoma-carcinoma sequence similar to colorectal adenocarcinoma.[8] AL may therefore also present as an adenocarcinoma. Occasionally, an AL may prove to be a neuroendocrine tumor.[9]

The diagnosis of AL is often incidental when patients, in their sixth to seventh decade of life, undergo an upper endoscopy or cross-sectional imaging for another clinical motive. They can also manifest clinically due to biliary and pancreatic outflow compression secondary to a mass effect of the neoplasm.

As most ALs are of neoplastic origin, resection is generally recommended. Factors such as age, comorbidities, anticipated life expectancy, tumor stage, and procedure-related risks have to be taken into account when managing these patients. Endoscopic papillectomy (EP), introduced by Suzuki and colleagues,[10] is an intervention associated with low morbidity and mortality and has become the preferred treatment over surgery for benign AL.

PRERESECTION EVALUATION

Careful evaluation of an AL is crucial to guide and ensure optimal management. This evaluation includes an endoscopic appraisal together with a staging investigation according to the TNM classification[11] for which endoscopic ultrasound (EUS) and magnetic resonance cholangiopancreatography (MRCP)[12] are appropriate investigational tools.

Role of Endoscopy

Endoscopy, using high-definition white light and dye-based or virtual chromoendoscopy, can help differentiate benign from malignant lesions and identify lesions with advanced histology that may be unsuitable for endoscopic resection.[13] When the major papilla is not correctly identified by standard gastroscopy, one option would be to perform cap-assisted endoscopy. Side-viewing duodenoscopy, however, is much preferred to evaluate AL and assess the opportunity for endoscopic resection.[12] Endoscopically, AL may be confined to the ampullary mound or can have an extrapapillary component and/or intraductal extension (IDE).[14] If the extrapapillary part involving the duodenal wall is greater than the size of the papillary adenoma, or there is a laterally spreading ampullary tumor with ≥10 mm extension beyond the ampullary mound, it is defined as a lateral spreading lesion of the papilla (LSL-P).[12] LSL-P are usually Paris type 0-IIa+Is.

Endoscopic features suggesting a benign AL include regular surface/margins, soft appearance, and mobility,[15] whereas ulceration, rigidity, friability, a depressed component, and nonlifting of LSL-P suggest local invasion.[16] Endoscopic biopsies and histologic examination may further increase the diagnostic accuracy of AL and are recommended before considering treatment.[12] They should be taken from 10- to 12-o'clock position of the ampulla to avoid the pancreatic orifice and the development of acute pancreatitis. Biopsies have a very high positive predictive value, but the negative predictive value is limited. They are particularly useful to confirm the presence of adenoma (with a sensitivity of more than 90%), but a diagnosis of adenocarcinoma can be missed in up to 30% of cases.[17] In addition, there are some rare inflammatory ("papillitis")[18] and tumor-like lesions, like hamartomatous lesions, adenomyomas, or adenomyomatous hyperplasia,[19] that should be differentiated from a dysplastic lesion. Diagnostic accuracy increases with more biopsies (at least 6) or repeating biopsies at least 1 week after sphincterotomy,[20,21] but complete removal and pathologic appraisal of the AL is crucial to confirm the diagnosis.

Role of EUS, CT, and MRI/MRCP

EUS and MRCP are recommended for helping in the diagnosis and staging of AL.[12] Both methods are important to specifically obtain/assess:

- histology of AL through EUS-guided tissue sampling, when standard histologic biopsies are not diagnostic[12];
- the presence and extent of IDE for which EUS appraisal is as good as ERCP[22];
- the presence of pancreas divisum for which EUS and MRCP are both appropriate modalities[23];
- local staging of ampullary cancers. EUS, sometimes combined with EUS-guided tissue sampling, can be of help to stage AL. For T staging, EUS has significantly higher accuracy compared with CT, and comparable or slightly but not significantly higher accuracy compared with MRCP.[24] A recent meta-analysis evaluated the performance of EUS and showed a pooled sensitivity and specificity of 77% (95% confidence interval [CI], 69% to 83%) and 78% (95% CI, 72% to 84%), respectively, for the diagnosis of a T1 tumor.[25] For N staging, MRCP is the best option, but the difference was not significantly different as compared with EUS or CT.[24] EUS has a statistically higher sensitivity for malignant lymph node diagnosis compared with CT.[22] The pooled sensitivity and specificity of morphologic criteria for lymph node involvement in EUS were 70% (95% CI, 62% to 77%) and 74% (95% CI, 67% to 80%), respectively.
- distant metastases by means of cross-sectional imaging investigations (CT and MRI).

Combining EUS with EP/ERCP in the same session has shown to be effective and safe,[26] increases patient comfort and reduces costs.

Role of ERCP

Although potentially useful to increase the accuracy of biopsies after having performed a biliary sphincterotomy and to be able to obtain brush cytology[27] or to evaluate the CBD with IDE to assess IDE, the risks involved and limited additional diagnostic value preclude the use of ERCP as a standard diagnostic staging technique.

Role of Colonoscopy

All patients with AL, regardless if they are sporadic or in the context of familial adenomatous polyposis (FAP), should be offered a screening colonoscopy before considering endoscopic ampullary resection to exclude colonic polyps as these patients have an increased risk for development of colorectal neoplasia.[28]

INDICATIONS FOR EP

EP is generally indicated for resection of histology-proven AL up to 20 to 30 mm in diameter, with benign endoscopic characteristics and with up to 20 mm IDE. Surgery should be considered in cases considered not feasible for endoscopic resection including the presence of a periampullary diverticulum, size > 4 cm, endoscopic features of malignancy, IDE of greater than 20 mm, or malignant AL of stage T1 or higher.[12] AL of 3 to 4 cm in size should be considered on a case-by-case basis.

TECHNIQUE
Equipment

EP is performed using a duodenoscope for optimal viewing of the ampullary region and optimal manipulation of instruments with the help of the elevator. Luminal insufflation is preferably achieved with carbon dioxide because it causes less luminal distension, less abdominal pain and bloating at the end of the procedure. Moreover, if there is a duodenal perforation, CO_2 insufflation potentially reduces the risk of tension pneumoperitoneum and the degree of extramural contamination.[29,30]

An electrosurgical generator with the possibility of providing alternating cycles of high-frequency short pulse cutting current and coagulation current is required. Both pure cutting and blended currents have been used. In our practice, we advocate the use of the endocut mode with standard settings for polypectomy (eg, Endocut Q, effect 3, cut duration 1, cutting interval 6; ERBE VIO 200D, Tübingen, Germany) for tissue transection and reduce intraprocedural and early postprocedural bleeding.[12,31]

Equipment that should always be readily available includes sphincterotomes, hydrophilic guidewires, injection catheters, polypectomy snares, coagulation forceps, endoscopic clips, biliary stents (short plastic 10Fr and fully-covered metal stents 8 and 10 mm diameter), pancreatic stents (short 5Fr with no internal flange but with a flange or a pigtail on the duodenal side[32]), retrieval nets, fluids and dyes, and diluted epinephrine for submucosal injection.

No superiority has been shown of a specific polypectomy snare although in most reports standard braided stainless steel wires have been used. No comparisons between snare shapes have been made either. In our practice, depending on the local situation, we tend to use either a large, flexible, oval snare (AcuSnare, Cook Medical) or a stiff hexagonal snare (Captivator, Boston Scientific).[14,31]

For submucosal lifting, ESGE suggests the use of injectates that are more viscous than normal saline and whose safety has been proven such as succinylated gelatin (gelofusine), hydroxyethyl starch, or glycerol.[33] The blue dyes indigo carmine and methylene blue can be used to enhance endoscopic demarcation of the margins of the AL, to define the extent of the submucosal cushion, and to check that one is cutting in the correct tissue plane. Diluted epinephrine (1:100.000) can be added to the submucosal solution to help reduce intraprocedural bleeding and to prolong the lifting time of the mucosa.

Sedation/Anesthesia

The type and depth of sedation (conscious sedation, deep sedation, or anesthesia) depend on patient's comorbidities, and type and extent of the AL. If a prolonged therapeutic procedure is anticipated in case of resection of a large AL, a deeper sedation (propofol) is preferable.

Endoscopic Technique

The duodenoscope should be inserted and placed in a stable position facing the ampulla. Margins and feasibility for en-bloc resection should be well assessed.

Despite lack of clear evidence, some endoscopists, especially when an EUS or MRCP was not performed, obtain a cholangiogram and a pancreatogram before EP, to rule out deep IDE.

For lesions confined to the papillary mound, no submucosal injection is indicated as it might hamper the resection: the center of the AL may not lift and is tethered down by the biliary and pancreatic ducts (**Fig. 1** and Video 1). Injection may create a "dome" effect, hinder snare placement and en-bloc resection[34]; and the risk of postresection pancreatitis may increase.[12] Moreover, it is not proven that it reduces the depth of thermal injury to the duodenal wall.[35]

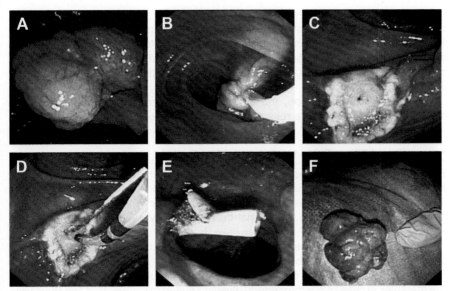

Fig. 1. (A) Papillary adenoma. (B) En-bloc snare resection of an ampullary adenoma without submucosal lifting. (C) Resection plane immediately after papillectomy. (D) Selective cannulation of the pancreatic duct. (E) Placement of a protective stent in the pancreatic duct. (F) Captured resection specimen to be sent off for pathologic evaluation.

En-bloc resection should be achieved in lesions up to 20 mm and may be attempted in lesions with 20–30 mm, if the adenoma does not extend > 1 cm beyond the papillary mound.[12]

For en-bloc resections, we use the wildly adopted fulcrum technique,[31] which consists of the following steps:

1. Open fully, or almost fully, the snare partially inside the working channel;
2. Anchor the tip of the snare proximal/cranial of the lesion and align it slightly to the right of the long axis of the infundibulum for better snare control and to avoid snare disimpaction;
3. Slowly push the snare out of the working channel and position it to fully grasp the papilla;
4. .Gently push the duodenoscope distally and slowly open the elevator slowly, while at the same time, apply a gentle force to keep the snare tip impacted in the duodenal wall above;
5. Slowly close the snare while maintaining its position parallel to the duodenal wall. When the snare is completely closed, the papilla/lesion should move independently of the duodenal wall. To confirm it, the snare should be moved back and forth with the elevator open;
6. .After completing these steps and ensuring there is no invasive disease and no deeper tissues are captured, the resection is performed by closing the snare with the elevator opened;

Balloon-catheter–assisted EP has been described to assist en-bloc resection mainly of flat papillary tumors.[36] A balloon catheter linked to a snare is inserted into the bile duct via the accessory channel of the duodenoscope and a snare resection is performed after pulling the inflated balloon toward the duodenal lumen.

After resection, the specimen should be captured for pathology, either using the snare or a retrieval net. An antiperistaltic agent, such as glucagon 1 mg or buscopan 10 to 20 mg i.v., can be administered before the ampullectomy to prevent distal migration of the specimen after resection. The specimen should ideally be pinned on a cork board to allow better histology assessment for lateral and deep margins, especially if larger than 15 mm.

Immediately after resection, the duodenoscope is reinserted for inspection to ensure hemostasis, complete resection, and exclude deep injury.

Pancreatic and Biliary Sphincterotomy and Stenting

Sphincterotomy before resection is generally not recommended. It does not confer any advantage for successful post-EP cannulation or stenting rates, may lower the rate of en-bloc and single-session resection due to scarring,[37] may hamper complete pathologic assessment due to thermal injury, and may even increase the risk of adverse events.[38]

After the specimen has been retrieved and the resection plane is inspected, the pancreatic duct (PD) should be cannulated and stented to reduce the risk of iatrogenic pancreatitis, papillary stricture formation, and offer safer usage of adjunctive coagulative therapies in case of postprocedural bleeding during follow-up.[39,40] The PD is visualized as a slit-like opening at the 5- to 6-o'clock position (**Fig. 2**). To facilitate PD identification after resection, some endoscopists prefer to inject a small amount of methylene blue into the PD before resection.[31] After resection also secretin can be administrated in case of difficult PD identification.[31]

Within 5 to 10 days after PD stent placement, patients should undergo a plain abdominal radiograph according to guidelines.[32] Retained stents should be removed promptly.

Usually, the rate of post-EP cholangitis is very low, and biliary cannulation, sphincterotomy, and stenting should only be attempted in case of a suspicion of delayed biliary drainage, intraprocedural bleeding or high risk of early postprocedural bleeding,

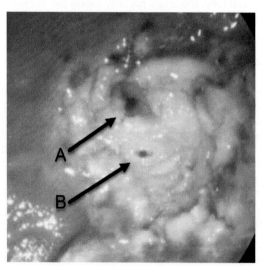

Fig. 2. Postpapillectomy anatomy showing the common bile duct orifice (A) and the pancreatic duct orifice (B).

biliary IDE (irrespective of having undergone treatment or not), or small perforations at the level of the papillectomy.[12] In case of bleeding or perforation, we prefer to insert a fully-covered metal stent. In case of IDE that is potentially amenable to endoscopic resection, an extended biliary sphincterotomy should be performed to facilitate complete resection using a smaller snare or argon plasma coagulation (APC).

Special Situations

Lateral spreading lesions of the papilla

In case of treating LSL-P endoscopically, some particular technical aspects must be considered.

We start approaching the lateral spreading component of the adjacent duodenal wall first by performing endoscopic mucosal resection (EMR) using submucosal injection in line with the recommendation for EMR in the gastrointestinal tract. Subsequently, the papilla is isolated, allowing en-bloc EP (**Fig. 3**).

Piecemeal resection is usually required for lesions measuring more than 2 cm. Major drawbacks of this technique are incomplete pathologic assessment and a higher risk for recurrence.

ALs with IDE

Classically, ALs with IDE were referred for surgery because of a significantly low rate of curative endoscopic resection and a high rate of rescue surgery.[41] Nonetheless, complementary endoscopic techniques, such as thermal ablation by cystotome or intraductal radiofrequency ablation (RFA), have been developed and are a feasible option for cases with an AL $\leq$ 20-mm IDE.[12]

Intraductal thermal ablation by a wire-guided cystotome (6Fr to 10Fr), using soft coagulation (effect 4–5) or forced coagulation (effect 3, 80W) is safe and has been successfully used to treat AL with IDE.[42]

More recently, RFA has been introduced as an ancillary technique to eradicate remnant endobiliary adenomatous tissue.[43] A recent study by Tringali and colleagues[44] prospectively evaluated patients with IDE of adenomatous ALs. They reported a technical success of 100% with 67% of patients free of recurrence after a median follow-up of 21 months. Another study by Hoon Choi and colleagues,[45] with a median follow-up period of 253 days, showed a 10% risk of recurrence needing additional surgery.

Biliary strictures and pancreatitis are common (up to 30%) after RFA for IDE[43–45] for which reason both temporary biliary and pancreatic stents should be placed prophylactically.[12]

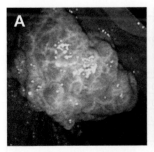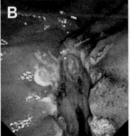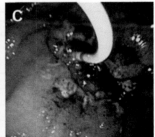

Fig. 3. (*A*) papillary adenoma with distal extension along the duodenal wall. (*B*) Resection plane after papillectomy and resection of the distal extension of the adenoma after submucosal lifting with saline and methylene blue (note the blue-stained submucosal plane). (*C*) Placement of a protective pancreatic stent.

Ampullary carcinoma

Several studies have reported that EP can be curative in case of early stages of adeno-carcinoma (Tis and T1) that are well-differentiated, with clear margins of resection and without lymphovascular invasion.[46–48] Nonetheless, to date there is insufficient evidence to recommend EP as the preferred therapy for T1 tumors although EP is regarded as a viable option for TisN0M0 lesions according to recent guidelines.[12]

Postprocedure Instructions

No clear guidelines exist on the immediate postprocedural care after EP. Given the risks associated with EP, in our unit, patients are admitted overnight and are kept nil by mouth for at least 6 hours before starting clear fluids. We should administer intravenous proton pump inhibitors for 24 hours, followed by oral PPI twice daily for a minimum of 4 weeks. If there are no symptoms or signs suggesting a complication, patients are discharged.

A plain abdominal film needs to be obtained 5 to 10 days after the procedure to document spontaneous PD stent migration. If the PD stent has not migrated spontaneously, it must be removed promptly by regular gastroduodenoscopy. A CBD stent can be removed at the first surveillance endoscopy 3 months after EP.

SPECIFIC CONSIDERATIONS IN THE FAP POPULATION

Although the majority of AL is sporadic, a genetic predisposition in the setting of adenomatous polyposis syndromes, including FAP and MUTYH-associated polyposis, must be suspected in case of diagnosis at a younger age. FAP represents the strongest hereditary predisposition with a 120-fold increased relative risk of ampullary adenocarcinoma and a 300-fold risk of duodenal adenocarcinoma compared with the general population,[49] with an absolute lifetime risk of developing duodenal adenocarcinoma or ampullary carcinoma of about 5%.[50] Duodenal and periampullary cancers have become a leading cause of death for FAP patients since prophylactic colectomy became the standard of care.[51] Fortunately, screening and early resection of AL have become more widespread. ESGE suggests starting endoscopic duodenal surveillance at age 25 years and continuing at intervals determined by the characteristics of previously found polyps[52] and the Spigelman score.[53] Spigelman score assesses the severity of duodenal polyposis according to number, size, histology, and grade of dysplasia of duodenal adenomas (**Table 1**). The surveillance interval should be based on both Spigelman stage and separate judgment of the ampulla (**Table 2**).

Table 1
Assessment of Spigelman score based on findings at duodenoscopy and pathologic examination

Findings at Duodenoscopy	1 Point	2 Points	3 Points
Number of adenomas	1–4	5–20	>20
Size, mm	1–4	5–10	>10
Histology[a]	Tubular	Tubulovillous	Villous
Dysplasia[a]	Low grade	NA	High grade

[a] Based on pathology obtained for complete removal of duodenal polyps or prior pathology results.

Table 2
Determination of the surveillance interval based on Spigelman score and stage

Spigelman Score	Spigelman Stage	Surveillance Score[a]
0 point	0	5 y
1–4 points	I	5 y
5–6 points	II	3 y
7–8 points	III	1 y
9–12 points	IV	6 mo, consider (endoscopic or surgical) treatment

[a] Additional adjustment based on inspection of the ampullary region: normal ampulla, surveillance interval of 5 y; adenomatous change less than 10 mm in the ampulla, 3 y; if $\geq$ 10 mm, 1 y is proposed for endoscopic surveillance interval or treatment (preferred).

Biopsies should only be taken if the AL seems not amenable to endoscopic removal because of size or suspicion of invasive growth.

In patients with ampullary adenomas associated with FAP, low-risk lesions are often monitored without immediate resection. This differs from the approach in sporadic AL and is based on the assumption that AL in FAP is less aggressive, although it is not clear whether the duration of progression from adenoma to advanced adenoma is truly longer.[54] It is hypothesized that specific histologic features and differences in the adenoma-carcinoma sequence, compared with sporadic lesions, lead to a slower progression.[54] Another consideration is the presence of multiple duodenal lesions in FAP, making it impossible to completely eradicate all the adenomatous tissue with only high-grade dysplastic lesions being removed in such cases. ESGE suggests treatment only for patients with ampullary adenomas $\geq$ 10 mm, showing excessive growth or suspicion of invasive growth.[52] The modality of treatment (endoscopic vs surgical) follows the same prerequisites as for sporadic AL. Although feasible and safe, there is a higher recurrence rate, partially explained by their underlying genetic predisposition.[54] The benefit of endoscopic management in patients with FAP is that it avoids additional surgery in patients who have likely undergone previous abdominal surgery, decreasing the risk of postoperative short-term and long-term adverse events including the development of a mesenteric desmoid tumor.[54]

Three small observational studies[55–57] have studied the effect of endoscopic ampullectomy in FAP patients: complication rates were high (19%–20% pancreatitis, 4%–13% bleeding, 8% abdominal pain) and recurrence occurred in up to 67% of the cases after a follow-up ranging from 53 to 85 months with no evidence of ampullary cancer. In one of the studies,[55] 2 patients (13%) needed surgery after several repeated endoscopic resections.

EXPERT TIPS ON MINIMIZING COMPLICATIONS AND THEN MANAGING COMPLICATIONS

Literature reports suggest a reduced rate of overall complications with EP compared with surgical treatment. Nevertheless, also after EP, the complication rate is significant. In our experience, 25.3% of patients suffered a procedure-related complication.[14] A recent systematic review reported an overall adverse event rate of 24.9% (95% CI, 21.2% to 29%).[16] Fortunately, complications are usually mild to moderate and can be treated conservatively. They can be divided into early complications including pancreatitis, bleeding and perforation, and delayed complications, such as papillary and biliary stenosis or duodenal luminal stenosis. EP-related mortality is rare and reported to be 0.3%.

Postprocedural Pancreatitis

Postprocedural pancreatitis is caused by temporary edema of the pancreatic orifice and obstruction as a result from the electrocautery and reported to be the most common adverse event occurring in 11.9% of cases (95% CI, 10.5% to 13.6%). Preventive measures include administration of 100 mg rectal indomethacin or diclofenac immediately before EP in all patients without a contraindication.[12,32] PD stent placement is recommended to reduce the pancreatitis risk,[12,58] except in cases of complete pancreas divisum. In case of minor ampullectomy, PD stent placement is only indicated in the setting of (in-)complete pancreas divisum. Despite the absence of sound scientific evidence, it is considered reasonable to place a PD stent after ID-RFA[43] or APC.[41] When prophylactic PD stenting is not possible after EP, high volume hydration using lactated Ringer's solution can be considered to reduce the risk of post-ERCP pancreatitis.[12] Management of postampullectomy pancreatitis follows the same recommendations for treating acute pancreatitis of other etiologies. Of interest, a PD wire-guided resection technique[59,60] has been developed to secure PD stenting to prevent postprocedural pancreatitis. For this, the PD is cannulated with a guidewire first, after which a snare loop is passed over that guidewire to capture the EL. Immediately after snare resection, a PD stent is placed over the indwelling guidewire. Although conceptually attractive, this technique is limited in its use because of decreased endoscopic maneuverability.

Bleeding

Bleeding is the second most frequent complication (10.6%; 95% CI, 5.2% to 13.6%) and is a significant adverse event in case of LSL-P,[61] because of high vascularization of the duodenal wall. Bleeding can present intraprocedural or delayed, usually in the first 12 hours after resection, but sporadically much later, as in colonic resections. The size of the lesion/resection is one of the most important risk factors for delayed bleeding. In case of intraprocedural bleeding, soft coagulation (80 W, effect 4) with the tip of snare or with coagulation forceps can be attempted. APC (with a 7Fr diameter device and a setting of 50–60W) can also be used safely, not only for immediate bleeding control but also for preventing postprocedure bleeding.[62] In case of a delayed bleeding presenting with melena in a hemodynamically stable patient, a conservative approach can be attempted, with admission and supportive care, as the bleeding usually settles spontaneously. If hematemesis or hematochezia occurs in an unstable patient, urgent endoscopy is indicated. Standard hemostasis techniques, such as epinephrine injection, electrocoagulation or clipping, noncontact hemostatic techniques, and APC, preferably using a duodenoscope, should be attempted to control the bleed. One study reported successful endoscopic hemostasis using fibrin glue in refractory bleeding.[63] Before applying these techniques, it is important to identify the PD orifice and ideally place a prophylactic PD stent in order to protect it from inadvertent closure (**Fig. 4**).

In Case of an Uncontrolled Major Bleeding, Angiographic Embolization and/or Surgery Is Indicated

Perforation
Perforation, an adverse effect related to electrocautery, is reported after EP in 3.1% of cases (95% CI, 2.2% to 4.2%). Careful inspection of the defect, endoscopically and fluoroscopically, is crucial to detect deep tissue injury. Owing to retroperitoneal

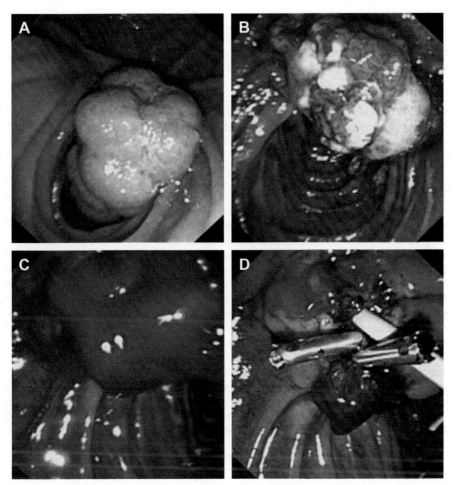

Fig. 4. (*A*) Papillary adenoma. (*B*) Immediately after papillectomy with specimen that needs to be retrieved without signs of a postpapillectomy bleeding. (*C*) Reintroduction of endoscope, however, shows an (arterial) postpapillectomy bleed. (*D*) Successful clipping of the bleeding spot AFTER securing pancreatic duct patency and drainage with a pancreatic stent.

location, it can almost always be managed conservatively. If diagnosed during the procedure, apart from administrating intravenous antibiotics, an attempt to close it with endoclips and biliary stenting with a fully covered self-expandable metallic stent should be performed. To avoid accidental clipping of the PD orifice, it is pivotal to assure a good anatomic overview or, even better, to place a protective pancreatic stent before closing the perforation. The patient should be kept NPO and admitted for clinical observation. If a suspicion of perforation develops after the procedure, an abdominal CT scan should be performed.

Cholangitis

Cholangitis is reported to occur in 2.7% of cases (95% CI, 1.9% to 4%).[16] It can be caused by bacterial translocation, which usually resolves quickly by the administration of antibiotics. In some cases, intraductal remnant adenoma or a blood clot causes ductal outflow obstruction requiring re-ERCP.

Duodenal Luminal Stenosis

Duodenal luminal stenosis occurs only after resection of LSL-P with extensive duodenal circumferential or longitudinal involvement. These cases can be managed with early pre-emptive dilation starting 3 to 4 weeks after the resection.[64]

Biliary and Pancreatic Orifice Stenosis

Biliary and pancreatic orifice stenosis occur in 2.4% of cases (95% CI, 1.6% to 3.4%). PD stent placement can prevent pancreatic stricture formation.[65] Sphincterotomy, balloon dilation, and serial stent placement result in stricture resolution in most of the cases.

OUTCOMES

In a systematic review, it is reported that complete endoscopic resection (or technical success), defined as the absence of any adenomatous remnant from the resection margins at the end of the procedure, was achieved in 94.2% of cases (95% CI, 90.5% to 96.5%).[16] Curative endoscopic resection was achieved in 87.1% of cases (95% CI, 90.5% to 96.5%). The only predictive factor of a curative resection was en-bloc resection, which was achieved in 82.4% of cases (95% CI, 74.7% to 88.1%). EP is considered to be curative if there are no histologic features of locoregional persistence and pathology confirms AL with low-grade dysplasia or high-grade dysplasia with free lateral and in-depth margins (R0).[12] If resection margins are positive (R+), complementary techniques such as APC or EMR need to be considered. Tis ampullary cancer with free margins after EP can be considered curative.[12] If pathology after EP reveals a malignant lesion of the ampulla including stage T1, pancreaticoduodenectomy (including lymphadenectomy) is recommended as the preferred treatment because the risk of lymph node metastasis is significant.[12]

Regarding LSL-P, endoscopic treatment has shown comparable outcomes regarding endoscopic curative resection and recurrence rate to those for adenoma confined to the ampulla,[14,61,66] but the risk of bleeding should be taken into consideration.[12]

Well-designed, prospective studies comparing EP and surgical treatment (either pancreaticoduodenectomy or transduodenal ampullectomy) of AL are not available.

FOLLOW-UP

Long-term endoscopic follow-up is recommended and should be performed using a duodenoscope with biopsies of the scar and any abnormal areas, at 3, 6, and 12 months, are thereafter yearly for at least 5 years (**Fig. 5**).[12] As aforementioned, in case of very large, circumferential LSL-P, earlier follow-up, at 3 to 4 weeks, is advised to evaluate for duodenal stricture and early treatment with balloon dilation when indicated.

Despite complete endoscopic resection at the index procedure, recurrence has been reported in 11.8% of cases (95% CI 8.4% to 16.5%).[16] Recurrence is defined as the discovery of a lesion after at least one surveillance endoscopy with biopsies showing no residual adenomatous tissue.[67] It is more frequently reported in the first 14 months of FU.[68] Younger age (<48 years), female sex, polyposis syndrome, larger lesions (>24 mm), high-grade dysplasia, and IDE have been implied as risk factors for recurrence. A small number of patients have shown delayed recurrence and adenocarcinoma even after 5 years, which questions whether certain patients should be followed up lifelong, but specific data guiding proper patient selection are lacking.[14,69,70]

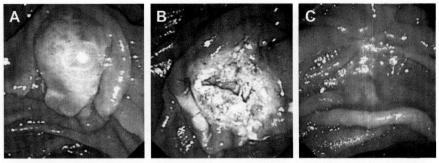

Fig. 5. (*A*) Papillary adenoma. (*B*) Immediately after papillectomy. (*C*) Follow-up endoscopy after 2 years showing no signs of recurrence.

Any recurrence should be carefully assessed before retreatment. Usually, recurrence is relatively minor and can be treated with snare excision or cold avulsion followed by snare tip soft coagulation or other ablation techniques.[12] In a systematic review, complete excision of the AL regardless of number of sessions and including recurrent lesions was achieved in 80.9% of cases (95% CI, 73% to 87%).[16]

SUMMARY

ALs are rare but responsible for 20% of all rumor-related obstructions of CBD. The incidence of AL has remained stable in old age groups, but is increasing among young adults. Most ALs are sporadic but a genetic predisposition, namely FAP, should be suspected if diagnosed at a younger age (<50 years).

EP is regarded as the first-line curative treatment for sporadic-proven AL of the major papilla with up to 20 to 30 mm in diameter, with benign endoscopic characteristics, and with up to 20 mm IDE. AL sized between 3 and 4 cm should be considered on a case-by-case basis. In the FAP population, endoscopic treatment is only indicated for ampullary adenomas ≥ 10 mm.

Preresection endoscopic evaluation of AL is pivotal for selecting the appropriate candidates for EA and improving outcome and generally includes side-viewing endoscopy, biopsies, EUS, and/or MRCP.

EP is an advanced procedure that requires specific endoscopic expertise and skills, appropriate equipment, and an experienced support team. The optimal technique of EP depends on the characteristics of the lesion, its size, the presence and extent of IDE, and the presence and extent of extrapapillary extension along the duodenal wall.

Complete endoscopic resection and curative resection rates are very high.

Complications can occur in up to a quarter of cases but are usually mild to moderate and can usually be managed conservatively. The most frequent early adverse events are postprocedural pancreatitis and bleeding.

Long-term monitoring after EP up to 5 years is recommended due to risk of recurrence.

CLINICS CARE POINTS

- Preresection evaluation of an AL involves a primary evaluation with standard gastroscopy, complemented with a side-viewing *duodenoscopy* and *biopsies*. Endoscopic biopsies should be taken from 10- to 12-o'clock position of the ampulla to avoid the pancreatic orifice.

- *EUS* and *MRCP* are complementary procedures useful for staging, namely to evaluate possible IDE and the presence of pancreas divisum or perform a local staging in case of ampullary cancer. EUS tissue sampling can also be performed if standard biopsies are inconclusive.

- All patients with AL should perform a *colonoscopy* before considering endoscopic resection, to exclude colonic polyps.

- EP is the first-line treatment for histology-proven ampullary lesions of the major papilla up to 20 to 30 mm in diameter, with benign endoscopic characteristics and with up to 20 mm IDE. Surgery should be considered in cases considered not feasible for endoscopic resection including the presence of a periampullary diverticulum, size > 4 cm, endoscopic features of malignancy, IDE of greater than 20 mm or malignant AL of stage T1 or higher. AL of 3 to 4 cm in size should be considered on a case-by-case basis.

- The following *equipment* should be available to perform EP: duodenoscope, CO_2 insufflation, electrosurgical generator with the possibility of providing alternating cycles of high-frequency short pulse cutting current and coagulation current, sphincterotomes, hydrophilic guidewires, injection catheters, polypectomy snares (no superiority has shown between different snares), coagulation forceps, endoscopic clips, biliary stents (short plastic 10Fr and fully-covered metal stents 8 and 10 mm diameter), pancreatic stents (short 5Fr with no internal flange but with a flange or a pigtail on the duodenal side), and submucosal lifting solutions (with injectates, blue dyes, diluted epinephrine).

- EP should be done under sedation and, for lesions confined to the papillary mound, en-bloc resection should be attempted by resecting with a snare without mucosal injection and by using the fulcrum *technique.* Variations of this technique will depend on the specific characteristics of the AL (eg, LST of the papilla).

- *Acute pancreatitis* is the most common complication. Its risk can be reduced by the administration of 100 mg rectal indomethacin or diclofenac immediately before EP when there is no contraindication and the placement of prophylactic pancreatic duct stenting whenever there is no pancreas divisum.

- *Bleeding* is the second most frequent adverse event and can generally be managed with standard endoscopic hemostasis techniques.

- EP has very good outcomes. Nonetheless, as there is a risk of recurrence, long-term *monitoring* after EP is advised. It should be based on duodenoscopy evaluation with biopsies of the scare and of any abnormality. The reevaluation should be done at regularly basis (first 3 months, at 6 and 12 months, and after, in a yearly basis for a minimum of 5 years).

DISCLOSURE

M.J. Bruno is a consultant for, and the recipient of industry-initiated and investigator-initiated studies from Boston Scientific, Cook Medical, and Pentax Medical and the recipient of support for investigator-initiated studies from Mylan and ChiRoStim.

SUPPLEMENTARY DATA

Supplementary data related to this article can be found online at https://doi.org/10.1016/j.giec.2022.01.005.

REFERENCES

1. Ramai D, Ofosu A, Singh J, et al. Demographics, tumor characteristics, treatment, and clinical outcomes of patients with ampullary cancer: a Surveillance, Epidemiology, and End Results (SEER) cohort study. Minerva Gastroenterol Dietol 2019;65(2). https://doi.org/10.23736/S1121-421X.18.02543-6.

2. Rostain F. Trends in incidence and management of cancer of the ampulla of Vater. WJG 2014;20(29):10144.

3. Hester CA, Dogeas E, Augustine MM, et al. Incidence and comparative outcomes of periampullary cancer: A population-based analysis demonstrating improved outcomes and increased use of adjuvant therapy from 2004 to 2012: HESTER et al. J Surg Oncol 2019;119(3):303–17.

4. Palazzo L. Staging of ampullary carcinoma by endoscopic ultrasonography. Endoscopy 1998;30(Suppl 1):A128–31.

5. Van Dyke AL, Shiels MS, Jones GS, et al. Biliary tract cancer incidence and trends in the United States by demographic group, 1999-2013. Cancer 2019; 125(9):1489–98.

6. El Hajj II, Coté GA. Endoscopic Diagnosis and Management of Ampullary Lesions. Gastrointest Endosc Clin N America 2013;23(1):95–109.

7. Fischer HP, Zhou H. Pathogenesis of carcinoma of the papilla of Vater. J Hepatobiliary Pancreat Surg 2004;11(5):301–9.

8. Seifert E, Schulte F, Stolte M. Adenoma and carcinoma of the duodenum and papilla of Vater: a clinicopathologic study. Am J Gastroenterol 1992;87(1):37–42.

9. Ruff SM, Standring O, Wu G, et al. Ampullary Neuroendocrine Tumors: Insight into a Rare Histology. Ann Surg Oncol 2021. https://doi.org/10.1245/s10434-021-10371-w.

10. Suzuki K, Kantou U, Murakami Y. Two cases with ampullary cancer who underwent endoscopic excision. Prog Dig Endosc 1983;23:236–9.

11. Amin MB, Greene FL, Edge SB, et al. The Eighth Edition AJCC Cancer Staging Manual: Continuing to build a bridge from a population-based to a more "personalized" approach to cancer staging. CA Cancer J Clin 2017;67(2):93–9.

12. Vanbiervliet G, Strijker M, Arvanitakis M, et al. Endoscopic management of ampullary tumors: European Society of Gastrointestinal Endoscopy (ESGE) Guideline. Endoscopy 2021;53(04):429–48.

13. Park JS, Seo DW, Song TJ, et al. Usefulness of white-light imaging-guided narrow-band imaging for the differential diagnosis of small ampullary lesions. Gastrointest Endosc 2015;82(1):94–101.

14. van der Wiel SE, Poley JW, Koch AD, et al. Endoscopic resection of advanced ampullary adenomas: a single-center 14-year retrospective cohort study. Surg Endosc 2019;33(4):1180–8.

15. Binmoeller KF, Boaventura S, Ramsperger K, et al. Endoscopic snare excision of benign adenomas of the papilla of Vater. Gastrointest Endosc 1993;39(2):127–31.

16. Spadaccini M, Fugazza A, Frazzoni L, et al. Endoscopic papillectomy for neoplastic ampullary lesions: A systematic review with pooled analysis. United Eur Gastroenterol j 2020;8(1):44–51.

17. Yamaguchi K, Enjoji M, Kitamura K. Endoscopic biopsy has limited accuracy in diagnosis of ampullary tumors. Gastrointest Endosc 1990;36(6):588–92.

18. Lee HS, Jang JS, Lee S, et al. Diagnostic Accuracy of the Initial Endoscopy for Ampullary Tumors. Clin Endosc 2015;48(3):239.

19. Handra-Luca A, Terris B, Couvelard A, et al. Adenomyoma and Adenomyomatous Hyperplasia of the Vaterian System: Clinical, Pathological, and New Immunohistochemical Features of 13 Cases. Mod Pathol 2003;16(6):530–6.

20. Bourgeois N, Dunham F, Verhest A, et al. Endoscopic biopsies of the papilla of Vater at the time of endoscopic sphincterotomy: difficulties in interpretation. Gastrointest Endosc 1984;30(3):163–6.

21. Chathadi KV, Khashab MA, Acosta RD, et al, ASGE Standards of Practice Committee. The role of endoscopy in ampullary and duodenal adenomas. Gastrointest Endosc 2015;82(5):773–81.

22. Ridtitid W, Schmidt SE, Al-Haddad MA, et al. Performance characteristics of EUS for locoregional evaluation of ampullary lesions. Gastrointest Endosc 2015;81(2): 380–8.

23. Shen Z, Munker S, Zhou B, et al. The Accuracies of Diagnosing Pancreas Divisum by Magnetic Resonance Cholangiopancreatography and Endoscopic Ultrasound: A Systematic Review and Meta-analysis. Sci Rep 2016;6(1):35389.

24. Manta R, Conigliaro R, Castellani D, et al. Linear endoscopic ultrasonography vs magnetic resonance imaging in ampullary tumors. World J Gastroenterol 2010; 16(44):5592–7.

25. Trikudanathan G, Njei B, Attam R, et al. Staging accuracy of ampullary tumors by endoscopic ultrasound: Meta-analysis and systematic review: EUS for staging ampullary tumors. Dig Endosc 2014;26(5):617–26.

26. Gornals JB, Esteban JM, Guarner-Argente C, et al. Endoscopic ultrasound and endoscopic retrograde cholangiopancreatography: Can they be successfully combined? Gastroenterol Hepatol 2016;39(9):627–42.

27. Bardales RH, Stanley MW, Simpson DD, et al. Diagnostic value of brush cytology in the diagnosis of duodenal, biliary, and ampullary neoplasms. Am J Clin Pathol 1998;109(5):540–8.

28. Lagarde S, Dauphin M, Delmas C, et al. Increased risk of colonic neoplasia in patients with sporadic duodenal adenoma. Gastroenterol Clin Biol 2009;33(5): 441–5.

29. Bourke MJ. Endoscopic resection in the duodenum: current limitations and future directions. Endoscopy 2013;45(2):127–32.

30. Paspatis GA, Arvanitakis M, Dumonceau JM, et al. Diagnosis and management of iatrogenic endoscopic perforations: European Society of Gastrointestinal Endoscopy (ESGE) Position Statement – Update 2020. Endoscopy 2020;52(09): 792–810.

31. Poley J, Campos S. Methods and outcome of the endoscopic treatment of ampullary tumors. Ther Adv Gastrointest Endosc 2020;13:1–13.

32. Dumonceau JM, Kapral C, Aabakken L, et al. ERCP-related adverse events: European Society of Gastrointestinal Endoscopy (ESGE) Guideline. Endoscopy 2020;52(02):127–49.

33. Ferlitsch M, Moss A, Hassan C, et al. Colorectal polypectomy and endoscopic mucosal resection (EMR): European Society of Gastrointestinal Endoscopy (ESGE) Clinical Guideline. Endoscopy 2017;49(03):270–97.

34. Menees SB, Schoenfeld P, Kim HM, et al. A survey of ampullectomy practices. World J Gastroenterol 2009;15(28):3486–92.

35. Hyun JJ, Lee TH, Park JS, et al. A prospective multicenter study of submucosal injection to improve endoscopic snare papillectomy for ampullary adenoma. Gastrointest Endosc 2017;85(4):746–55.

36. Aiura K, Imaeda H, Kitajima M, et al. Balloon-catheter-assisted endoscopic snare papillectomy for benign tumors of the major duodenal papilla. Gastrointest Endosc 2003;57(6):743–7.

37. Desilets DJ, Dy RM, Ku PM, et al. Endoscopic management of tumors of the major duodenal papilla: Refined techniques to improve outcome and avoid complications. Gastrointest Endosc 2001;54(2):202–8.

38. Lee SK, Kim MH, Seo DW, et al. Endoscopic sphincterotomy and pancreatic duct stent placement before endoscopic papillectomy: are they necessary and safe procedures? Gastrointest Endosc 2002;55(2):302–4.
39. Harewood GC, Pochron NL, Gostout CJ. Prospective, randomized, controlled trial of prophylactic pancreatic stent placement for endoscopic snare excision of the duodenal ampulla. Gastrointest Endosc 2005;62(3):367–70.
40. Napoléon B, Alvarez-Sanchez MV, Leclercq P, et al. Systematic pancreatic stenting after endoscopic snare papillectomy may reduce the risk of postinterventional pancreatitis. Surg Endosc 2013;27(9):3377–87.
41. Bohnacker S, Seitz U, Nguyen D, et al. Endoscopic resection of benign tumors of the duodenal papilla without and with intraductal growth. Gastrointest Endosc 2005;62(4):551–60.
42. Pérez-Cuadrado-Robles E, Piessevaux H, Moreels TG, et al. Combined excision and ablation of ampullary tumors with biliary or pancreatic intraductal extension is effective even in malignant neoplasms. United Eur Gastroenterol j 2019;7(3): 369–76.
43. Camus M, Napoléon B, Vienne A, et al. Efficacy and safety of endobiliary radiofrequency ablation for the eradication of residual neoplasia after endoscopic papillectomy: a multicenter prospective study. Gastrointest Endosc 2018;88(3): 511–8.
44. Tringali A, Matteo MV, Orlandini B, et al. Radiofrequency ablation for intraductal extension of ampullary adenomatous lesions: proposal for a standardized protocol. Endosc Int Open 2021;09(05):E749–55.
45. Choi YH, Yoon SB, Chang JH, et al. The Safety of Radiofrequency Ablation Using a Novel Temperature-Controlled Probe for the Treatment of Residual Intraductal Lesions after Endoscopic Papillectomy. Gut and Liver 2021;15(2):307–14.
46. Petrone G, Ricci R, Familiari P, et al. Endoscopic snare papillectomy: a possible radical treatment for a subgroup of T1 ampullary adenocarcinomas. Endoscopy 2013;45(5):401–4.
47. Yamamoto K, Itoi T, Sofuni A, et al. Expanding the indication of endoscopic papillectomy for T1a ampullary carcinoma. Dig Endosc 2019;31(2):188–96.
48. Alvarez-Sanchez MV, Oria I, Luna OB, et al. Can endoscopic papillectomy be curative for early ampullary adenocarcinoma of the ampulla of Vater? Surg Endosc 2017;31(4):1564–72.
49. Offerhaus GJ, Giardiello FM, Krush AJ, et al. The risk of upper gastrointestinal cancer in familial adenomatous polyposis. Gastroenterology 1992;102(6):1980–2.
50. Brosens LAA. Prevention and management of duodenal polyps in familial adenomatous polyposis. Gut 2005;54(7):1034–43.
51. de Campos FGCM, Perez RO, Imperiale AR, et al. Evaluating Causes of Death in Familial Adenomatous Polyposis. J Gastrointest Surg 2010;14(12):1943–9.
52. van Leerdam ME, Roos VH, van Hooft JE, et al. Endoscopic management of polyposis syndromes: European Society of Gastrointestinal Endoscopy (ESGE) Guideline. Endoscopy 2019;51(09):877–95.
53. Spigelman AD, Williams CB, Talbot IC, et al. Upper gastrointestinal cancer in patients with familial adenomatous polyposis. Lancet 1989;2(8666):783–5.
54. Angsuwatcharakon P, Ahmed O, Lynch PM, et al. Management of ampullary adenomas in familial adenomatous polyposis syndrome: 16 years of experience from a tertiary cancer center. Gastrointest Endosc 2020;92(2):323–30.
55. Gluck N, Strul H, Rozner G, et al. Endoscopy and EUS are key for effective surveillance and management of duodenal adenomas in familial adenomatous polyposis. Gastrointest Endosc 2015;81(4):960–6.

56. Ma T, Jang EJ, Zukerberg LR, et al. Recurrences are common after endoscopic ampullectomy for adenoma in the familial adenomatous polyposis (FAP) syndrome. Surg Endosc 2014;28(8):2349–56.

57. Ouaïssi M, Panis Y, Sielezneff I, et al. Long-Term Outcome After Ampullectomy for Ampullary Lesions Associated With Familial Adenomatous Polyposis. Dis Colon Rectum 2005;48(12):2192–6.

58. Gambitta P, Aseni P, Villa F, et al. Safety of Endoscopic Snare Ampullectomy for Adenomatous Ampullary Lesions: Focus on Pancreatic Stent Placement to Prevent Pancreatitis. Surg Laparosc Endosc Percutan Tech 2021. https://doi.org/10.1097/SLE.0000000000000909.

59. Moon JH, Cha SW, Cho YD, et al. Wire-guided endoscopic snare papillectomy for tumors of the major duodenal papilla. Gastrointest Endosc 2005;61(3):461–6.

60. Kobayashi M, Ryozawa S, Iwano H, et al. The usefulness of wire-guided endoscopic snare papillectomy for tumors of the major duodenal papilla. PLoS One 2019;14(1):e0211019.

61. Klein A, Qi Z, Bahin FF, et al. Outcomes after endoscopic resection of large laterally spreading lesions of the papilla and conventional ampullary adenomas are equivalent. Endoscopy 2018;50(10):972–83.

62. Nam K, Song TJ, Kim RE, et al. Usefulness of argon plasma coagulation ablation subsequent to endoscopic snare papillectomy for ampullary adenoma. Dig Endosc 2018;30(4):485–92.

63. Mutignani M, Seerden T, Tringali A, et al. Endoscopic hemostasis with fibrin glue for refractory postsphincterotomy and postpapillectomy bleeding. Gastrointest Endosc 2010;71(4):856–60.

64. Klein A, Tutticci N, Bourke MJ. Endoscopic resection of advanced and laterally spreading duodenal papillary tumors. Dig Endosc 2016;28(2):121–30.

65. Catalano MF, Linder JD, Chak A, et al. Endoscopic management of adenoma of the major duodenal papilla. Gastrointest Endosc 2004;59(2):225–32.

66. Yamamoto K, Sofuni A, Tsuchiya T, et al. Clinical Impact of Piecemeal Resection Concerning the Lateral Spread of Ampullary Adenomas. Intern Med 2019;58(7):901–6.

67. Li S, Wang Z, Cai F, et al. New experience of endoscopic papillectomy for ampullary neoplasms. Surg Endosc 2019;33(2):612–9.

68. Laleman W, Verreth A, Topal B, et al. Endoscopic resection of ampullary lesions: a single-center 8-year retrospective cohort study of 91 patients with long-term follow-up. Surg Endosc 2013;27(10):3865–76.

69. Ridtitid W, Tan D, Schmidt SE, et al. Endoscopic papillectomy: risk factors for incomplete resection and recurrence during long-term follow-up. Gastrointest Endosc 2014;79(2):289–96.

70. Tringali A, Valerii G, Boškoski I, et al. Endoscopic snare papillectomy for adenoma of the ampulla of vater: Long-term results in 135 consecutive patients. Dig Liver Dis 2020;52(9):1033–8.

Biliary Endoscopy in Altered Anatomy

Linda Y. Zhang, MBBS[a],*, Shayan Irani, MD[b], Mouen A. Khashab, MD[a]

KEYWORDS

- Altered anatomy ERCP • Gastrectomy • Roux-en-y gastric bypass
- Whipple surgery • Enteroscopy-assisted ERCP • Laparoscopy-assisted ERCP
- EUS-Directed trans-gastric ERCP

KEY POINTS

- Biliary endoscopy in altered anatomy requires not only familiarity with the various surgeries and alterations in the UGI tract, but also high technical expertise and thorough understanding of available endoscopes and devices
- Before any endoscopy on patients with altered anatomy, one must thoroughly review the patient's surgical history including the nature and length of any enteric limbs and presence/type of biliary reconstruction
- The length of bowel to traverse, the presence of an intact papilla versus bilioenteric anastomosis, and the intended biliary intervention (eg, cholangioscopy) determine endoscope choice
- Various techniques have been developed to aid biliary intervention in patients with altered anatomy, each with different success rates, risks, and benefits
- The selection of biliary access approach will depend on the patient's anatomy, operator experience, and procedural availability

INTRODUCTION

Endoscopic retrograde cholangiopancreatography (ERCP) is the standard treatment of biliary disease with high success rates of greater than 90% in patients with standard anatomy. However, alterations in upper gastrointestinal anatomy can significantly complicate endoscopic biliary intervention. The past decade has seen significant advances in the endoscopic management of patients with altered anatomy. This review article will provide tips and tricks for successful biliary access in the most common surgical alterations with a focus on the management of biliary diseases following Roux-en-Y (RY) reconstructions.

[a] Department of Gastroenterology & Hepatology, Johns Hopkins Medical Institutions, Baltimore, MD, USA; [b] Digestive Disease Institute, Virginia Mason Medical Center, Seattle, WA, USA
* Corresponding author.
E-mail address: Lzhan170@jh.edu

Gastrointest Endoscopy Clin N Am 32 (2022) 563–582
https://doi.org/10.1016/j.giec.2022.02.001
1052-5157/22/© 2022 Elsevier Inc. All rights reserved.

PREPROCEDURE EVALUATION

Before any endoscopy on patients with altered anatomy, one must thoroughly review the surgical history. If possible, the nature and length of any enteric limbs and presence/type of biliary reconstructions should be determined (**Table 1**). The time interval between surgery and ERCP should be balanced with the procedural indication. For example, avoiding deep enteroscopy on fresh surgical anastomoses (<2 weeks) if an alternative is available seems prudent. Radiologic studies will help guide the pretest probability of a disease process being present, the expected difficulty in reaching the major papilla or bilioenteric anastomosis, and cannulation once reached. This will also help to plan interventions (eg, cholangioscopy), which will influence endoscope choice. Further, cross-sectional imaging can help to determine the feasibility of EUS-guided drainage if the major papilla or the anastomosis cannot be reached. If the patient has had prior endoscopic intervention, the report should be obtained and note made of the endoscope and equipment which resulted in successful access.

The 3 major considerations when performing biliary endoscopy in altered anatomy are: (1) how to access the afferent limb and reach the ampulla or bilioenteric anastomosis, (2) how to cannulate the bile duct, and (3) once the bile duct is accessed, how to perform the planned intervention. An understanding of available endoscopes and device compatibility is vital (**Table 2**). Ideally, required endoscopes and equipment should be determined before the procedure. One or more alternative plans should be determined in advance, in case of failure. An upfront discussion should be carried out with the patient and family detailing the overall likelihood of success, whether multiple procedures are anticipated, and alternatives if the planned technique is unsuccessful, including conversion to EUS-guided biliary drainage, or subsequent referral to interventional radiology or surgery.

PATIENTS WITH ALTERED ANATOMY RESULTING IN MINIMAL EFFECT ON ENDOSCOPIC BILIARY ACCESS

Certain surgeries will result in minimal effect on endoscopic biliary access including esophagectomy and nondiverting bariatric surgeries (eg, sleeve gastrectomy). A Billroth I procedure consists of distal gastrectomy and anastomosis of the gastric remnant to the duodenum (**Fig. 1**). It is the only postgastrectomy reconstruction strategy that restores a physiologic digestive tract. A careful clinical history should be obtained to identify the possibility of anastomotic strictures which may require dilation before endoscope passage or consideration of endotracheal intubation if retained gastric contents are suspected. These surgeries should otherwise have minimal effect on endoscopic biliary intervention. Although there is some loss of scope stability due to a shorter position, ERCP can generally be performed using a duodenoscope and conventional devices with similar success rates compared with patients with normal anatomy.[1]

PATIENTS WITH ALTERED ANATOMY AND NATIVE MAJOR PAPILLA

This category includes patients with partial or complete gastric resections and reconstruction without resection, for example, gastric bypass.

Billroth II

In a Billroth II reconstruction, an end-to-side gastrojejunal anastomosis is created, leading to 2 visible lumens from the remnant stomach: one leading to the intact major papilla and closed proximal duodenal stump (afferent limb) and the other leading to the

Table 1
Summary of surgeries and recommended approach for biliary access

Surgery	Biliary Drainage	Recommended Approach
Esophagectomy	Intact papilla	Duodenoscope
Nondiverting bariatric surgeries (sleeve gastrectomy, band gastroplasty)	Intact papilla	Duodenoscope
Billroth I gastric resection	Intact papilla	Duodenoscope
Billroth II gastric resection	Intact papilla, inverted access	Colonoscope Duodenoscope possible but may require forward-viewing scope first EA-ERCP
Subtotal/total gastrectomy with Roux-en-Y anastomosis	Intact papilla, inverted access	Colonoscope with clear cap EA-ERCP EUS-guided approach
Roux-en-Y gastric bypass	Intact papilla in excluded duodenum	EDGE LA-ERCP EA-ERCP
Whipple pancreaticoduodenectomy	Bilioenteric anastomosis	Colonoscope or EA-ERCP Duodenoscope possible but may require forward-viewing scope first EUS-guided approach
Roux-en-Y hepaticojejunostomy	Bilioenteric anastomosis Intact papilla for pancreatic access	Colonoscope or EA-ERCP EUS-guided approach

[a]Clear distal attachment recommended for all forward-viewing endoscopes.

alimentary (efferent) limb (**Fig. 2**). The Polya and Hofmeister methods differ in the diameter of the anastomosis, and a Braun procedure may be performed to divert bile away from the remnant stomach. In this variation, a side-to-side jejunojejunostomy is created between the afferent and efferent limbs.

The afferent limb usually enters the stomach at a more acute angle, while the efferent limb enters en face (**Fig. 3**). Maneuvering the endoscope from the neutral position in a sharp upwards angulation typically allows the intubation of the afferent limb. The distance from the gastrojejunal anastomosis to the major papilla is typically short, (average 30–50 cm), and usually accessible with a forward-viewing endoscope or duodenoscope. The Braun variation may result in sharper luminal angulations and a longer afferent limb with the potential to loop back to the stomach if the wrong jejunal limb is intubated.[2]

The afferent limb is more readily accessed by a forward-viewing scope. However, forward-viewing endoscopes have challenges including the absence of an elevator, smaller working channel, and difficulty obtaining an en face view of the papilla. In contrast, a duodenoscope facilitates easier cannulation and subsequent intervention through the intact major papilla but can result in challenging the intubation of the afferent loop. Helpful maneuvers to facilitate duodenoscope intubation of the afferent limb include starting with the patient in the left lateral position or leaving a guidewire with a forward-viewing as a guide. Visible bile and the observation of peristalsis toward

Table 2
Summary of available endoscopes and compatible devices

Endoscope	Working Length (cm)	Instrument Channel Diameter (mm)	Compatible Devices	Pros	Cons
Therapeutic duodenoscope	124	4.2	All ERCP accessories	Elevator facilitates biliary cannulation, device exchange	Increased stiffness may increase the risk of perforation Side-viewing
Adult colonoscope	168	3.7	Most ERCP accessories Up to 10-Fr stents Cholangioscopy	Forward viewing	Lack of elevator Increased length limits use of devices
Pediatric colonoscope	168	3.2	Most ERCP accessories Up to 7-Fr stents	Forward viewing Facilitates small bowel passage and intubation of afferent limb	Lack of elevator Increased length limits use of devices Smaller instrument channel
Single-balloon enteroscope	200	2.8	Limited long ERCP accessories Up to 7-Fr stents	Forward viewing Facilitates deep intubation	Lack of elevator Increased length significantly limits the use of devices Small channel size
Double-balloon enteroscope	200	2.8	Limited long ERCP accessories Up to 7-Fr stents	Forward viewing Facilitates deep intubation	Lack of elevator Increased length significantly limits use of devices Small channel size
Short-type balloon enteroscope	152	3.2	Most ERCP accessories Up to 7-Fr stents	Forward viewing Facilitates deep intubation Improved channel size	Lack of elevator Will not allow cholangioscopy

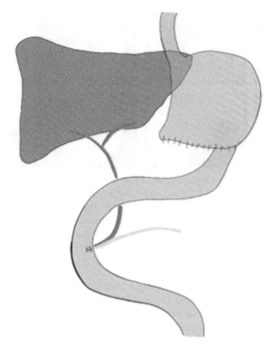

Fig. 1. Billroth I anatomy.

the endoscope may be helpful indicators of correct afferent limb intubation, but neither is always reliable. Instead, each limb should be traversed as far as able or until the major papilla is reached. Fluoroscopy can be very helpful in guiding one to the right upper quadrant. A simple mucosal biopsy can be taken just beyond the anastomosis to mark the efferent limb if initially accessed, preventing repeated passage into the same limb. For difficult afferent limb intubations, a tattoo can be performed on endoscope withdrawal if future procedures are anticipated.

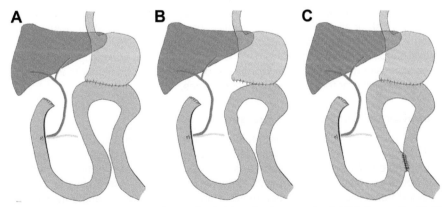

Fig. 2. Billroth II anatomy (*A*) Polya method, (*B*) Hofmeister method, (*C*) Polya method with Braun anastomosis.

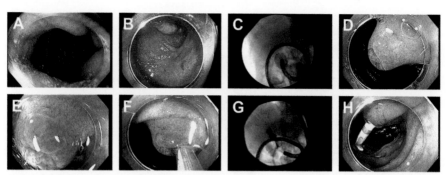

Fig. 3. ERCP using a pediatric colonoscope in Billroth II anatomy (*A*) gastrojejunal anastomosis, (*B*) and (*C*) endoscopic and fluoroscopic view of scope at the blind end of afferent limb, (*D*) intact major papilla, (*E*) clear cap is used to improve access to the major papilla, (*F*) cannulation toward a 6 o'clock orientation, (*G*) cholangiogram demonstrating a large stone in the distal common bile duct, (*H*) plastic biliary stent placed. In this patient, a subsequent procedure is planned using an adult colonoscope to allow cholangioscopy.

It is important to note the inverted bile duct orientation in Billroth II anatomy (**Fig. 4**). In contrast to conventional 11 to 12 o'clock orientation, biliary access in Billroth II anatomy is typically toward the 5 to 6 o'clock position. As most standard sphincterotomes tend to have an upward curve, a straight or rotatable catheter is generally preferred in this situation.

One meta-analysis reported improved afferent loop intubation with the forward-viewing endoscope compared with side-viewing (90.3% vs 86.8%) but similar rates of selective biliary cannulation (91.1% vs 92.3%).[3] Thus, both a duodenoscope and a forward-viewing endoscope with a clear cap could be considered equivalent first choices. Balloon-assisted enteroscopy, including short-type enteroscopes and those with a larger working channel designed specifically for ERCP, have been used in Billroth II patients with high rates of success.[4–6] However, a large systematic review reported higher rates of bowel perforation with side-viewing duodenoscopes (3.6%) and balloon-enteroscopes (4.1%) compared with forward-viewing endoscopes (1.7%).[7] A randomized controlled trial found forward-viewing endoscopes to be more successful in obtaining afferent loop intubation without perforation, a complication which was reported in 18% of the side-viewing cohort.[8] A retrospective series including 146 patients with Billroth II gastrectomy reported a 7.6% rate of perforation, and 11.6% risk of all AEs, which was significantly higher than in other postsurgical anatomy including post-Whipple and RY gastric bypass (RYGB).[9]

Novel endoscopes include dual lumen[10] or multiple bending endoscopes.[11] However, the success rate of these thus far has not been shown to be higher than conventional side-viewing or forward-viewing endoscopes.

Gastric resection with Roux-en-Y reconstruction

In an RY reconstruction, the distal stomach is resected, and a duodenal stump is created (**Fig. 5**). The jejunum is transected approximately 40 cm distal to the ligament of Treitz. An end-to-side gastrojejunal anastomosis is then created between the distal small bowel and the remnant stomach. Intestinal continuity is restored by the creation of a side-to-side jejunojejunal anastomosis. Hence, the postgastric anatomy consists of a blind limb (usually <10 cm long) and an alimentary limb. The length of a nonbariatric roux limb (gastrojejunal anastomosis to jejunojejunal anastomosis) is usually at

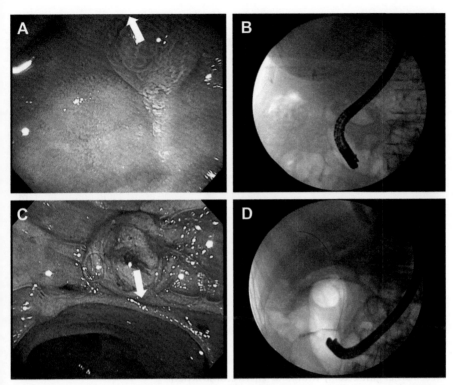

Fig. 4. Bile duct orientation (*A*) endoscopic view of the major papilla in normal anatomy with the orientation of the bile duct toward 11 o'clock, (*B*) fluoroscopic view of the duodenoscope at the major papilla in normal anatomy, (*C*) endoscopic view of the major papilla in Billroth II anatomy showing reversed orientation in the 5 o'clock direction, (*D*) fluoroscopic view of the duodenoscope at the major papilla in Billroth II anatomy.

least 40 cm to lower incidence of postoperative complications including bile reflux and gastritis of the remnant stomach[12].

Biliary access is challenging in RY anastomoses due to multiple reasons: the long roux and afferent limbs, acute angulation at the jejunojejunal anastomosis, and an inverted intact major papilla. Fortunately, in nonbariatric RY anastomoses, the jejunal limb tends to be shorter, Hence, biliary access can usually be accomplished with forward-viewing endoscopes including colonoscopes or enteroscopes, although a side-viewing duodenoscope may also reach the papilla in rare cases. Again, a clear cap is recommended for all forward-viewing endoscopes. Special note should be made on the scope length and instrument channel width when determining equipment use. for example, a 3.2 mm channel on pediatric colonoscopes will only accommodate 7-Fr stents, whereas a 3.7 mm channel on adult colonoscopes will allow cholangioscopy and 10-Fr stents.

Roux-en-Y gastric bypass

RYGB is the second most common surgical treatment for morbid obesity across the world[13]. In contrast to gastric resection with RY anastomosis, in RYGB a small gastric pouch is anastomosed side-to-side to the jejunum and the remnant stomach is left in situ (**Figs. 6** and **7**). A long roux limb, usually between 75 and 150 cm, leads to

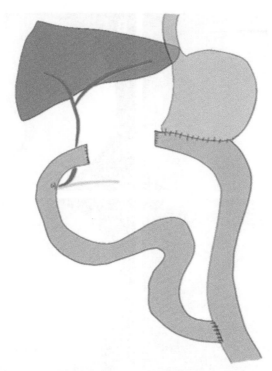

Fig. 5. Partial gastrectomy with Roux-en-Y reconstruction.

the jejunojejunostomy. The duodenum and the major papilla are then typically a further 30 to 60 cm distal to this.

Biliary intervention is not uncommonly required for patients following bariatric surgery as rapid weight loss is a risk factor for the development of gallstones.[14] However, given the long jejunal limbs leading to the native major papilla, ERCP is usually not possible using duodenoscopes. Thus, various specialized procedures have been adopted including enteroscopy-assisted ERCP (EA-ERCP), laparoscopic-assisted ERCP (LA-ERCP), and EUS-Directed trans-Gastric ERCP (EDGE) (**Fig. 8**).

Enteroscopy-assisted endoscopic retrograde cholangiopancreatography

Various enteroscopes have been used to assist with ERCP in patients with RYGB. Balloon enteroscopes facilitate deep enteral intubation by sequential balloon inflation and deflation to pleat jejunal folds. Similarly, a spiral enteroscope uses a rotating overtube to facilitate deep intubation. Despite this, EA-ERCP is time-consuming and associated with modest success rates especially with combined roux and biliopancreatic limbs exceeding 150 cm.[15] In addition, the length and working channel diameter on enteroscopes limits biliary intervention even when the major papilla is reached. A large multicenter retrospective comparative study reported similar rates of technical success across single-balloon, double-balloon and spiral enteroscopy with an overall technical success of 63% and AE rate of 12.4%.[16] Shorter balloon enteroscopes have been introduced with a working channel of up to 3.2 mm which allow the use of most standard ERCP devices but are not available in the United States. A more recent meta-analysis evaluating double-balloon enteroscopy reported pooled procedural success rate of 93% across all surgically altered anatomy, remaining at 92%

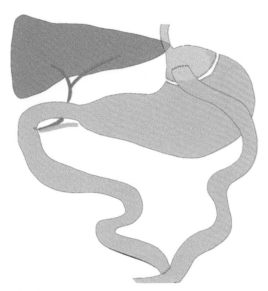

Fig. 6. Roux-en-Y gastric bypass.

even when patients with Billroth II were excluded given the shorter biliopancreatic limb.[17] No difference was noted between short-type and long-type double-balloon enteroscopes.

Laparoscopy-assisted endoscopic retrograde cholangiopancreatography

In LA-ERCP, a surgical port of minimum 15 mm diameter is placed into the excluded stomach and secured with sutures, followed by percutaneous passage of the duodenoscope via the port. To facilitate duodenoscope passage into the second portion of the duodenum, the port should be placed as far from the pylorus as possible. The use of a duodenoscope allows standard ERCP devices to be used. Following the completion of the ERCP, the gastrostomy is generally closed, but if further procedures are anticipated, access can be maintained via the placement of a large diameter gastrostomy tube.[18] LA-ERCP offers high rates of procedural success, with the largest study including 579 patients reporting the procedural success of 98% and AE rate of 18%.[19] However, LA-ERCP does carry disadvantages including the relative invasiveness of the procedure, associated pain, future risk of adhesions, and in one study almost a 10% need for conversion to open surgery.[20] LA-ERCP is more time-consuming and cumbersome requiring coordination between the surgical and endoscopy teams.

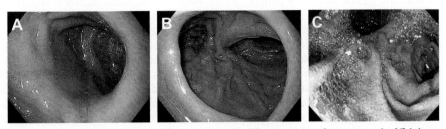

Fig. 7. Roux-en-Y gastric bypass (*A*) gastric pouch, (*B*) gastrojejunal anastomosis, (*C*) jejunojejunal anastomosis.

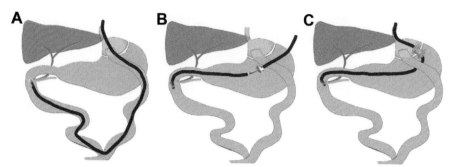

Fig. 8. Biliary access in Roux-en-Y gastric bypass anatomy (*A*) enteroscopy-assisted ERCP, (*B*) laparoscopic-assisted ERCP (*C*) EUS-Directed trans-gastric ERCP (EDGE).

Furthermore, if a gastrostomy tube is placed, there are associated risks of gastrostomy site infection, bleeding, or chronic fistulas. The ideal scenario for LA-ERCP may be in patients who require concurrent cholecystectomy, in institutions whereby coordinating surgical and endoscopic schedules are feasible.

Endoscopic ultrasound-directed trans-gastric endoscopic retrograde cholangiopancreatography

The EDGE procedure uses a lumen-apposing metal stent (LAMS) to create a tract from the gastric pouch or proximal jejunal limb to the excluded stomach under EUS-guidance. The LAMS then functions as a conduit to allow scope passage for not only ERCP but also the treatment of other pathology in and around the excluded stomach and duodenum in patients with RYGB.[21] EDGE was originally performed as a two-stage procedure to allow the gastrogastric fistula to mature before duodenoscope passage. The concern, understandably, was that stent migration during the index procedure would result in a free perforation. Furthermore, endoscopic closure of a defect in the excluded stomach may not be feasible. However, two-stage procedures are not feasible in the setting of urgent indications such as ascending cholangitis, bile leak, or malignant biliary obstruction. Short-interval (2–4 day) dual-session EDGE may reduce the risk of LAMS dislodgement although evidence is limited.[22] Single-stage EDGE was thus introduced. A recent multicenter study evaluated 128 patients undergoing single-session EDGE and reported an overall LAMS migration rate of 8.6% including 2.3% which required surgical rescue.[23] They identified smaller diameter (15 mm) LAMS as a predictor of intraprocedural stent migration. Importantly, no sutured stents migrated whereas 27.3% of nonsutured stents did.

In our own practice, we almost exclusively perform single-stage EDGE (**Fig. 9**). In brief, a therapeutic linear echoendoscope is first used to identify the excluded stomach from the gastric pouch (or jejunum if required). The excluded stomach is punctured with a EUS needle and the correct position is confirmed using contrast injection under fluoroscopy. Once the excluded stomach is distended with a saline/contrast mixture, a cautery-enhanced LAMS is placed freehand creating a gastrogastrostomy (or jejunogastrostomy). A 20 mm LAMS is preferred. Ideally, the LAMS should be positioned in the proximal excluded stomach as this facilitates duodenoscope passage to the ampulla. The LAMS is then dilated to 18 mm and the proximal flange is fixed to the gastric pouch with endoscopic sutures. The duodenoscope is then able to traverse through the LAMS to the second portion of the duodenum and ERCP can be performed using standard equipment. We routinely remove the LAMS and perform primary closure of the gastrogastric fistula at 4 weeks. For patients requiring multiple procedures, for example, complex bile duct stones or benign biliary strictures, the LAMS can remain in situ until necessary therapy has been completed.

EDGE is a purely endoscopic procedure that carries high rates of procedural success. A large multicenter study including 178 patients who underwent EDGE reported technical success of 98%.[24] A recent systematic review confirmed these findings with an overall technical success rate of 96.8%.[25] Although the overall AE rate was 27.8%, the rate of severe AE was only 0.6%. There is a risk of persistent fistula, which increases the risk of acid reflux and ulcers. This also functionally reverses the RYGB, thus theoretically can cause weight regain, although this has not been demonstrated to date.[25,26] In patients undergoing objective testing, the persistent fistula rate is up to 10%.[25] However, in this study, all patients who underwent attempted endoscopic treatment had successful fistula closure.

Despite its advantages, EDGE is a technically challenging procedure with potentially dire AEs. Thus, EDGE should be performed at specialized centers with extensive therapeutic EUS experience and adequate surgical backup.

PATIENTS WITH ALTERED ANATOMY AND BILIOENTERIC ANASTOMOSES
Pancreaticoduodenectomy (Whipple procedure)

The Whipple resection or pancreaticoduodenectomy is the most common operation for diseases involving the head of the pancreas or proximal duodenum including the periampullary area (**Fig. 10**). There are 2 variations: standard or pylorus-preserving Whipple. The standard resection involves a gastric antrectomy, cholecystectomy, and removal of the distal common bile duct, head of pancreas, duodenum, proximal jejunum, and regional lymph nodes. Reconstruction then consists of a

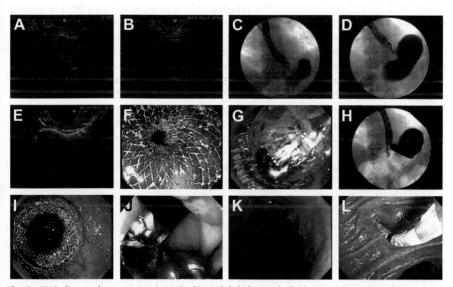

Fig. 9. EUS-directed trans-gastric ERCP (EDGE) (*A*) the excluded stomach is identified on EUS, (*B*) the excluded stomach is punctured with a 19-gauge needle, (*C*) contrast is injected to confirm puncture into the excluded stomach, (*D*) a saline and contrast mixture is infused to distend the excluded stomach, (*E*, *F*) a 20 mm lumen apposing metal stent (LAMS) is placed, (*G–I*) LAMS dilated to 18 mm using through-the-scope balloon, (*J*) proximal flange secured using 2 interrupted endoscopic sutures, (*K*) duodenoscope advanced through the LAMS into the excluded stomach (*L*) the major papilla is accessed for ERCP.

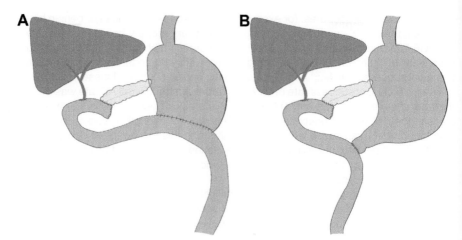

Fig. 10. Whipple pancreaticoduodenectomy (A) classic Whipple, (B) pylorus-preserving Whipple.

gastrojejunostomy, hepaticojejunostomy and pancreaticojejunostomy. The pylorus-preserving pancreaticoduodenostomy is increasingly favored to preserve physiologic gastric emptying. In this technique, resection commences in the duodenum 1–3 cm distal to the pylorus. In general, the pancreatic and biliary anastomoses are located 45 to 60 cm from the gastrojejunal or duodenojejunal anastomosis. The pancreatico-jejunostomy is at the blind end of the afferent limb and the hepaticojejunostomy is located 5 to 10 cm downstream. The relatively short pancreatobiliary limb is usually accessible via both side-viewing and forward-viewing endoscopes.

At the gastrojejunal or duodenojejunal anastomosis, similar to other surgically altered anatomy, the afferent limb is usually at a sharp angulation (**Fig. 11**). The chosen limb should be traversed to the maximal extent possible, using fluoroscopy to guide progress to the right upper quadrant. Once the blind end is reached, a careful pullback should allow the identification of the biliary anastomosis. The absence of an ampulla frequently results in an air cholangiogram on fluoroscopy. Sometimes contrast injection into the afferent jejunal lumen and placing the patient in Trendelenburg position can result in filling of the bile duct or pancreatic duct, provided the anastomosis is patent.

Enteroscopy-assisted ERCP offers procedural success of 83.1% to 96.4% in post-Whipple anatomy,[27–29] with no significant difference between the use of short-type or standard balloon enteroscopes.[28,29] While guidelines are not specific on endoscope preference in post-Whipple anatomy, EA-ERCP should be considered,[30] and the use of a clear cap is recommended with forward-viewing endoscopes.[1,31]

Roux-en-Y hepaticojejunostomy

In RY hepaticojejunostomy, the stomach and duodenum are left intact, the distal bile duct is transected, and the proximal bile duct is anastomosed to a loop of jejunum (**Fig. 12**). Biliary access requires passage of the endoscope past an intact major papilla which only communicates with the pancreatic duct and a blind end of the distal common bile duct. The jejunojejunostomy is typically 15 to 20 cm downstream from the ligament of Treitz, with the afferent limb usually identified by a sharp angulation (**Fig. 13**). Once the end of the afferent limb is reached, the bilioenteric anastomosis

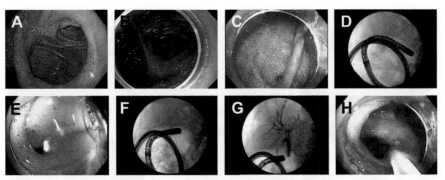

Fig. 11. ERCP using a pediatric colonoscope in classic Whipple anatomy (*A*) gastrojejunal anastomosis, afferent limb sharply angulated upwards, (*B*) jejunojejunal anastomosis, (*C*) blind end of afferent limb, pancreaticojejunal anastomosis visualized at the 6 o'clock position, (*D*) an air cholangiogram is seen on fluoroscopy, (*E*) hepaticojejunal anastomosis, (*F*) bile duct cannulated with guidewire through the hepaticojejunal anastomosis, (*G*) balloon dilation of the narrowed hepaticojejunal anastomosis, (*H*) improved appearance following dilation.

is usually an end-to-side anastomosis at or near the blind end. Depending on the level of resection, there may be one opening leading to the common hepatic duct or 2 openings leading to the left and right hepatic ducts. Similar to postpancreaticoduodenectomy, an air cholangiogram may be seen or contrast injection into the jejunal lumen may help identify the position of the anastomosis.

As the stomach is left intact in RY hepaticojejunostomy, significant looping of the endoscope may be experienced. Thus, colonoscopes or enteroscopes are generally

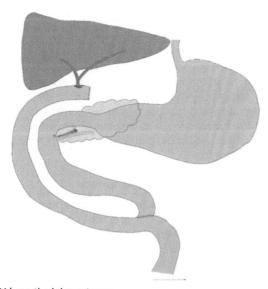

Fig. 12. Roux-en-Y hepaticojejunostomy.

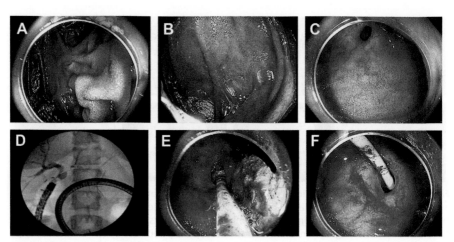

Fig. 13. ERCP using a pediatric colonoscope in Roux-en-Y hepaticojejunostomy (A) jejunoje-junal anastomosis, (B) tattoo marking the afferent limb, (C) hepaticojejunal anastomosis, (D) cholangiogram demonstrates a filling defect in the common hepatic duct, (E) balloon sweep with stone removal, (F) plastic biliary stent placed.

preferred. Procedural success with EA-ERCP is 75.9% to 92.2%,[32–34] and is higher than what can be achieved with a pediatric colonoscope (58.5%).[34]

NOVEL TECHNIQUES

Interventional EUS is increasingly used with ERCP in the treatment of complex biliary disease. In addition to the already discussed EDGE procedure, EUS-biliary drainage can be achieved in several ways including transmural access via a hepaticogastrostomy, EUS-guided antegrade intervention, EUS-guided rendezvous ERCP, or EUS-directed trans-Enteric ERCP (EDEE).

Endoscopic ultrasound-guided hepaticogastrostomy

In this procedure, the left intrahepatic bile duct branch is identified from the proximal stomach (or jejunum if the stomach has been resected), punctured, and injected with contrast to confirm appropriate position (**Fig. 14**). The tract is then dilated using either a catheter or a balloon followed by the placement of a stent to create the hepaticogastrostomy. Endoscopic ultrasound-guided hepaticogastrostomy (EUS-HG) can be effectively and safely performed for the treatment of benign and malignant conditions in patients with altered anatomy.[35,36]

Endoscopic ultrasound-guided antegrade intervention

In this technique, the left intrahepatic bile duct branch is punctured, and a guidewire advanced to the papilla or anastomosis.[37,38] The tract may then be dilated to facilitate necessary therapy. For example, a transpapillary stent can then be placed antegrade across a biliary stricture. Alternatively, choledocholithiasis can be pushed out of the papilla/anastomosis using a stone extraction balloon after dilating the papilla/anastomosis. If further intervention is anticipated, a stent can be placed to secure the hepaticogastrostomy for future access.

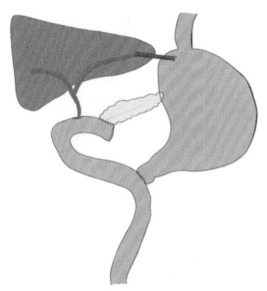

Fig. 14. EUS-guided hepaticogastrostomy in a pylorus-preserving Whipple surgery.

Endoscopic ultrasound-guided rendezvous endoscopic retrograde cholangiopancreatography

A rendezvous technique can be used if the papilla or biliary anastomosis cannot be identified endoscopically. In this method, an intrahepatic bile duct is punctured under EUS-guidance and a guidewire is advanced across the papilla or anastomosis (**Fig. 15**). The echoendoscope is then withdrawn leaving the guidewire in place. An endoscope is then passed to the papilla or anastomosis and a snare or forceps is used to grasp the guidewire and pull it through the endoscope.

Endoscopic ultrasound-directed transenteric endoscopic retrograde cholangiopancreatography

The above EUS approaches may not be feasible in all patients with surgically altered anatomy. For example, a transhepatic approach (eg, hepaticogastrostomy) may not be feasible if there is insufficient intrahepatic biliary dilation, there has been total gastrectomy, liver resection, or liver transplant. In these cases, a de novo gastroenteric or enteroenteric anastomosis between the proximal gastrointestinal tract to the pancreatobiliary or afferent loop can be created using LAMS (**Fig. 16**). Identification of the afferent limb can be achieved via percutaneous drain placement (followed by contrast injection via the drain) or when reached endoscopically contrast can be injected (for a pure endoscopic approach). This allows a "short-cut" to the biliary tree for subsequent ERCP with reported high rates of technical success and low AE rate.[39] This technique, termed EUS-directed trans-enteric ERCP (EDEE), is particularly useful in patients whereby repeated access is anticipated, such as in benign biliary strictures or complex stone disease.

Overall, EUS-guided biliary intervention offers a higher degree of clinical efficacy and shorter procedure time when compared with enteroscopy-assisted ERCP in patients with altered anatomy.[38] A higher rate of AEs, although mostly mild/moderate, should be noted and pending further evidence, EUS-biliary intervention should be limited to highly specialized centers and reserved for patients failing other methods.

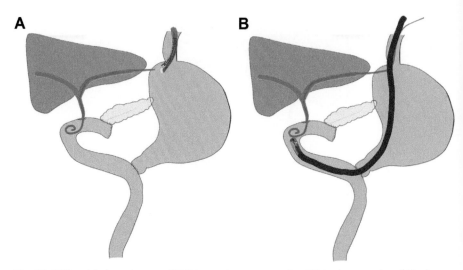

Fig. 15. EUS-guided rendezvous ERCP in a pylorus-preserving Whipple procedure (*A*) a linear EUS is used to identify, puncture and place a wire through the left intrahepatic system and through the hepaticojejunal anastomosis, (*B*) the EUS scope is removed, leaving the wire in position. A duodenoscope or forward-viewing endoscope is then advanced to afferent limb and the wire is grasped.

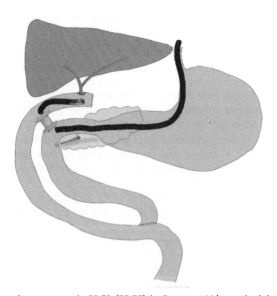

Fig. 16. EUS-directed trans-enteric ERCP (EDEE) in Roux-en-Y hepaticojejunostomy.

SUMMARY

Endoscopic biliary interventions are increasingly available for patients with surgically altered gastrointestinal anatomy. While significant advances have been made, there is potential for further improvement. Specifically designed devices are desired. Further, standardization of procedural technique and reporting of outcomes or AEs are needed to not only improve the quality of the procedures but also to assist with the development of training programs. Importantly, biliary endoscopy in altered anatomy requires not only familiarity with the various surgeries and alterations in the UGI tract, but also high technical expertise and a thorough understanding of available endoscopes and devices. The selection of biliary access approach will depend on the patient's anatomy, operator experience, and procedural availability. A multidisciplinary approach is warranted, with close collaboration with surgeons and interventional radiologists when needed.

DISCLOSURES

L Zhang reports no relevant disclosures. S. Irai is a consultant for Boston Scientific and Gore Medical. M Khashab is a consultant for Boston Scientific, Olympus America, Medtronic, Apollo Endosurgery, Pentax, and GI Supply. He receives royalties from UpToDate and Elsevier.

CLINICS CARE POINTS

Before procedure:
- Review surgical reports
  - If possible, determine lengths of reconstructed limbs
  - Native papilla versus bilioenteric anastomosis
- Review clinical information
  - Detailed patient history
  - Review all available radiology
  - Laboratory results
- Determine the goals of the procedure
  - One procedure versus multiple
  - Determine "Plan B"
- Detailed discussion with patient and family: expected procedural success, potential future procedures, alternative management in case of failure

During procedure:
- Involve anesthesia team: low threshold for general anesthesia given expected prolonged duration of procedure
- Consider patient position: supine ideal if manual pressure is required, changing to left lateral or prone may help manipulate angulation or biliary cannulation
- Endoscope and accessory choice
  - Forward versus side-viewing
  - Length of scope: is balloon-enteroscopy required?
  - If forward-viewing, consider the use of clear cap
  - Prepare necessary devices in advance and ensure compatible with chosen scope

- Accurate documentation to facilitate subsequent procedures: in particular, indicate the orientation of afferent limb, estimated distance, consider placing tattoo at the entrance to biliary limb

REFERENCES

1. ASGE Technology Committee, Enestvedt BK, Kothari S, Pannala R, et al. Devices and techniques for ERCP in the surgically altered GI tract. Gastrointest Endosc 2016;83(6):1061–75.
2. Wu WG, Gu J, Zhang WJ, et al. ERCP for patients who have undergone billroth II gastroenterostomy and braun anastomosis. World J Gastroenterol 2014;20(2):607–10.
3. Park TY, Bang CS, Choi SH, et al. Forward-viewing endoscope for ERCP in patients with billroth II gastrectomy: A systematic review and meta-analysis. Surg Endosc 2018;32(11):4598–613.
4. Shimatani M, Hatanaka H, Kogure H, et al. Diagnostic and therapeutic endoscopic retrograde cholangiography using a short-type double-balloon endoscope in patients with altered gastrointestinal anatomy: A multicenter prospective study in japan. Am J Gastroenterol 2016;111(12):1750–8.
5. Shimatani M, Tokuhara M, Kato K, et al. Utility of newly developed short-type double-balloon endoscopy for endoscopic retrograde cholangiography in postoperative patients. J Gastroenterol Hepatol 2017;32(7):1348–54.
6. Yane K, Katanuma A, Maguchi H, et al. Short-type single-balloon enteroscope-assisted ERCP in postsurgical altered anatomy: Potential factors affecting procedural failure. Endoscopy 2017;49(1):69–74.
7. Park TY, Song TJ. Recent advances in endoscopic retrograde cholangiopancreatography in billroth II gastrectomy patients: A systematic review. World J Gastroenterol 2019;25(24):3091–107.
8. Kim MH, Lee SK, Lee MH, et al. Endoscopic retrograde cholangiopancreatography and needle-knife sphincterotomy in patients with billroth II gastrectomy: A comparative study of the forward-viewing endoscope and the side-viewing duodenoscope. Endoscopy 1997;29(2):82–5.
9. Tokuhara M, Shimatani M, Mitsuyama T, et al. Evaluation of complications after endoscopic retrograde cholangiopancreatography using a short type double balloon endoscope in patients with altered gastrointestinal anatomy: A single-center retrospective study of 1,576 procedures. J Gastroenterol Hepatol 2020;35(8):1387–96.
10. Wang S, Liu W, Sun S, et al. Clinical evaluation of double-channel gastroscope for endoscopic retrograde cholangiopancreatography in patients with billroth II gastrectomy. Prz Gastroenterol 2016;11(3):163–9.
11. Koo HC, Moon JH, Choi HJ, et al. The utility of a multibending endoscope for selective cannulation during ERCP in patients with a billroth II gastrectomy (with video). Gastrointest Endosc 2009;69(4):931–4.
12. Nishizaki D, Ganeko R, Hoshino N, et al. Roux-en-Y versus billroth-I reconstruction after distal gastrectomy for gastric cancer. Cochrane Database Syst Rev 2021;9(9):CD012998.
13. Angrisani L, Santonicola A, Iovino P, et al. Bariatric surgery survey 2018: Similarities and disparities among the 5 IFSO chapters. Obes Surg 2021;31(5):1937–48.
14. Haal S, Guman MSS, Boerlage TCC, et al. Ursodeoxycholic acid for the prevention of symptomatic gallstone disease after bariatric surgery (UPGRADE): A multicentre, double-blind, randomised, placebo-controlled superiority trial. The Lancet Gastroenterol Hepatol 2021;6(12):993–1001.
15. Schreiner MA, Chang L, Gluck M, et al. Laparoscopy-assisted versus balloon enteroscopy-assisted ERCP in bariatric post-roux-en-Y gastric bypass patients. Gastrointest Endosc 2012;75(4):748–56.

16. Shah RJ, Smolkin M, Yen R, et al. A multicenter, U.S. experience of single-balloon, double-balloon, and rotational overtube-assisted enteroscopy ERCP in patients with surgically altered pancreaticobiliary anatomy (with video). Gastrointest Endosc 2013;77(4):593–600.
17. Anvari S, Lee Y, Patro N, et al. Double-balloon enteroscopy for diagnostic and therapeutic ERCP in patients with surgically altered gastrointestinal anatomy: A systematic review and meta-analysis. Surg Endosc 2021;35(1):18–36.
18. Tekola B, Wang AY, Ramanath M, et al. Percutaneous gastrostomy tube placement to perform transgastrostomy endoscopic retrograde cholangiopancreaticography in patients with roux-en-Y anatomy. Dig Dis Sci 2011;56(11):3364–9.
19. Abbas AM, Strong AT, Diehl DL, et al. Multicenter evaluation of the clinical utility of laparoscopy-assisted ERCP in patients with roux-en-Y gastric bypass. Gastrointest Endosc 2018;87(4):1031–9.
20. Kedia P, Tarnasky PR, Nieto J, et al. EUS-directed transgastric ERCP (EDGE) versus laparoscopy-assisted ERCP (LA-ERCP) for roux-en-Y gastric bypass (RYGB) anatomy: A multicenter early comparative experience of clinical outcomes. J Clin Gastroenterol 2019;53(4):304–8.
21. Krafft MR, Hsueh W, James TW, et al. The EDGI new take on EDGE: EUS-directed transgastric intervention (EDGI), other than ERCP, for roux-en-Y gastric bypass anatomy: A multicenter study. Endosc Int Open 2019;7(10):E1231–40.
22. Krafft MR, Fang W, Nasr JY. Shortened-interval dual-session EDGE reduces the risk of LAMS dislodgement while facilitating timely ERCP. Dig Dis Sci 2021; 66(8):2776–85.
23. Shinn B, Boortalary T, Raijman I, et al. Maximizing success in single-session EUS-directed transgastric ERCP: A retrospective cohort study to identify predictive factors of stent migration. Gastrointest Endosc 2021;94(4):727–32.
24. Runge TM, Chiang AL, Kowalski TE, et al. Endoscopic ultrasound-directed transgastric ERCP (EDGE): A retrospective multicenter study. Endoscopy 2021;53(6): 611–8.
25. Prakash S, Elmunzer BJ, Forster EM, et al. Endoscopic ultrasound-directed transgastric ERCP (EDGE): A systematic review describing the outcomes, adverse events, and knowledge gaps. Endoscopy 2022;54(1):52–61.
26. Krafft MR, Lorenze A, Croglio MP, et al. Innocent as a LAMS": Does spontaneous fistula closure (secondary intention), after EUS-directed transgastric ERCP (EDGE) via 20-mm lumen-apposing metal stent, confer an increased risk of persistent fistula and unintentional weight gain? Dig Dis Sci 2021. https://doi.org/10.1007/s10620-021-07003-4. Advance online publication.
27. Park BK, Jeon TJ, Jayaraman V, et al. Endoscopic retrograde cholangiopancreatography in patients with previous pancreaticoduodenectomy: A single-center experience. Dig Dis Sci 2016;61(1):293–302.
28. Itokawa F, Itoi T, Ishii K, et al. Single- and double-balloon enteroscopy-assisted endoscopic retrograde cholangiopancreatography in patients with roux-en-Y plus hepaticojejunostomy anastomosis and whipple resection. Dig Endosc 2014;26(Suppl 2):136–43.
29. Tanisaka Y, Ryozawa S, Mizuide M, et al. Status of single-balloon enteroscopy-assisted endoscopic retrograde cholangiopancreatography in patients with surgically altered anatomy: Systematic review and meta-analysis on biliary interventions. Dig Endosc 2021;33(7):1034–44.
30. Liao WC, Angsuwatcharakon P, Isayama H, et al. International consensus recommendations for difficult biliary access. Gastrointest Endosc 2017;85(2):295–304.

31. Testoni PA, Mariani A, Aabakken L, et al. Papillary cannulation and sphincterotomy techniques at ERCP: European society of gastrointestinal endoscopy (ESGE) clinical guideline. Endoscopy 2016;48(7):657–83.

32. Wu WG, Qin LC, Song XL, et al. Application of single balloon enteroscopy-assisted therapeutic endoscopic retrograde cholangiopancreatography in patients after bilioenteric roux-en-Y anastomosis: Experience of multi-disciplinary collaboration. World J Gastroenterol 2019;25(36):5505–14.

33. Sato T, Kogure H, Nakai Y, et al. Double-balloon endoscopy-assisted treatment of hepaticojejunostomy anastomotic strictures and predictive factors for treatment success. Surg Endosc 2020;34(4):1612–20.

34. Azeem N, Tabibian JH, Baron TH, et al. Use of a single-balloon enteroscope compared with variable-stiffness colonoscopes for endoscopic retrograde cholangiography in liver transplant patients with roux-en-Y biliary anastomosis. Gastrointest Endosc 2013;77(4):568–77.

35. Hathorn KE, Canakis A, Baron TH. EUS-guided transhepatic biliary drainage: A large single-center U.S. experience. Gastrointest Endosc 2021;95(3):443–51.

36. Minaga K, Takenaka M, Ogura T, et al. Endoscopic ultrasound-guided biliary drainage for malignant biliary obstruction with surgically altered anatomy: A multi-center prospective registration study. Therap Adv Gastroenterol 2020;13. 1756284820930964.

37. Mukai S, Itoi T, Sofuni A, et al. EUS-guided antegrade intervention for benign biliary diseases in patients with surgically altered anatomy (with videos). Gastrointest Endosc 2019;89(2):399–407.

38. Khashab MA, El Zein MH, Sharzehi K, et al. EUS-guided biliary drainage or enteroscopy-assisted ERCP in patients with surgical anatomy and biliary obstruction: An international comparative study. Endosc Int Open 2016;4(12):E1322–7.

39. Ichkhanian Y, Yang J, James TW, et al. EUS-directed transenteric ERCP in non-roux-en-Y gastric bypass surgical anatomy patients (with video). Gastrointest Endosc 2020;91(5):1188–94.e2.

Future of Cholangioscopy

Jorge D. Machicado, MD, MPH[a], Isaac Raijman, MD, FACG, AGAF, FACP[b],
Raj J. Shah, MD, MASGE, AGAF, FACG[c],*

KEYWORDS

- Cholangioscopy • Biliary tract disease • Biliary stricture • Bile duct stones
- Cholangiocarcinoma • Endoscopic retrograde cholangiopancreatography

KEY POINTS

- Cholangioscopy allows direct visualization of the biliary tree and is an adjunct to endoscopic retrograde cholangiopancreatography.
- Peroral cholangioscopy has evolved in recent years with the development of digital single-operator cholangioscopy (SOC) and refinements of compatible accessories.
- Cholangioscopy is mostly used for difficult bile duct stones and indeterminate biliary strictures, but the number of diagnostic and therapeutic applications is expanding.
- Future improvements on the configuration and visualization of SOC platforms and the introduction of real-time artificial intelligence algorithms are necessary to expand the clinical applicability of cholangioscopy at nonexpert hands.

INTRODUCTION

Cholangioscopy was first reported in the 1970s with the goal of reducing reliance on the 2- dimensional black and white imaging produced by endoscopic retrograde cholangiopancreatography (ERCP).[1] This technology has evolved over the past 2 decades with the development of high-quality video cholangioscopes and refinements of compatible accessories. These technologic improvements have resulted in greater availability and utilization of cholangioscopy in endoscopy units worldwide. This review, highlights the current status of cholangioscopy, including the different platforms, devices, indications, and practical technical aspects. In addition, the authors present their personal view on the future directions of cholangioscopy that could serve to reduce the present unmet needs and to further guide developments of the technology.

[a] Division of Gastroenterology and Hepatology, University of Michigan, 1500 East Medical Center Drive, Floor 3, Reception D, Ann Arbor, MI 48109, USA; [b] Texas Digestive Disease Consultants, 4100 South Sheperd Drive, Houston, TX 77098, USA; [c] Pancreas and Biliary Endoscopy, Division of Gastroenterology and Hepatology, University of Colorado Anschutz Medical Campus, 1635 Aurora Court, Mail Stop F735, Aurora, CO 80045, USA
* Corresponding author.
E-mail address: raj.shah@cuanschutz.edu

Gastrointest Endoscopy Clin N Am 32 (2022) 583–596
https://doi.org/10.1016/j.giec.2022.03.002
1052-5157/22/© 2022 Elsevier Inc. All rights reserved.
giendo.theclinics.com

PRESENT OF CHOLANGIOSCOPY
Cholangioscopy Access

Cholangioscopy can be performed via the percutaneous or peroral routes (**Fig. 1**). The percutaneous approach first requires placement of a percutaneous transhepatic biliary drain (PTBD). After maturation and serial dilations of the tract over the span of weeks, a short cholangioscope is inserted through a percutaneous tract sheath (typically 12F catheter) under fluoroscopic guidance, and subsequent interventions are performed.[2] Given the time required for tract maturation and the problems that are inherent to a percutaneous drain, the peroral route is preferred. This is conventionally done through a transpapillary approach at the time of ERCP, and this article will mainly discuss this method. However, peroral access can also be achieved through endoscopic ultrasound (EUS)-guided hepaticogastrostomy or choledochoduodenostomy when the transpapillary approach is not feasible.[3]

Peroral Cholangioscopy Platforms

Direct peroral cholangioscopy (DPOCS) is performed by advancing an ultraslim (5–6 mm outer diameter) forward-viewing endoscope directly into the bile duct. Although this method provides a large working channel for interventions and excellent image quality with capability for narrow band imaging (NBI), the challenges include overcoming the angle between the duodenum and the common bile duct, advancing the endoscope over small-caliber ducts, and maintaining endoscope stability inside the biliary tree. Despite some technique modifications and endoscope developments,

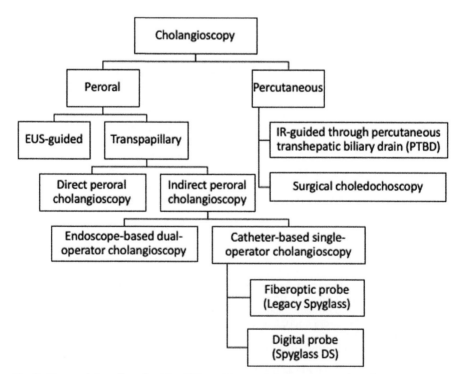

Fig. 1. Nomenclature flowchart for different types of cholangioscopy based on access route. EUS, endoscopic ultrasound; IR, interventional radiology.

DPOCS remains challenging and is only done by skilled endoscopists in a few centers worldwide.

Indirect peroral cholangioscopy consists of advancing a cholangioscope through the duodenoscope working channel into the bile duct. This was first done with the endoscope-based dual-operator system, also known as the mother-daughter system, in which 1 operator handles the duodenoscope, and the other advances a baby cholangioscope (2.4–3.5 mm outer diameter). These reusable mother-daughter cholangioscopes provide high quality images and NBI function; however, they are fragile, require high capital investment, have limited tip deflection (up/down only), and are not currently under development.

In 2007, a catheter-based single-operator cholangioscopy (SOC) system was introduced for clinical use, which overcame some of the limitations of dual-operator cholangioscopy; it was less fragile, had 4-way tip deflection, and a second operator was not necessary. This was initially composed by a reusable fiberoptic probe that was inserted over a disposable plastic delivery catheter (Legacy SpyGlass, Boston Scientific, Marlborough, MA). This platform widened the clinical utilization of cholangioscopy, followed by an exponential increase in the number of annual research studies describing its different applications.[4] However, this early system had suboptimal image quality and field of view, limited fiberoptic probe durability, small working channel, and difficult set up. A newer SOC platform that uses high-resolution digital CMOS technology (SpyGlass DS Direct Visualization System) was released for clinical use in 2015. Compared with the fiberoptic system, the digital SOC is an all-inclusive endoscope that provides better image quality, wider field of view, brighter light source, improved tip maneuverability, and easier set up.[5] In 2018, a third-generation catheter with higher resolution and improved visibility was released (SpyScope DSII). This 214 cm long catheter has an outer diameter of 3.5 mm and contains 2 independent light-emitting diodes (LEDs), 2 channels for irrigation, and a 1.2 mm diameter working channel for accessory devices and aspiration. This disposable digital-based platform has become the preferred modality for cholangioscopy worldwide. A historic timeline of the development of cholangioscopy is presented in **Fig. 2**.

Set up of Catheter-Based Single-Operator Cholangioscopy

The catheter's handle is strapped just below the duodenoscope working channel with a silicone belt. The connection cable is attached to the processor (SpyGlass DS digital

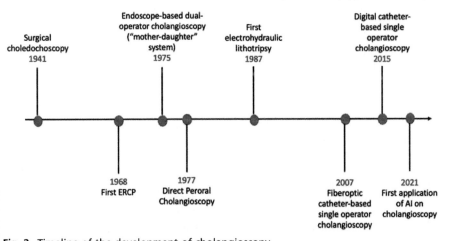

Fig. 2. Timeline of the development of cholangioscopy.

controller), which generates light and receives video signals that are then processed as images in an attached monitor. The irrigation pump is connected to the proper port, and sterile water or normal saline can be used for irrigation. The suction tubing is attached to the suctioning port, ideally with a 10 cc syringe, and the suction valve is kept closed unless suction is needed. A Y adaptor is placed at the handle wire port to improve suction force. The catheter is then inserted through the duodenoscope working channel.

Technique of Catheter-Based Single-Operator Cholangioscopy

Patients should receive antibiotics before cholangioscopy to prevent risk of cholangitis. Biliary sphincterotomy and/or balloon dilation are required to facilitate passage of the 10-French SOC catheter. An initial cholangiogram provides procedural guidance to the target area of interest; however, endoscopists should avoid excessive contrast injection that may interfere with intraductal visualization. The SOC catheter can be advanced through the biliary orifice over a short or long guidewire, or by the freehand technique. The duodenoscope elevator and big dial can assist advancing the catheter into the bile duct. To advance the catheter into the desired ductal location, manipulation of the SOC 4-way steering dials and gentle pushing of the duodenoscope may be required. Once the target location is reached, the SOC dials can be partially or fully locked for stabilization and fine tip movements. If the catheter was advanced with the assistance of a guidewire, this is then removed to enhance suctioning and passage of instruments. Irrigation should be kept as low as possible to permit visualization. It is best to start the visualization by first suctioning contrast and debris before starting irrigation. Periodic suctioning with the duodenoscope and the SOC catheter can then be applied. Fluoroscopy is intermittently used throughout the procedure, especially when advancing the cholangioscope into the intrahepatic ducts. The bile duct should be systematically assessed, but full visualization may be difficult in markedly dilated ducts, or when scope passage is hindered by a narrow duct or severe stricture. Similar set up and technique are used for SOC through single-use disposable duodenoscopes.[6]

Compatible Tools with Catheter-Based Single-Operator Cholangioscopy

A dedicated biopsy forceps has been available for tissue acquisition since the first-generation SOC (SpyBite legacy). A new generation biopsy forceps recently became available (SpyBite Max), with design enhancements including serrated teeth and elongated fenestration holes, aiming theoretically for larger tissue specimens. Both forceps types are 286 cm long, 1 mm diameter, and have a jaw opening of 4.1 mm. For cholangioscopy-directed biopsies, the target site is localized with cholangioscopy, and 1 to 2 miniature biopsies are obtained per pass. A new 9 mm snare is available to remove intraductal foreign bodies (eg, migrated stents, clips) and to resect polypoid lesions. A dedicated 15 mm retrieval basket is also available to retrieve small stones.

For the treatment of difficult biliary stones, electrohydraulic lithotripsy (EHL) and laser lithotripsy (LL) probes can be advanced through the working channel of the SOC. The EHL probe is a 1.9-French catheter and 375 cm long, with 2 coaxially insulated electrodes ending in an open tip. The probe is connected to a power source (Autolith Touch EHL generator), that when activated with a foot pedal, sparks energy at the fiber tip and produces high amplitude intraductal hydraulic pressure under water immersion. The optimal effect is achieved when the tip of the fiber is 1 to 2 mm en face from the stone and when the fluid media contain electrolytes (normal saline). The generator allows selecting the number of pulses per second (1–15) and the power settings (low, moderate, or high). The authors recommend starting with 3 to 5 pulses per second at a low power, to reduce the risk of ductal injury and to prolong the life of the fiber. For LL, a laser beam is transmitted by a quartz fiber advanced through the working channel. A 300 cm long x 365 μm diameter fiber designed for biliary indications is commonly used (Lumenis, SlimLine SIS GI), and is plugged to a holmium laser system (Lumenis, VersaPulse). Smaller fibers, such as 265 μm size, can permit better tip cholangioscope deflection and targeting. Repetitive laser pulses lead to gaseous ion collection and free electrons of high kinetic energy (vapor bubble) that expand quickly and result in stone fragmentation. Power is usually set at 0.6 to 1.2 J at 6 to 15 Hz for total laser energy of 12 kJ.

Traditional Clinical Applications

Cholangioscopy can be used for various diagnostic and therapeutic purposes. **Box 1** presents a nonexhaustive list of the current indications for cholangioscopy. Most of the time, cholangioscopy is used for the management of difficult biliary stones (see Simon Phillpotts and colleagues' article, "Endoscopic Management of Complex Biliary Stones," in this issue) and for assessment of indeterminate biliary strictures (see Zaheer Nabi and D. Nageshwar Reddy's article, "Multidisciplinary Approach to Indeterminate Biliary Strictures," in this issue). In a recent systematic review of 1762 subjects from 35 studies evaluating the role of cholangioscopy in the treatment of difficult biliary stones (eg, stone diameter greater than 1 cm or greater than the downstream duct, barrel shape, intraductal location), cholangioscopy with EHL or LL achieved overall stone fragmentation success of 91.2% over an average of 1.3 sessions.[7] Similar high efficacy (approximately 90%) has also been demonstrated in prospective studies and randomized controlled trials (RCTs).[7–10] There are no RCTs directly comparing outcomes of EHL and LL in biliary stones, so currently the decision of cholangioscopy-lithotripsy technique is based on the endoscopist's experience and resource availability. In a systematic review, both EHL and LL appear equally effective and safe; however, LL seems to achieve higher duct clearance in a single session and

---

Box 1
Indications of cholangioscopy

Common indications
    Management of biliary stones (EHL, LL, basket extraction)
    Evaluation of indeterminate biliary strictures (visual inspection and targeted biopsies)
    Selective guidewire passage through tight strictures or angulated intrahepatic ducts
    Selective guidewire access of the cystic duct to facilitate transpapillary gallbladder stenting

Miscellaneous diagnostic indications
    Determining the extent of cholangiocarcinomas (visual inspection and mapping biopsies)
    Detection of stones missed during cholangiography
    Surveillance of choledochal cysts
    Assessment of intraductal extension of ampullary adenomas

Miscellaneous therapeutic indications
    Targeting ablation of cholangiocarcinomas with PDT or RFA, and assessing response
    Laser dissection/ablation of biliary strictures or complete biliary obstruction
    Cholangioscopy-based radiation-free ERCP
    Retrieval of intraductal migrated stents
    Resection of biliary polypoid lesions

Abbreviations: EHL, eletrohydraulic lithotripsy; ERCP, endoscopic retrograde cholangiopancreatography; LL, laser lithotripsy; PDT, photodynamic therapy; RFA, radiofrequency ablation.

to require shorter procedure duration.[7] Additional advantages with LL include that probes appear to be more durable, and because of their ability to alter retropulsion, less likely to bounce stones away, although it requires more accurate targeting en face with the stone. In contrast, EHL is more widely available in clinical practice and does not require special electricity, protective eyewear, or formal training in laser safety (**Fig. 3**).

Direct visual evaluation with cholangioscopy provides the ability for predicting histology of biliary strictures and obtaining targeted biopsies for histologic diagnosis. Several cholangioscopy findings such as dilated and tortuous blood vessels, nodularity, raised lesion, infiltrative stricture, ulcerations, friability, and papillary or villous mucosal projections, can be found in malignant strictures and should prompt targeted biopsies (**Fig. 4**).[11,12] The ability of cholangioscopy patterns to differentiate malignant from benign biliary strictures is highly variable, with sensitivity ranging from 74% to 100% and specificity from 47% to 98% across studies.[13–16] These diagnostic parameters are higher with the newer digital SOC than with the fiberoptic platform.[17] Despite these improvements, there remains significant interobserver variation among expert endoscopists at interpreting cholangioscopic features.[16] Furthermore, visual impression can be misleading in the setting of primary sclerosing cholangitis, stent-associated changes, distal strictures, and benign extrinsic compression (**Fig. 5**). For these reasons, one cannot yet rely on cholangioscopic predictions alone and histologic diagnosis remains crucial for treatment decisions. The sensitivity and specificity of ERCP methods for tissue acquisition are improved with cholangioscopy-targeted biopsies.[18] In a recent systematic review of 15 studies, cholangioscopy-targeted biopsies were highly specific (99.1%), but had suboptimal sensitivity (71.9%).[19] To maximize diagnostic accuracy (approximately 90%), a minimum of 3 biopsies is recommended.[20,21] Further refinements in specimen collection and processing techniques are needed to reduce false-negative results with cholangioscopy-targeted biopsies. The addition of rapid on-site evaluation (ROSE) using touch imprint cytology has not been shown to be superior to 3 standard biopsies without ROSE in a recent RCT, so the authors do not advocate its use until more data are available.[21] It remains unclear if the new-generation biopsy forceps (SpyBite Max) improves the diagnostic accuracy of cholangioscopy-targeted biopsies.

EXPANDING DIAGNOSTIC INDICATIONS

After extracting bile duct stones during ERCP, final occlusion cholangiograms can miss residual stones, especially in the presence of a dilated bile duct, significant

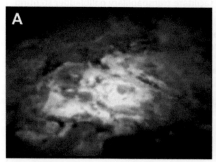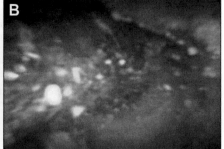

Fig. 3. Cholangioscopy-assisted electrohydraulic lithotripsy (EHL) of large stone. (*A*) Cholangioscopy visualization of large stone and positioning of EHL probe in preparation for lithotripsy. (*B*) Stone fragments following EHL.

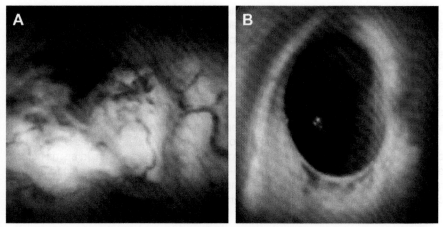

Fig. 4. Cholangioscopy evaluation of biliary strictures. (*A*) Cholangioscopy revealing abnormal tumor vessels, irregular surface, and nodules, with biopsies consistent with chol-angiocarcinoma. (*B*) Cholangioscopy revealing a short, smooth, diaphragm-like stricture without malignant features.

pneumobilia, or following lithotripsy. Previous literature, including 2 prospective studies, demonstrated that cholangioscopy detects residual stones in approximately 10% to 30% of patients after stone removal, which are otherwise missed by conventional cholangiography.[22–24] However, the clinical significance of detecting and removing these residual stones is unclear. Another setting in which cholangioscopy can be helpful is when a bile duct stone has been suggested during intraoperative cholangiogram or other imaging modality, but no stone is found during the ERCP. Other patients who may benefit from cholangioscopy are those in whom lithotripsy

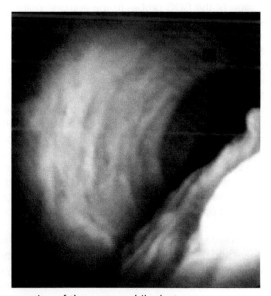

Fig. 5. Extrinsic compression of the common bile duct.

was carried out in the hilum. These patients have an increased risk of intrahepatic stone fragment entrapment and increased risk of ductal occlusion and infection.

One of the challenges of ERCP can be placement of a guidewire in a duct of interest, either because of a tight stricture or the anatomic characteristics of the upstream duct. Prior retrospective studies have demonstrated that cholangioscopy can successfully assist guidewire advancement into the ducts of interest when conventional ERCP methods have failed. This can be particularly helpful for wire access of the cystic duct, tight anastomotic biliary strictures, and angulated intrahepatic ducts, allowing selective cholangiography and conventional ERCP maneuvers.[25,26]

In patients with extrahepatic cholangiocarcinoma, mapping biopsies are useful to determine the lateral extent of lesions and to guide the surgical plan. In a small cross-over RCT of 28 patients, cholangioscopy-guided mapping biopsies obtained a higher rate of successful biopsies than cholangiography-guided biopsies.[27] This may be challenging in the case of tight strictures through which the SOC catheter cannot pass.

NOVEL THERAPEUTIC APPLICATIONS

Cholangioscopy can assist in the treatment of malignant and benign biliary strictures. In the case of unresectable cholangiocarcinomas, photodynamic therapy (PDT) and radiofrequency ablation (RFA) administered during ERCP have shown promising results. In a few case reports and retrospective studies, cholangioscopy served as an adjunct of cholangiography to target intraductal PDT/RFA and to assess treatment response in real time.[28–31] Commercially available PDT and RFA probes do not fit in the working channel of SOC catheters, so the treatment administration is still done under cholangiography visualization, and cholangioscopy is used immediately before and after therapy. For recalcitrant benign biliary strictures, laser dissection/ablation guided by cholangioscopy has been shown to be technically feasible, safe, and effective for short-term stricture resolution, in 2 small retrospective case series.[32,33] This is performed using cut power settings lower than with lithotripsy and by applying gentle short laser strokes from proximal to distal in 3 quadrants, until improved luminal patency allows passage of the SOC probe. In the authors' opinion, the continuous Thulium laser is a preferred technology for soft tissue dissection and ablation. Cholangioscopy with laser has also been used for recanalization of complete biliary obstruction not accessible by a guidewire for conventional interventions.[34]

The use of fluoroscopy in ERCP carries the risk of radiation exposure and causes access issues when a fluoroscopy suite is not available. In a recent prospective study, cholangioscopy-based radiation-free ERCP was shown to be a feasible, safe, and effective alternative for the management of noncomplex choledocholithiasis.[35] When using this approach, cholangioscopy serves to locate the stone(s) and confirm clearance after removal with conventional methods. In addition, either EHL or LL can be used when stones are large. Although fluoroscopy-based ERCP remains the gold standard for choledocholithiasis, cholangioscopy-based ERCP seems useful when fluoroscopy is not available or when radiation needs to be minimized (eg, pregnancy). An international multi-center RCT is ongoing comparing conventional fluoroscopy-based ERCP with cholangioscopy directed access for noncomplex biliary stone management.

The therapeutic armamentarium of cholangioscopy has expanded with the availability of the Spyglass snare and basket. Proximally migrated plastic or metallic stents can be removed using the Spyglass forceps, snare, or basket, as recently demonstrated in a case series and case reports.[36,37] The Spyglass snare also serves to resect intraductal premalignant, malignant, or indeterminate polyps using cold snare polypectomy.[38]

Although not studied yet, deep intraductal biopsies may be possible using the cold snare. Following cholangioscopy-assisted lithotripsy, stone fragments can be removed using the novel Spyglass basket, avoiding the exchange of the SOC catheter for conventional ERCP instruments for stone extraction.[37] These baskets can also assist in retrieving small bile duct stones that are otherwise difficult to remove with conventional ERCP methods (**Fig. 6**).[39]

USE OF ARTIFICIAL INTELLIGENCE

Artificial intelligence (AI) is being rapidly introduced to all aspects of gastrointestinal endoscopy. The application of AI tools has been recently evaluated on cholangioscopy-based images to overcome some of the challenges on diagnosing indeterminate biliary strictures and to assist novice and less frequent cholangioscopy users. In a retrospective single center study of 85 patients, interpretation of cholangioscopy images using convolutional neural networks (CNNs) was highly sensitive (95%), specific (92%), and accurate (AUC 1.00) in differentiating benign from malignant lesions.[40] In a more recent multicenter retrospective study of 528 patients, a cholangioscopy-based CNN model showed high sensitivity (81%), specificity (91%), and accuracy (AUC 0.86), in distinguishing indeterminate biliary strictures.[41] Although AI appears to improve the predictive accuracy of cholangioscopy on classifying biliary strictures, these findings require further validation before clinical implementation. Incorporating real-time AI algorithms in cholangioscopy may decrease the interobserver variability on image interpretation, may improve the diagnostic accuracy of biliary strictures among both nonexperts and experts, and may allow wider proficient implementation of the technology.

FUTURE IMPROVEMENTS

Additional technologic improvements are necessary to optimize the access and visualization of the SOC system. The present catheter maneuverability and tip deflection are limited, especially once devices are within the working channel tip. These issues impact advancing the catheter efficiently into areas of interest, passage of devices, and preventing positioning some lesions optimally for interventions. The diameter of

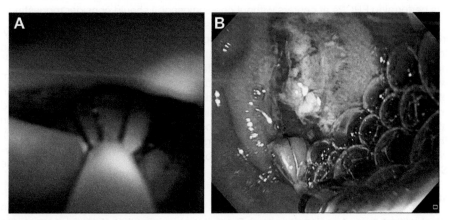

Fig. 6. Cholangioscopy-guided basket retrieval of a common bile duct stone. (*A*) Positioning of cholangioscopy-guided basket around stone. (*B*) Endoscopic visualization of stone removal with the Spyglass basket.

the SOC probe prohibits its access through severe strictures or intrahepatic ducts, so a smaller diameter cholangioscope catheter would be helpful for these indications. With a working channel of 1.2 mm, the range of accessories that can be inserted through the SOC is limited (dedicated miniature forceps, snare, basket, EHL/LL probes) especially considering that more power could be delivered using a larger laser fiber to facilitate large stone fragmentation. A larger working channel would expand the diagnostic and therapeutic potential of SOC, allowing one to obtain regular larger biopsies or to perform balloon dilation across a stenosis to permit SOC passage across it or even place a small caliber stent for ductal decompression. This would also facilitate the passage of accessories through the angulation between the elevator and the biliary orifice. The location of the working channel at the 6 o'clock position limits the ability to access the upper visual quadrants, and perhaps greater rotation of the catheter would overcome this problem. In addition to refinements in the design of the SOC catheter, there is also a need for image enhancement that can improve the resolution, automated lighting, depth of view, and field of view of SOC to be even more comparable to a video image. The present SOC system lacks the ability to perform NBI or magnification, which may be able to increase the diagnostic accuracy of SOC for indeterminate biliary strictures, especially magnification for identifying suspected tumor vessels.[42] The role of chromocholangioscopy with dye solution, autofluorescence imaging (AFI), and near-infrared fluorescence, needs to be further studied using SOC.[43,44]

Novel cholangioscopy platforms are being developed and hopefully will overcome some of the issues illustrated in this article. The future of SOC is promising, and the incorporation of breakthrough scientific discoveries will continue expanding its use. The addition of nanotechnology could help treating biliary diseases by reprogramming gene expression or regulation. The use of navigation systems in the SOC catheter may decrease the reliance of contrast during cholangioscopy and may allow more efficient fluoroscopy-free ERCPs. External 3-dimensional image reconstruction of the biliary tree based on cholangioscopy could help mapping the extension of cholangiocarcinomas and guiding surgical planning or stenting strategy.

EXPANDING CHOLANGIOSCOPY UTILIZATION

Cholangioscopy is still not available at many endoscopy units worldwide. Endoscopists performing ERCPs at centers without cholangioscopy should consider requesting their hospital administration about investing to start that practice. The cost of purchasing the necessary equipment for cholangioscopy is variable and ranges from $50,000 to $90,000.[45] This cost is offset by avoiding unnecessary surgeries, decreasing the need for transferring patient care to other facilities, and reducing the additional work-up and consequences of undiagnosed biliary neoplasias. No cost-effectiveness studies are available to guide administrators on purchasing the equipment for cholangioscopy, so the decision should be based on local patterns and availability of trained endoscopists. Training on cholangioscopy is beyond the intention of this article; however, endoscopists performing cholangioscopy should be proficient with ERCPs of complexity level 3 to 4 based on the grading system of the American Society of Gastrointestinal Endoscopy.[46]

SUMMARY

What is the future of cholangioscopy? The authors envision that cholangioscopy will become a conventional tool in the shelf of any biliary endoscopist. Although some complex cholangioscopy cases will still need referral to expert centers, high-volume biliary endoscopists at community and private practice settings will be able to manage large stones and to conduct the initial work-up of biliary strictures using cholangioscopy. If local availability and experience are not present, referral to a center that has experience with the technology earlier rather than later can improve patient outcomes and satisfaction. However, future technologic improvements and the introduction of real-time AI algorithms will optimize the outcomes of cholangioscopy even in nonexpert hands. The number of tools and applications of cholangioscopy will continue expanding; however, prospective studies and RCTs to further assess these will be needed. It is an incredibly exciting time to be a biliary endoscopist with an increasing armamentarium of devices and techniques to enhance patient options in an attempt to improve quality of life.

CLINICS CARE POINTS

1. Cholangioscopy has evolved over the last 5 decades. Currently, it is most frequently done using catheter-based, digital, single-operator, peroral cholangioscopy at the time of endoscopic retrograde cholangiopancreatography (ERCP).

2. The most common indications for cholangioscopy include difficult bile duct stones and indeterminate biliary strictures; however, the number of diagnostic and therapeutic applications is expanding.

3. The authors envision that cholangioscopy will eventually be available in the shelf of any biliary endoscopist. Endoscopists performing cholangioscopy should be proficient with ERCPs of complexity level 3 to 4.

4. Additional technologic improvements are necessary to optimize the access and visualization of cholangioscopy.

DISCLOSURE

I. Raijman is in the advisory board for Boston Scientific Corporation, Microtech, Pentax, and Olympus; and is co-owner of EndoRx. R.J. Shah is a consultant of Boston Scientific Corporation, Cook Endoscopy, and Olympus.

REFERENCES

1. Takekoshi T, Takagi K. Retrograde pancreatocholangioscopy. Gastroenterol Endosc 1975;17:678–83.
2. Gerges C, Vazquez AG, Tringali A, et al. Percutaneous transhepatic cholangioscopy using a single-operator cholangioscope (pSOC), a retrospective, observational, multicenter study. Surg Endosc 2021. https://doi.org/10.1007/s00464-020-08176-1.
3. Kawakami H, Itoi T, Ban T. Intrahepatic biliary stones extraction via an EUS-guided hepaticogastrostomy route confirmed by peroral transluminal video cholangioscopy (with video). J Hepatobiliary Pancreat Sci 2020;27(2):E11–2.
4. Subhash A, Abadir A, Iskander JM, et al. Applications, limitations, and expansion of cholangioscopy in clinical practice. Gastroenterol Hepatol (NY) 2021;17(3):110–20.
5. Shah RJ, Neuhaus H, Parsi M, et al. Randomized study of digital single-operator cholangioscope compared to fiberoptic single-operator cholangioscope in a novel cholangioscopy bench model. Endosc Int Open 2018;6(7):E851–6.

6. Reddy DN, Ramchandani M, Lakhtakia S, et al. Single-use duodenoscope in the management of an elderly patient with difficult bile duct stones: laser lithotripsy using a disposable cholangioscope. VideoGIE 2021;6(7):319–21.

7. McCarty TR, Gulati R, Rustagi T. Efficacy and safety of peroral cholangioscopy with intraductal lithotripsy for difficult biliary stones: a systematic review and meta-analysis. Endoscopy 2021;53(2):110–22.

8. Buxbaum J, Sahakian A, Ko C, et al. Randomized trial of cholangioscopy-guided laser lithotripsy versus conventional therapy for large bile duct stones (with videos). Gastrointest Endosc 2018;87(4):1050–60.

9. Bang JY, Sutton B, Navaneethan U, et al. Efficacy of single-operator cholangio-scopy-guided lithotripsy compared with large balloon sphincteroplasty in management of difficult bile duct stones in a randomized trial. Clin Gastroenterol Hepatol 2020;18(10):2349–2356 e3.

10. Angsuwatcharakon P, Kulpatcharapong S, Ridtitid W, et al. Digital cholangioscopy-guided laser versus mechanical lithotripsy for large bile duct stone removal after failed papillary large-balloon dilation: a randomized study. Endoscopy 2019;51(11):1066–73.

11. Kahaleh M, Gaidhane M, Shahid HM, et al. Digital single-operator cholangio-scopy interobserver study using a new classification: the Mendoza classification (with video). Gastrointest Endosc 2021. https://doi.org/10.1016/j.gie.2021.08.015.

12. Mounzer R, Austin GL, Wani S, et al. Per-oral video cholangiopancreatoscopy with narrow-band imaging for the evaluation of indeterminate pancreaticobiliary disease. Gastrointest Endosc 2017;85(3):509–17.

13. Navaneethan U, Njei B, Lourdusamy V, et al. Comparative effectiveness of biliary brush cytology and intraductal biopsy for detection of malignant biliary strictures: a systematic review and meta-analysis. Gastrointest Endosc 2015;81(1):168–76.

14. Sadeghi A, Mohamadnejad M, Islami F, et al. Diagnostic yield of EUS-guided FNA for malignant biliary stricture: a systematic review and meta-analysis. Gastroint-est Endosc 2016;83(2):290–298 e1.

15. Navaneethan U, Hasan MK, Lourdusamy V, et al. Single-operator cholangioscopy and targeted biopsies in the diagnosis of indeterminate biliary strictures: a systematic review. Gastrointest Endosc 2015;82(4):608–614 e2.

16. Stassen PMC, Goodchild G, de Jonge PJF, et al. Diagnostic accuracy and inter-observer agreement of digital single-operator cholangioscopy for indeterminate biliary strictures. Gastrointest Endosc 2021. https://doi.org/10.1016/j.gie.2021.06.027.

17. Mizrahi M, Khoury T, Wang Y, et al. Apple far from the tree": comparative effective-ness of fiberoptic single-operator cholangiopancreatoscopy (FSOCP) and digital SOCP (DSOCP). HPB (Oxford) 2018;20(3):285–8.

18. Gerges C, Beyna T, Tang RSY, et al. Digital single-operator peroral cholangioscopy-guided biopsy sampling versus ERCP-guided brushing for inde-terminate biliary strictures: a prospective, randomized, multicenter trial (with video). Gastrointest Endosc 2020;91(5):1105–13.

19. Badshah MB, Vanar V, Kandula M, et al. Peroral cholangioscopy with cholangioscopy-directed biopsies in the diagnosis of biliary malignancies: a sys-temic review and meta-analysis. Eur J Gastroenterol Hepatol 2019;31(8):935–40.

20. Tamada K, Kurihara K, Tomiyama T, et al. How many biopsies should be per-formed during percutaneous transhepatic cholangioscopy to diagnose biliary tract cancer? Gastrointest Endosc 1999;50(5):653–8.

21. Bang JY, Navaneethan U, Hasan M, et al. Optimizing outcomes of single-operator cholangioscopy-guided biopsies based on a randomized trial. Clin Gastroenterol Hepatol 2020;18(2):441–448 e1.
22. Itoi T, Sofuni A, Itokawa F, et al. Evaluation of residual bile duct stones by peroral cholangioscopy in comparison with balloon-cholangiography. Dig Endosc 2010; 22(Suppl 1):S85–9.
23. Sejpal DV, Trindade AJ, Lee C, et al. Digital cholangioscopy can detect residual biliary stones missed by occlusion cholangiogram in ERCP: a prospective tandem study. Endosc Int Open 2019;7(4):E608–14.
24. Huang SW, Lin CH, Lee MS, et al. Residual common bile duct stones on direct peroral cholangioscopy using ultraslim endoscope. World J Gastroenterol 2013;19(30):4966–72.
25. Bokemeyer A, Gross D, Bruckner M, et al. Digital single-operator cholangioscopy: a useful tool for selective guidewire placements across complex biliary strictures. Surg Endosc 2019;33(3):731–7.
26. Ridtitid W, Piyachaturawat P, Teeratorn N, et al. Single-operator peroral cholangioscopy cystic duct cannulation for transpapillary gallbladder stent placement in patients with acute cholecystitis at moderate to high surgical risk (with videos). Gastrointest Endosc 2020;92(3):634–44.
27. Ogawa T, Kanno Y, Koshita S, et al. Cholangioscopy- versus fluoroscopy-guided transpapillary mapping biopsy for preoperative evaluation of extrahepatic cholangiocarcinoma: a prospective randomized crossover study. Surg Endosc 2020. https://doi.org/10.1007/s00464-020-08141-y.
28. Choi HJ, Moon JH, Ko BM, et al. Clinical feasibility of direct peroral cholangioscopy-guided photodynamic therapy for inoperable cholangiocarcinoma performed by using an ultra-slim upper endoscope (with videos). Gastrointest Endosc 2011;73(4):808–13.
29. Patel J, Rizk N, Kedia P, et al. Cholangioscopy-assisted photodynamic therapy for cholangiocarcinoma. Gastrointest Endosc 2015;81(4):1012–3.
30. Brunaldi VO, Brunaldi JE, Vollet-Filho JD, et al. Photodynamic therapy of extrahepatic cholangiocarcinoma using digital cholangioscopy. Arq Bras Cir Dig 2020; 33(1):e1490.
31. Ogura T, Onda S, Sano T, et al. Evaluation of the safety of endoscopic radiofrequency ablation for malignant biliary stricture using a digital peroral cholangioscope (with videos). Dig Endosc 2017;29(6):712–7.
32. Lou J, Hu Q, Ma T, et al. A novel approach with holmium laser ablation for endoscopic management of intrahepatic biliary stricture. BMC Gastroenterol 2019; 19(1):172.
33. Han S, Shah RJ. Cholangiopancreatoscopy-guided laser dissection and ablation for pancreas and biliary strictures and neoplasia. Endosc Int Open 2020;8(8): E1091–6.
34. WA Y, AC K, U D, et al. 987 Cholangioscopy with laser recanalization to enable internal biliary drainage. Gastroenterol Endosc 2020;91(6 Supplement):AB90.
35. Barakat MT, Girotra M, Choudhary A, et al. A prospective evaluation of radiation-free direct solitary cholangioscopy for the management of choledocholithiasis. Gastrointest Endosc 2018;87(2):584–589 e1.
36. Al Lehibi A, Al Mtawa A, Almasoudi T, et al. Removal of proximally migrated biliary stents by using single-operator cholangioscopy. VideoGIE 2020;5(5):213–6.
37. Fejleh MP, Thaker AM, Kim S, et al. Cholangioscopy-guided retrieval basket and snare for the removal of biliary stones and retained prostheses. VideoGIE 2019; 4(5):232–4.

38. Bronswijk M, Reekmans A, Van der Merwe S. Digital cholangioscopy-guided cold snare resection of an inflammatory intraductal pseudopolyp. Dig Endosc 2021; 33(5):875–6.
39. Han S, Shah RJ. Cholangioscopy-guided basket retrieval of impacted stones. VideoGIE 2020;5(9):387–8.
40. Mascarenhas Saraiva M, Ribeiro T, Ferreira JPS, et al. Artificial intelligence for automatic diagnosis of biliary strictures malignancy status in single-operator cholangioscopy: a pilot study. Gastrointest Endosc 2021. https://doi.org/10.1016/j.gie.2021.08.027.
41. Ghandour B, Hsieh H-W, Akshintala V, et al. S1 machine learning for classification of indeterminate biliary strictures during cholangioscopy. Am Coll Gastroenterol 2021;116:S1.
42. Itoi T, Sofuni A, Itokawa F, et al. Peroral cholangioscopic diagnosis of biliary-tract diseases by using narrow-band imaging (with videos). Gastrointest Endosc 2007; 66(4):730–6.
43. Itoi T, Neuhaus H, Chen YK. Diagnostic value of image-enhanced video cholangiopancreatoscopy. Gastrointest Endosc Clin N Am 2009;19(4):557–66.
44. Glatz J, Garcia-Allende PB, Becker V, et al. Near-infrared fluorescence cholangiopancreatoscopy: initial clinical feasibility results. Gastrointest Endosc 2014;79(4): 664–8.
45. Committee AT, Komanduri S, Thosani N, et al. Cholangiopancreatoscopy. Gastrointest Endosc 2016;84(2):209–21.
46. Cotton PB, Eisen G, Romagnuolo J, et al. Grading the complexity of endoscopic procedures: results of an ASGE working party. Gastrointest Endosc 2011;73(5): 868–74.

Moving?

Make sure your subscription moves with you!

To notify us of your new address, find your **Clinics Account Number** (located on your mailing label above your name), and contact customer service at:

Email: journalscustomerservice-usa@elsevier.com

800-654-2452 (subscribers in the U.S. & Canada)
314-447-8871 (subscribers outside of the U.S. & Canada)

Fax number: 314-447-8029

Elsevier Health Sciences Division
Subscription Customer Service
3251 Riverport Lane
Maryland Heights, MO 63043

Printed and bound by CPI Group (UK) Ltd, Croydon, CR0 4YY

08/05/2025

01864723-0003